Praise for *Good Energy*

"A tour de force on how metabolism underpins most major diseases and what we can do to feel better and live longer. Everyone will benefit from reading *Good Energy*."

**—Mark Hyman, MD, author of the #1 *New York Times*
bestselling *Young Forever***

"In *Good Energy*, Dr. Means makes a bold case for why food—and particularly regenerative agriculture—must be at the very center of health care. Dr. Means makes it clear that we can't drug our way out of a broken food system."

**—Will Harris, regenerative agriculture leader and
owner of White Oak Pastures**

"In *Good Energy*, Casey and Calley Means powerfully explain how we can use metabolic health tools and strategies to support our own health and that of our children and families."

—Kelly LeVeque, nutritionist and author of *Body Love*

"*Good Energy* should be required reading for every medical student and health-care practitioner. As a system and as individuals, we must adopt a metabolic, mitochondria-focused lens for health and vitality. Autoimmunity—along with many other chronic illnesses—is closely tied to metabolic dysfunction and insulin resistance. Foundational to better energy and health outcomes is getting metabolic health and blood sugar under control. Dr. Means shows readers how."

—Terry Wahls, MD, author of *The Wahls Protocol*

"Dr. Casey Means brilliantly illuminates the pivotal role of disturbed metabolism in setting the stage for chronic degenerative diseases, and offers a comprehensive road map for enhancing and maintaining metabolic health. This book is a must-read for health care professionals and individuals alike who are seeking to understand and improve their overall health. With her insightful and loving guidance, Dr. Means is handing us the keys to the kingdom for prolonging our health span, making this book a game-changing, invaluable resource in our journey toward lasting wellness."

—**David Perlmutter, MD, author of the #1** *New York Times* **bestselling** *Grain Brain* **and** *Drop Acid*

"There's no life without energy. Our mitochondria know how to capture chemical energy and optimize it. But what if our cells are poisoned? Think cyanide; think heavy metals. Now think alcohol, sugar, trans fats, all the environmental toxins that inhibit your mitochondria from their capacity. Dr. Casey Means brings the problem of cellular energy front and center to explain what's really wrong in chronic disease, why medicines won't fix it, why she walked away from a promising surgical career, how to remake our entire health and health care paradigm to save lives and money, and who's blocking it. Part memoir, part manifesto, this book proves there isn't another voice in the zeitgeist as cogent, urgent, and powerful as Casey's. The gauntlet's been thrown down—consider yourself warned."

—**Robert H. Lustig, MD, author of** *Metabolical* **and professor emeritus of pediatrics, UCSF**

GOOD
ENERGY

The Surprising Connection Between
Metabolism and Limitless Health

Casey Means, MD
with Calley Means

Avery
an imprint of Penguin Random House
New York

AVERY

an imprint of Penguin Random House LLC
penguinrandomhouse.com

Most Avery books are available at special quantity discounts for bulk purchase for sales promotions, premiums, fundraising, and educational needs. Special books or book excerpts also can be created to fit specific needs. For details, write SpecialMarkets@penguinrandomhouse.com.

Library of Congress Cataloging-in-Publication Data

Names: Means, Casey, author. | Means, Calley, author.
Title: Good energy: the surprising connection between metabolism and limitless health / Casey Means, MD, with Calley Means.
Description: New York: Avery, an imprint of Penguin Random House, [2024] | Includes index.
Identifiers: LCCN 2023043612 (print) | LCCN 2023043613 (ebook) |
    ISBN 9780593712641 (hardcover) | ISBN 9780593712665 (epub)
Subjects: LCSH: Metabolic syndrome—Diet therapy—Popular works. |
    Energy metabolism—Popular works. | Self-care, Health—Popular works. |
    Aging—Nutritional aspects—Popular works. | Diet therapy—Popular works
Classification: LCC RC662.4 .M425 2024 (print) | LCC RC662.4 (ebook) |
    DDC 616.3/990654—dc23/eng/20231227
LC record available at https://lccn.loc.gov/2023043612
LC ebook record available at https://lccn.loc.gov/2023043613

Printed in the United States of America
3rd Printing

Book design by Silverglass Studio

For Gayle Means

Born 1949, died 2021 of pancreatic cancer
(a preventable metabolic condition)

CONTENTS

Everything Is Connected

I weighed eleven pounds, nine ounces at birth. My mom's doctors congratulated her for producing one of the largest babies in the hospital's history.

My mom had trouble losing the baby weight and continued to battle her weight for years after. Her primary care doctor told her this was normal. She just had a baby and was getting older, after all. They told her to "eat healthier."

In her forties, her cardiologist diagnosed her with elevated blood pressure. The doctor said this was very common for women her age and prescribed an angiotensin-converting enzyme (ACE) inhibitor to help relax her arteries.

In her fifties, her internal medicine doctor informed her she had high cholesterol (or more technically, high triglycerides, low HDL, and high LDL cholesterol). She was prescribed a statin and told this was almost a rite of passage for a person her age: statins are one of the most prescribed drugs in U.S. history, with over 221 million prescriptions doled out annually.

In her sixties, her endocrinologist said she had developed prediabetes. The doctor stressed that this, too, was very common and not of much concern. It's a "pre-disease," after all, right—and one that 50 percent of American adults qualify for. She left the office with her prescription of metformin, a drug that is prescribed over 90 million times per year in the United States.

In January 2021, when my mom was seventy-one years old, she was taking her daily hike with my dad near their home in Northern California. Suddenly, she felt a deep pain in her belly and experienced uncharacteristic fatigue. Concerned, she visited her primary care doctor, who conducted a CT scan and ran lab work.

One day later, she received a text message with her results: stage 4 pancreatic cancer.

Thirteen days later, she was dead.

Her oncologists at Stanford Hospital called her pancreatic cancer "unlucky." My mom—who at the time of her cancer diagnosis was seeing *five separate specialists* prescribing *five separate medications*—was frequently complimented by her doctors in the decade running up to her diagnosis for being "healthy" compared to most women her age. And, statistically, she was: the average American over sixty-five sees twenty-eight doctors in their lifetime. Fourteen prescriptions are written per American per year.

Obviously, something isn't right when it comes to the health trends of our children, our parents, and ourselves.

Among teens, 18 percent have fatty liver disease, close to 30 percent are prediabetic, and more than 40 percent are overweight or obese. Fifty years ago, pediatricians might go an entire career without seeing these conditions among their patients. Today, young adults exist in a culture where conditions such as obesity, acne, fatigue, depression, infertility, high cholesterol, or prediabetes are common.

Six out of ten adults are living with a chronic illness. About 50 percent of Americans will deal with mental illness sometime in life. Seventy-four percent of adults are overweight or have obesity. Rates of cancer, heart disease, kidney disease, upper respiratory infections, and autoimmune conditions are all going up at the exact time we are spending more and more to treat them. In the face of these trends, American life expectancy has been declining for the most sustained period since 1860.

We are convinced these increasing rates of conditions—both mental and physical—are part of being human. And we are told we can treat the increasing rates of chronic conditions with "innovations" from modern medicine. In the decades leading up to my mom's cancer diagnosis, she was informed her rising cholesterol, waistline, fasting glucose, and blood pressure levels were conditions that she could "manage" for life with a pill.

But instead of isolated conditions, all of the symptoms my mom experienced leading to her death were warning signs of the same thing: dysregulation in how her cells were producing and using energy. Even my enormous size at birth—which medically fit the criteria for fetal macrosomia (literally "big-bodied baby")—was a robust indicator of energy dysfunction in her cells and almost certainly a sign of undiagnosed gestational diabetes.

But through decades of symptoms, my mom—and most other adults in the modern world—are simply prescribed pills and not set on a path of curiosity about how these conditions are connected and how the root cause can be reversed.

There is a better way, and it starts with understanding that the biggest lie in health care is that the root cause of why we're getting sicker, heavier, more depressed, and more infertile is complicated.

This sounds radical until you realize that virtually no animals in the wild suffer from widespread chronic disease. There aren't rampant obesity, heart disease, or type 2 diabetes rates among lions or giraffes. But preventable lifestyle conditions are responsible for 80 percent of modern human deaths.

Depression, anxiety, acne, infertility, insomnia, heart disease, erectile dysfunction, type 2 diabetes, Alzheimer's disease, cancer, and most other conditions that torture and shorten our lives are actually rooted in the *same thing*. And the ability to prevent and reverse these conditions—and feel incredible *today*—is under your control and simpler than you think.

Good Energy

I want to share a vision of health that is big and bold. It predicates health and longevity on something simple, powerful, and absolutely fundamental. A single physiological phenomenon that can change almost everything about how you feel and function today and in the future. It's called Good

Energy, and the reason it has such a life-changing impact is that it governs the very essence of what (quite literally) makes you tick: whether your cells have the energy to do their jobs of keeping you nourished, clear-minded, hormonally balanced, immune protected, heart-healthy, structurally sound—and so much more. Having Good Energy is the core underlying physiological function that, more than any other process in your body, determines your predilection to great mental and physical health or to poor health and disease.

Good Energy is also known as metabolic health. Metabolism refers to the set of cellular mechanisms that transform food into energy that can power every single cell in the body. You might not have thought much about whether you have Good Energy or not. When cellular energy production is working well, you don't have to "think" about it or be conscious of it. It just is. Your body has an exquisite set of mechanisms that make Good Energy happen every second of every day; these cellular mechanisms create sustained and balanced energy, distribute it to every cell in your body, and clean up the residues from the process that would otherwise clog up the system.

When you hold the keys to this one critical bodily process, you can be an outlier—a truly positive kind of outlier. You can feel vital and enlivened and function with clarity of mind. You can enjoy balanced weight, a pain-free body, healthy skin, and a stable mood. If you're of childbearing age and hoping to have kids, you can enjoy the natural state of fertility that is your birthright. If you're getting older, you can live relieved of the nagging anxiety that precipitous physical or mental decline awaits you or that you'll develop a disease that "runs in the family."

When you lose the keys to Good Energy, however, so much starts to go wrong. Organs, tissues, and glands are, after all, mere collections of cells. Lose the capacity for properly and safely powering those cells and—no real surprise—the organs made up of them start to struggle and fail. This means that just about any disease can arise as a result—and today, given the pressures that Good Energy is under, that's exactly what is occurring.

The problem, simply stated, is a mismatch. The metabolic processes that run our bodies evolved over hundreds of thousands of years in a synergistic relationship with the environment around us. But those environmental conditions around the cells of our bodies have profoundly and rapidly changed in recent decades. Starting with our diet, yet including our movement patterns, our sleep patterns, our stress levels, and exposure to nonnatural chemicals, things are not as they once were. The environment for the cells of the average modern human is now radically different from what the cells expect and need. This evolutionary mismatch is tipping normal metabolic function into dysfunction: Bad Energy. And when small cellular disturbances happen in every cell, at every moment, the effect is outsized—rippling up into the tissues, organs, and systems of your body and negatively influencing how you feel, think, function, look, age, and even how well you combat pathogens and avoid chronic disease. In fact, almost every chronic health symptom that Western medicine addresses is the result of our cells being beleaguered by how we've come to live. It's a terrible trickle-up: Bad Energy leads to broken cells, broken organs, broken bodies, and the pain you feel.

We have two hundred different types of cells in the human body, and when Bad Energy shows up in different cell types, different symptoms can arise. For instance, if an ovarian theca cell is experiencing Bad Energy, it looks like infertility in the form of polycystic ovary syndrome (PCOS). If a blood vessel–lining cell is experiencing Bad Energy, it can look like erectile dysfunction, heart disease, high blood pressure, retinal problems, or chronic kidney disease (all issues resulting from poor blood flow to different organs). If a liver cell is experiencing Bad Energy, it can look like non-alcoholic fatty liver disease (NAFLD). In the brain, Bad Energy can look like depression, stroke, dementia, migraine, or chronic pain, depending on where these dysfunctional cellular processes are most prominently showing up. Recently, research has clearly shown us that every one of these conditions—and dozens more—is linked directly to metabolic issues, a problem with how our cells make energy: Bad Energy. The way we practice medicine, however, has not caught up with this root-cause understanding. We still "treat" the *organ-specific results* of the Bad Energy, *not* the Bad Energy itself. And we will never improve the failing health of our modern population if we don't address the correct issue (metabolic dysfunction), which is why the more we spend on health care, and the more we work as physicians, and the more access to health care and medications we provide to patients, the worse the outcomes get.

Compared to one hundred years ago, we are consuming astronomically more sugar (i.e., up to 3,000 percent more liquid fructose), working in more sedentary jobs, and sleeping 25 percent less. We're also exposed to over eighty thousand synthetic chemicals in our food, water, and air. As a result of all these factors and many others, our cells have stopped being able to make energy the way they should. Many aspects of our industrialized life over the past century share a unique and *synergistic* ability to attack the machinery inside the cells that produce chemical energy. The result: cellular dysfunction throughout our bodies, showing up as the explosion of chronic symptoms and diseases we are facing today.

Our body has simple ways to show us whether we have brewing metabolic dysfunction: increasing waist size, suboptimal cholesterol levels, high fasting glucose, and elevated blood pressure. My mom experienced all of them, and 93 percent of Americans are in the danger zone on at least one key metabolic marker.

Aside from some significant excess belly fat, my mom appeared healthy on the outside. She was vibrant, happy, and energetic, and actually looked years younger than her age. This is a funny thing about metabolic dysfunction: it doesn't necessarily show up everywhere all at once, and it can look very different in different individuals, based on which cell types show the manifestations most obviously.

Her case is only one example of something that is happening every day to millions of people and families. I am writing this book because her story is relevant to everyone. Disease isn't some random occurrence that might happen in the future. It is a result of the choices you make and how you feel today. If you are battling annoying and seemingly nonlethal health issues—like fatigue, brain fog, anxiety, arthritis, infertility, erectile dysfunction, or chronic pain—an underlying contributor to these conditions is generally the same thing that will lead to a "major" illness sometime later in life if nothing changes in how you care for your body. This information stings and can be scary, but it's crucial to convey: if you ignore the minor issues as signs of Bad Energy brewing inside your body today, you could get much louder signals in the future.

Waking Up

For most of my adult life, I was a vocal advocate for the modern health care system and collected credentials to rise within its ranks: a research internship at the National Institutes of Health (NIH) at age sixteen, president of my Stanford class at eighteen, best undergraduate human biology thesis award at age twenty-one, top of my Stanford Medical School class at twenty-five, a surgical resident in ear, nose, and throat (ENT) surgery at Oregon Health & Science University (OHSU) by age twenty-six, and winner of ENT research awards at thirty. I had been published in premier medical journals, presented my research at national conferences, spent thousands of lonely nights studying, and was the pride of my family. It was my entire identity.

But five years into surgical residency, I met Sophia.

Recurrent sinus infections had plagued this fifty-two-year-old woman, leading to a persistent foul smell in her nose and difficulty breathing. Over the past year, her physicians had prescribed steroid nasal sprays, antibiotics, oral steroid medication, and medicated nasal rinses. She'd undergone CT scans, in-office nasal endoscopy procedures, and a nasal polyp biopsy. Her recurrent infections caused her to miss work and lose sleep, and she was overweight and had prediabetes. She had also been taking medication for high blood pressure and dealt with back pain and depression, which she attributed to her health issues and getting older. She saw a different doctor and received a separate treatment plan for each issue.

None of Sophia's sinus medications were successfully solving the problem, so she came to my department for surgery. In 2017, I was a young doctor starting my fifth and final year of surgery training.

After Sophia was wheeled into the operating room, I inserted a rigid camera into her nose and used a small instrument to break up the bones and swollen tissue and vacuum them out of the sinus passages just millimeters from her brain. In the postoperative area, the anesthesiologists struggled to control her blood sugar and blood pressure with an insulin drip and intravenous antihypertensives.

"You saved me," she said while grasping my hand after the procedure. But looking into her eyes after the surgery, I didn't feel proud. I felt defeated.

At best, I had relieved the downstream symptoms of her chronic nasal inflammation, but I had done absolutely nothing to cure the underlying dynamics causing that inflammation. I also did absolutely nothing to help with her other health conditions. I knew she would return with many other symptoms and continue going through the revolving doors of several specialists for her health issues that weren't my focus. Was she leaving this post-op area "healthy" after I'd permanently altered her nasal anatomy? What were the chances that the factors driving her prediabetes, excess fat, depression, and high blood pressure (all conditions that I knew had some relationship to inflammation) had absolutely *nothing* to do with the recurrent inflammation in her nose?

Sophia was my second sinusitis surgery of the *day*, the fifth of my week. I'd performed hundreds of these operations during residency on angry, inflamed sinus tissue. But so many patients kept returning to the hospital for follow-up sinus procedures and treatments for other diseases—with diabetes, depression, anxiety, cancer, heart disease, dementia, hypertension, and obesity among the most common.

Despite surgically treating inflamed tissues of the head and neck day in and day out, not once—*ever*—was I taught what *causes* the inflammation in the human body or about its connection to the inflammatory chronic diseases so many Americans are facing today. Not once was I prompted to ask, *Huh*, why *all the inflammation*? My gut told me that all of Sophia's conditions could be related, but instead of tapping into that curiosity, I always stayed in the lane of my specialty, followed the guidelines, and reached for my prescription pad and scalpel.

Soon after my encounter with Sophia, I felt an overwhelming conviction that I couldn't cut into another patient until I figured out why—despite the monumental size and scope of our health care system—the patients and people around me were sick in the first place.

I wanted to understand why so many conditions were rising exponentially and in clear patterns indicating potential connections. And most important, I needed to figure out whether there was anything I could do as a physician to keep my patients *out* of the operating room. I had become a doctor to generate foundational, vibrant health for my patients—not to drug, cut, and bill as many bodies as I possibly could each day.

It was increasingly becoming clear to me that although I was surrounded by practitioners who got into medicine to help patients, the reality is that every institution that impacts health—from medical schools to insurance companies to hospitals to pharma companies—makes money on "managing" disease, not curing patients. These incentives were clearly creating an invisible hand that was guiding good people into allowing bad outcomes.

Striving to reach the top of the medical field had been my laser-focused path. If I stopped operating on patients, I had no backup plan and half a million dollars had gone toward my education. At that time, I still couldn't imagine what I'd do other than be a surgeon.

But these considerations all seemed so inconsequential compared to the one blaring fact I couldn't get out of my head: **The patients aren't getting better.**

In September 2018, on my thirty-first birthday and just months shy of completing my five-year residency, I walked into the chairman's office at OHSU and quit. With a wall full of awards and honors for my clinical and research performance and with prominent hospital systems pursuing me for mid-six-figure faculty roles, I walked out of the hospital and embarked on a journey to understand the real reasons why people get sick and to figure out how to help patients restore and sustain their health.

The insights I learned on this quest couldn't save my mom—her cancer had likely been growing quietly in her body long before I left conventional medical practice. I am writing this book because millions of people can improve and extend their lives right now with simple principles doctors aren't taught in medical school.

I am also convinced our lack of understanding about the root cause of disease represents a larger spiritual crisis. We have become disconnected from the awe about our bodies and life, separated from the production of the foods we eat, made more sedentary by our work and school, and detached from our core biological needs, like sunlight, quality sleep, and clean water and air. This has put our bodies into a state of confusion and fear. Our cells are dysregulated at scale, which of course impacts our brains and bodies, which determine our perception of the world. The medical system has capitalized on this fear and offers "solutions" to symptoms of this dysfunction. That's why the medical system is the largest and fastest-growing industry in the United States. We are locked into a reductionist, fragmented view of the body that breaks us into dozens of separate parts. This view does not foster human flourishing. In reality, the body is an awe-inspiring and interconnected entity that is constantly regenerating and exchanging energy and matter with the external environment every time we eat, breathe, or bask in sunlight!

There is no question that the American medical system has produced miracles in the past 120 years, but we have lost our way when it comes to preventing and reversing metabolic conditions that account for over 80 percent of health care costs and deaths today. The situation is dire, but this is a book of optimism and practicality. The fact that we can vigorously criticize and reform our health care system is one of its strengths. Throughout prior crucible moments, human ingenuity has created advancements and systems changes that few could imagine. The next revolution in health will come from understanding how the root of almost every disease relates to energy, and how less specialization, rather than more, is the answer. We will see that our ailments are connected rather than siloed, a reality that research is only recently allowing us to see clearly, now that we have tools and technology to truly understand what's happening inside our cells at the molecular level. And when we shift our framework to this energy-centric paradigm, we will rapidly heal our system and our bodies. Fortunately, improving Good Energy is easier and simpler than it seems—and you can take steps to prioritize it in your life. This book will show you how.

Part 1 explains the science of how our metabolism is at the root of disease and the incentives that lead our current system to ignore it. Part 2 provides mindsets and tactics you can start implementing to feel better today. Part 3 brings all of these concepts together into an actionable plan, and Part 4 presents thirty-three recipes that include Good Energy eating principles. Throughout the book, I'll use stories from my experience inside and outside the system and insights from metabolic health leaders.

Good Energy is the goal, and the state of mind—and what it can create—is incredible . . . a world where we are eating beautiful food, moving our bodies, interacting with nature, taking pleasure in the world around us, and feeling fulfilled, vibrant, and alive. The view is exciting, because living with Good Energy means good food, happy people, real connections, and expanding into the most beautiful expression of our precious lives.

It's true that the challenges we're up against on the quest for upleveling our health are enormous. Yet I have seen that all of this can start to change *right now*. It starts when you simply ask one question: What would it feel like to have Good Energy? I invite you to ask that question now: What would it feel like to have your body functioning optimally, for your body to just be at ease enjoying this human experience, for your mind to be working clearly and creatively, and to feel that your life is established on a steady and strong source of inner power? Imagine a powerful life force from within that allows you to take on each day with pleasure, energy, gratitude, and joy. Take a moment. Really feel it. Imagine it. Let yourself.

My hope for this book is to change your life by enabling you to feel better today and prevent disease tomorrow. It all begins by understanding and acting upon the science of Good Energy.

To view the scientific references cited in this chapter, please visit us online at caseymeans.com/goodenergy.

PART 1

THE TRUTH ABOUT ENERGY

CHAPTER 1

Siloed Health vs. Energy-Centric Health

At the end of medical school, I had to choose one of forty-two specialties: one part of the body to devote my life to.

Separation defines modern medicine. Starting from my first year of medical education, I funneled from a broad perspective on the body to increasingly narrower and narrower ones. When I picked a premed major in college, I left the study of physics and chemistry behind to focus solely on biology. In med school, I memorized all the facts on *human* biology, no longer focusing on other biologic systems like plants and animals. As a resident, I was focused on performing surgeries on one specific area: the head and neck, and thought little about the rest of the body.

Had I completed five years of that training, I would have been eligible to zero in even further on a subspecialty within that specialty. I could have become a rhinologist (focused solely on the nose), a laryngologist (focused solely on the larynx), an otologist (focused solely on the three tiny bones of the inner ear, plus the cochlea and eardrum), or a specialist in head and neck cancer (among other options). The primary goal for my career would have been to become better and better at treating a smaller and smaller part of the body.

If I were *really* good at what I did, maybe the medical establishment would even name a disease of a body part after me, as they did for the dean of Stanford Medical School—a world-renowned otologist named Dr. Lloyd B. Minor, who focused his entire career on about three square inches of the body. In the condition named after him, Minor's syndrome, microscopic changes in the inner ear bones are thought to lead to various balance and otologic symptoms. Dean Minor represented a physician's ultimate model of success: stay focused on your specialty and climb the ladder. You also protect yourself that way: for the average clinician, staying in your lane ensures you don't incur liability for incorrectly treating something out of your scope of practice.

By my fifth year, I was the chief resident in otology, a subspecialty of head and neck surgery, focusing on those three square inches of the body around the ear that control hearing and balance. I frequently saw patients like Sarah, a thirty-six-year-old woman who visited the otology clinic gripped with intractable migraine, with attacks occurring more than ten times per month. Since dizziness and auditory symptoms can be a feature of this debilitating neurological condition, sufferers often find their way to this specialized department as they make their way through a labyrinth of providers. After a decade of bad migraine episodes, Sarah's world had shrunk dramatically in scope. As she was living on disability and largely housebound, her existence revolved around her condition. She was so light-sensitive that she always wore wraparound sunglasses and walked with a cane due to her inflammatory arthritis. A support dog always stood by her side.

Reviewing her hundred pages of faxed medical charts, I discovered she had seen eight medical specialists in the past year to address a larger cluster of persistent and painful symptoms. A neurologist had prescribed medications for her migraine attacks. A psychiatrist had prescribed a selective serotonin reuptake inhibitor (SSRI) for her depression. A cardiologist had prescribed hypertension medication. A palliative care specialist had prescribed additional remedies for the unremitting pain throughout her joints. Despite all these interventions and medications, Sarah was still suffering.

Carefully paging through the documents, I felt stunned. What could I *possibly* offer this woman that she had not already tried?

As part of my routine migraine intake questions, I asked if she had had any success with trying a migraine elimination diet. She had not heard of it. That surprised me. Printed handouts on that very subject were readily available in our clinics to give to patients like her. But nutritional intervention hadn't registered as important enough for my colleagues to mention. Instead, she had been sent for testing, undergone expensive CT scans, and was prescribed psychoactive and other medications—one on top of the other. She visibly balked when I described the hopeful possibilities of a diet that would eliminate migraine trigger foods. If such a mundane thing as *food* could have helped, her body language suggested, the medical professionals would have told her long ago. She wanted to try another medication.

Sarah's case was not the first time I had encountered such a scenario. Patients often came in with stubborn cases of chronic disease, toting stacks of paperwork. But Sarah was cruelly young for this amount of suffering, and she'd bounced between so many different specialists so quickly that her case made the system failure especially upsetting. She was sick and getting sicker, living with not just one chronic illness but multiple ones. Unbeknownst to her, but evident to me, her life span was almost certainly shortening. She was frustrated with the care she'd received, yet she was still reliant on it—clinging to it, even.

I tried to hide my discomfort. How could I dole out another prescription without encouraging Sarah to try some simple strategies with significant data to back them up? My stomach churned at the knowledge that another prescription drug would not be the magic bullet that would radically change her life. She and I could go through the charade of engendering hope in a new medication, scheduling a follow-up six weeks out to see how it worked, and leaving our meeting feeling satisfied that we'd done the best we could. But at some level, we both knew a "medication deficiency" was not why Sarah had illness expressed throughout her entire body.

I could do what the other doctors entrusted with her care had done—and what I was explicitly expected to do: name the condition according to symptom-based criteria, rule out serious life-threatening issues, attach a prescription, input billing codes, and move on. That would be practicing respectable medicine. But Sarah, and the other complex cases like hers, made me want to work differently, to look upstream, and question why those symptoms might be there.

PEELING BACK THE LAYERS: WHAT CAUSES DISEASE?

Invisible Inflammation: Everywhere, All at Once

When in doubt, always start by asking questions. And the obvious one in Sarah's case was the following: Were her different conditions so separate after all, or did something connect them that my colleagues and I couldn't see?

Looking through her labs, I noticed one of her inflammatory markers was high. I vaguely recalled learning in med school that this marker was high in conditions like diabetes and obesity. I noted that Sarah also had inflammatory arthritis. Chronic inflammation was at play here. So I asked another question: Could inflammation have a role in causing migraine? Surprisingly, a quick PubMed search offered over a thousand scientific papers connecting the two.

I knew well that inflammation refers to the swelling, heat, redness, pus, or pain created when immune cells rush to a site of injury or infection. All these symptoms are helpful: they indicate that a robust and coordinated defense is occurring to contain, resolve, and heal damaged or endangered tissue. The immune system is always looking for anything foreign, unwanted, or injurious and will jump to respond this way within seconds of detecting something wrong. After the problem is resolved, the immune system turns off the inflammation, and everything returns to normal. The heat, redness, swelling, and pain go away.

But Sarah's physical checkup and other lab markers were confounding. She had no injury, no overt infection I could see. Nothing was temporary about the phenomenon in this case. Her inflammatory response was switched on—and left on—to the point that it was causing collateral damage to her body. Why would the immune system stay so activated and remain in such a persistent state of alarm and defense—chronically inflamed—outside of acute situations, even to the extent of causing collateral damage to the body's tissues?

When I reflected on what I was treating as an ENT surgeon, something struck me: it was almost *all* inflammation. In medicine, the suffix *-itis* means *inflammation*, and our practice was made up of sinusitis, tonsillitis, pharyngitis, laryngitis, otitis, chondritis, thyroiditis, tracheitis, adenoiditis, rhinitis, epiglottitis, sialadenitis, parotitis, cellulitis, mastoiditis, osteomyelitis, vestibular neuritis, labyrinthitis, glossitis, and more. I was an inflammation physician, and I didn't even realize it! As an ENT, my job revolved around putting out inflammation wherever it appeared in the ear, nose, or throat. Often the process included using oral, nasal, intravenous, inhaled, and topical *anti-inflammatory* medications: Flonase spray, compounded steroid nasal irrigations, prednisone creams, IV Solu-Medrol, and inhaled nebulizers of steroids—all kinds of things to address the immune system getting so revved up in these bodies.

Suppose the medications failed, as was the case with my sinusitis patient Sophia. In that case, we might go to the next level in surgery: creating holes in a patient's body to reduce obstruction caused by inflammation and let inflammatory fluid drain. Sometimes we would intervene mechanically to force the anatomy out of the way of swelling. We might insert tubes through the eardrum to let fluid drain, drill through the skull bones to release trapped pus, or insert a balloon to enlarge an airway narrowed by chronic inflammation.

The medications and surgery would temporarily turn the inflammation off or minimize its effects—like subduing the invader with a tactical jujitsu move to the floor—but the tissues would often swell again or the pus would collect once more in whatever area was blocked. It wasn't in our job description as medical professionals to look for *why* inflammation kept returning.

But once I began peeling back the onion, the *whys* wouldn't stop. Why were the immune systems of my patients like Sophia and Sarah so chronically revved up? Why were cells that should be healthy sending out "fear" signals to recruit helper immune cells to come to their aid? I couldn't see or detect an obvious threat like a cut or an infection, nor could my patients. So why were these cells so frightened on the microscopic level?

I reflected on Sarah's labs and the inflammatory marker that I knew was strongly associated with chronic diseases like diabetes, obesity, and autoimmune diseases. And suddenly it struck me. Could *all* her symptoms—not just those under my purview as an ENT—be driven by inflammation? Is one mechanism driving so many different disease states? Was every part of her body responding fearfully to the same *invisible* threats? From my point of view today, that truth seems utterly self-evident. Research has shown that chronic inflammation is a crucial instigator of all kinds of diseases and conditions outside of the ear, nose, and throat—from cancer and cardiovascular disease to autoimmune diseases to respiratory infections to gastrointestinal conditions to skin disorders to neurological disorders. Yet it was not part of the institutional medical culture to focus on those connections nor to go deeper to ask *why* all that inflammation is there.

Then I began to realize how much I knew. Ever since I had fulfilled my required histology coursework and gazed at hundreds of slides of human tissue and flesh under a microscope, I had been in awe of the nearly forty trillion cells that make up the human body. I felt awe at their complexity and tiny importance as life's very foundation and how all that we are is a collection of cells. They hold so much information inside. Each cell is a little universe of buzzing work and activity. And the result of all that activity, simply put, is our lives.

Our cells cannot talk or tell us what they fear. But incredibly, if we look from the perspective of the cell, the answers to the *whys* are there—complex, yes, but not nearly as baffling, complicated, or specialized as some might want us to believe.

After I left my position as a chief resident at OHSU, an opportunity for discovery opened before me. Free to fill the gaps my conventional education had left—and feeling infinitely healthier and more energized—I excitedly leaped into advanced training in nutritional biochemistry, cell biology, systems and network biology, and functional medicine, expanding and revolutionizing my understanding of health and disease. I got to know dozens of physicians who, like me, had exited prestigious institutions in pursuit of better medicine in the quest of learning to help patients actually *heal* rather than be managed. Reinspired and reinvigorated, I soon opened a small medical practice in the Pearl District neighborhood of Portland, happily settling into a coworking space with sunny windows and many plants. I let a few friends and colleagues know I was doing something different: instead of offering sick care, I focused on generating health. Instead of managing diseases from the pinnacle of medicine as an esteemed surgeon, I would work to restore and maintain good health from the pyramid's base, via having deep conversations and creating personalized plans. Together, my patients and I would build the foundations of a solid and healthy body from the ground up. Word got out: my schedule was quickly full.

Many patients came to see me with clusters of chronic and intractable-seeming conditions like Sarah's and Sophia's. But this time, we started treating the problem from a different place: the foundational cellular level. I put the onus on giving the cells what they needed to do their jobs and removing what was blocking them, with a focus on nutritional changes, lifestyle changes, and overall cellular support. The results my patients achieved were different, too—often, transformative. Stubborn problems—weight gain, lousy sleep, unshakable pain, chronic conditions, high cholesterol, and even reproductive issues—began to resolve, sometimes in weeks, sometimes months. Inflammation began to disappear, never to return. Patients often reduced, and even eliminated, their medication regimen. Hope and optimism about what life could feel like returned in the dedicated people I was fortunate to help. Often, the results came from doing far *less*. They occurred from doing the opposite of what I had always learned, which was to add the next medication and add the next intervention.

I learned many things through practicing medicine in this new way. Not the least was that inflammation—which leads to disease, pain, and suffering—takes root because core dysfunctions occur inside our cells, impacting how they function, signal, and replicate themselves. Something became blatantly clear: if we truly want to restore general health in the body and mind, we must look one layer deeper than the mechanism of inflammation alone and into the very center of the cells themselves.

Trouble Where It's Hard to See: Metabolism, Mitochondria, and Malfunction

After years of my digging for it, the answer to what is causing inflammation inside patients like Sarah turned out to be remarkably simple: the chronic inflammation is often a response to our body's cells feeling threatened by being persistently underpowered due to Bad Energy processes.

Immune cells rush to areas of the body that are in danger, thus producing inflammation.

An *underpowered* cell—metabolically dysfunctional, struggling to make energy, and sputtering along through its daily work—is a cell that is threatened and at risk. This flailing cell will send out chemical alarm signals and recruit the immune system to help it. In their efforts to help, the immune cells cause immense collateral damage—creating a literal war within the body to protect itself from itself—that results in worse symptoms. This is a key reason why chronic inflammation typically goes in lockstep with metabolic dysfunction and widespread symptoms.

Diving into the world of cellular biology sounds like an intimidating prospect. But there's one simple measure that can powerfully reframe how we understand health and disease: how well or poorly the mitochondria in the cell are making energy.

Likely you have heard the word "mitochondria," and perhaps you know it from high school biology as "the powerhouse of the cell." Mitochondria convert food energy into cellular energy. These tiny organelles are transformers: they take breakdown products of the food we eat and are tasked to convert it into a currency of energy that our cells can use to do their many jobs. Different types of cells in the body—liver, skin, brain, ovarian, eye, and so forth—have vastly different amounts of mitochondria inside them. Some cells have hundreds of thousands inside; others have just a handful, depending on what kind of work that cell must do and what its energy needs are to power that work.

When the body is in a healthy state, fatty acids from dietary fats, and glucose (sugar) from dietary carbohydrates, are broken down in digestion. Then they enter the bloodstream and are transported into individual cells. Glucose is further broken down inside the cell. These molecules are transported inside the mitochondria and through a series of chemical reactions generate electrons (charged particles). These electrons get carried and passed through specialized mitochondrial machinery to ultimately synthesize adenosine triphosphate (ATP). This is the most important molecule in the human body: it is the energy currency that "pays" for all the activity inside our cells, and therefore pays for our lives.

There's a lot of ATP, as it turns out. Trillions upon trillions of chemical reactions happen in our bodies every second, the result of which bubbles up into our lives! All these activities run on energy—namely, the ATP that the mitochondria produce—and they require enough at all times. Without all this hubbub, we'd fall apart, literally; we'd be decomposing on the ground with no energetic force holding us together.

Even though ATP is a microscopic molecule, the average human produces about eighty-eight cumulative pounds of it per day—constantly making, using, and recycling it so fast that we never even notice. Each of our thirty-seven trillion cells is like a little city—continually bustling with action, transactions, and production—and contained by its cell membrane. While the processes that our cells engage in every second are far too many to count, the main things that a cell needs for optimal functioning can be grouped into seven categories of activity, and all require ATP—and therefore Good Energy—to occur properly.

1. **Make Proteins:** Cells are responsible for synthesizing approximately seventy thousand different types of proteins needed for all aspects of building and operating our bodies. Proteins come in all shapes, sizes, and functions and have an array of responsibilities. They can be receptors on the surface of cells, channels through which things like glucose can flow into and out of the cell, structural scaffolding inside the cell to give it shape and help it move, regulators that sit on the DNA and activate or suppress genes, signaling molecules like hormones and neurotransmitters that transmit information to other cells, and anchors that keep neighboring cells attached together. Moreover, several different proteins can bind together to form specialized machines in the cell, such as the rotary turbine called ATP synthase that lives inside the mitochondria and is the final step in making ATP. These are just a few of the things that proteins do, but, simply put, they are structural, mechanical, and signaling workhorses in the cell.

2. **Repair, Regulate, and Replicate DNA:** Cells are responsible for replicating their DNA to ensure that each new cell has a complete copy of the genetic material during the process of cell division. Cells also repair

any damage to the DNA to prevent mutations that could lead to cancer and other diseases. In addition to this, cells have complex mechanisms for modifying the folding and three-dimensional structure of the genome through *epi*genetic changes, which regulate which genes are expressed in a given cell type and at what time. Our cells are constantly turning over and replacing themselves, and the DNA replication and cell division processes allow for this.

3. **Cell Signaling:** Inside a cell, all activity is coordinated via cell signaling—microscopic biochemical messages constantly being transported around the inside and outside of the cell to give instructions and information about what needs to be done, where things need to go, and what needs to turn on and off. For instance, in the body's effort to bring blood sugar back down to normal after a meal, the body will produce insulin. The insulin binds to the surface of cells, kicking off a series of signals inside the cell that prompts the cell to send glucose channels to the cell membrane to allow glucose to flow in. Cells also constantly communicate with other cells in the body through various signaling pathways, in which they receive and transmit information through chemical signals, like hormones, neurotransmitters, and electrical impulses.

4. **Transport:** Just as trucks transport cargo all over the country, cells must move molecular materials all around the inside of the cell for things to function properly. Each cell is capable of packaging, labeling, and shipping molecules throughout its microscopic environment with incredible precision. For instance, when the cell makes a batch of the neurotransmitter serotonin (which helps regulate mood, among other things), it packages it in a cellular bag called a vesicle and sends the vesicle on a motor protein (like a little car) to the cell membrane to act on neighboring neurons. This process creates your thoughts and feelings. Some cells—like immune cells—must also transport *themselves* around the body at times. When an immune cell is triggered by an inflammatory chemical signal to go to the scene of a threatening situation, it might launch itself out of the bone marrow into the bloodstream, as if it were jumping on the freeway. Once it

reaches the organ in danger, it will crawl through the organ by extending fingerlike projections until it reaches the site of threat where it needs to do its work.

5. **Homeostasis:** Cells are constantly working to maintain healthy operating conditions, like pH, salt concentration, gradients of charged molecules that can generate electrical impulses, and temperature. This maintenance of an optimal environment in which the body's chemical reactions can take place is called homeostasis.

6. **Cell Waste Cleanup and Autophagy:** Cells are also able to recycle their own components through a process called autophagy (literally "self-eating"), which is a way for cells to clear out damaged parts and proteins and recycle the raw materials. When the mitochondria undergo this recycling and renewal, it is called mitophagy, a critical component of maintaining healthy mitochondrial populations within cells. More dramatically, cells can also incite their own death to make way for healthier cells, a critical process called apoptosis.

7. **Metabolism:** And of course, the production of energy itself. Even *this* requires energy to work!

Every one of these activities requires ATP—made by well-functioning mitochondria—to occur. When the suitable materials are available in the correct amounts, the mitochondria produce sufficient energy for the cell's activities. This trickles up to health throughout the body. Organs are, in simple terms, aggregations of cells. Groups of healthy, energized cells that can carry out all their duties become healthy organs that carry out their jobs. Every cell has the blueprint it needs to work; it simply needs the resources. But when the mitochondria do not have the right conditions or they get inundated with the wrong materials in the wrong amounts, they don't produce enough ATP for the cells to do their jobs. This cellular level problem of Bad Energy not only directly trickles up to problems in the organs but leads cells to sound an alarm bell: *Something's not right, we need help.* Our immune system—always ready to help—is there in a flash.

But in this case, the problem is not an infection or a wound that immune cells can mop up and be done with: it's something more pro-found, a fundamental problem with how the cells function. And it's some-thing the immune cells can't solve, because the thing that is robbing the mitochondria of doing its job, resulting in cells not being able to do their work, is *outside of us*. It's the environment in which our bodies now exist, an environment that—from our cells' perspective—is virtually unrecognizable from a hundred years ago.

Our modern diets and lifestyles are synergistically ravaging our mito-chondria. Our mitochondria and the greater cells that house them co-evolved over eons in relationship with our environment. Their mechanisms work in connection with a combination of inputs and information that come from the outside world into our bodies and ultimately into them. Certain kinds of nutrients, sunlight, and information from bacteria in the gut, among other things, all help trigger or supply the cells and their power-houses with what they require to work. But many of those inputs and in-formation streams have changed radically, resulting in blocks to proper mitochondrial function and downright damage to it.

A mighty immune cell trying to support a cell that is ailing and threat-ened from its mitochondrial dysfunction is rendered completely impotent. The immune cell cannot halt the damaging factors and the lack of re-sources resulting from the unnatural environment of our modern indus-trial world. An immune cell can't stop you from drinking a soda, filter your water, turn off the stress-inducing notifications on your phone, pre-vent you from eating hormone-disrupting pesticides and microplastics, or get you to go to sleep earlier. So the immune cell will use the tools at its disposal: it will recruit more immune cells, send out more inflammatory signals, and just keep fighting until things resolve. But the problems don't resolve, because the damaging environmental inputs never resolve. This is the root of chronic inflammation.

A group of cells not working due to mitochondrial dysfunction and the immune system's overzealous—yet helpless—response to infiltrate that area and support it results in organ dysfunction, which manifests as a symptom. Most of the chronic symptoms we battle today are simply differ-ent expressions of this same disaster happening in other parts of the body:

the mitochondria are hurt by the way we're living, a poorly powered cell becomes dysfunctional, the immune system tries to help but can't, and, in trying, the immune system makes the issue worse.

How exactly does the environment we live in today ravage our mitochondria? The answer comes down to ten main factors (which we will discuss more in Part 2), all of which are tightly interlinked:

1. **Chronic Overnutrition:** Chronic overnutrition, which refers to consuming more calories and macronutrients than the body needs over an extended period, can lead to mitochondrial dysfunction in several ways. We eat approximately 20 percent more calories than we did one hundred years ago, and 700 to 3,000 percent more fructose, all of which the body must process. Imagine being asked to do 700 to 3,000 percent more work than you normally do daily—you'd collapse! The cell simply cannot process all the material coming in from too much food, so things back up, damaging by-products are produced in excess, and many processes in the cell, including the efforts of mitochondria, get gummed up. This strain leads to the inside of the cell filling with toxic fats, which block the cell's ability to do its normal signaling and activity. Additionally, when mitochondria are taxed with the burden of trying to convert so much excess food to energy, they produce and release reactive molecules called free radicals. Free radicals are molecules with a negatively charged, highly reactive electron that seeks to neutralize itself by binding to other structures in the mitochondria and cell and, in doing so, causes significant damage. The body has several mechanisms for safely neutralizing free radicals, including the production of antioxidants, which bind and quell free radicals. However, when the production of these damaging molecules exceeds the body's capacity to handle them, as is the case with chronic overnutrition, a damaging imbalance called oxidative stress can occur that hurts the mitochondria and surrounding cellular structures. Normally, a low and controlled level of free radicals is healthy and they act as signaling molecules in the cell. But when the level gets out of control and oxidative stress takes hold, it's a chain reaction of damage.

Healthy levels of free radicals represent a cozy campfire; oxidative stress is a destructive forest fire.

A key reason why we are chronically consuming far too much food energy is because of the wide accessibility of ultra-processed, industrially manufactured foods, which impair our body's self-regulatory satiety mechanisms and directly trigger hunger and cravings. These ultra-processed industrial foods are chemically engineered to be addictive and make up nearly 70 percent of calories that people in the United States consume today.

2. **Nutrient Deficiencies:** The lack of certain micronutrients, such as vitamins and minerals, can lead to mitochondrial dysfunction. The final steps in making energy in the mitochondria involve electrons moving through five protein structures called the electron transport chain, which ultimately powers a small molecular motor that churns out ATP. These five protein complexes all need micronutrients to activate them to work, like little locks and keys. Unfortunately, we have the most micronutrient-depleted diet we've ever had in history. As much as half of all people in the United States are deficient in at least some critical micronutrients. This is partly because of soil depletion (from modern industrial farming practices like pesticide use and mechanized tilling) and the lack of diversity in our diets. At least 75 percent of people are not eating the recommended amounts of vegetables and fruits. Most of our calories come from refined forms of commodity crops like wheat, soy, and corn, all of which are micronutrient deficient and doubly cause problems by flooding our bodies with a dense excess of carbohydrates and inflammatory fats. For example, a deficiency in coenzyme Q10 (CoQ10), a micronutrient that is essential for the function of the electron transport chain, has been shown in research studies to lead to decreased ATP synthesis. Other micronutrients involved in key mitochondrial processes involve selenium, magnesium, zinc, and several B vitamins.

3. **Microbiome Issues:** A healthy, flourishing gut microbiome, fed with microbiome-supportive foods and free of microbiome-harming

chemicals, produces thousands of "post-biotic" chemicals that travel into our bodies from our gut and act as important signaling molecules, some of which directly affect the mitochondria. Post-biotic molecules, such as short-chain fatty acids (SCFAs), are essential for the proper function of mitochondria and to protect mitochondria against oxidative stress. When microbiome imbalance—called dysbiosis—takes hold, the production of these helpful chemicals gets derailed, depriving mitochondria of this signaling and support. Dysbiosis can be triggered by excess refined sugar and ultra-processed foods, pesticides, medications like nonsteroidal anti-inflammatory medications (NSAIDs, like Advil), antibiotics, chronic stress, lack of sleep, alcohol consumption, physical inactivity, smoking, and infections, among other factors.

4. **Sedentary Lifestyle:** Lack of physical activity can lead to decreased mitochondrial function and a reduction in the number and size of mitochondria in cells. Movement is a powerful signal to the cells that they need to produce more energy for the muscles to do work, and as such, physical activity has a relationship with stimulating the function and number of mitochondria in cells in a positive way through the upregulation of several genes and hormonal pathways. Additionally, exercise stimulates our body to generate antioxidant molecules. When we're sedentary, we have less protection from free radicals, which can then damage the mitochondria, and the positive signals for the mitochondria are absent, leading to worse mitochondrial function.

5. **Chronic Stress:** Prolonged stress can lead to mitochondrial dysfunction through several mechanisms. The first is that it activates the release of the stress hormone cortisol, which is a steroid hormone that can directly damage the mitochondria. Cortisol is known to inhibit the expression of genes involved in the production of new mitochondria, thus reducing the number of mitochondria in the cell, leading to less energy production. Excess cortisol also generates increased free radicals, in part by inhibiting the production of antioxidants.

6. **Medications and Drugs:** Many medications hurt the function of mitochondria. These include several antibiotics, chemotherapy drugs,

antiretroviral drugs, statins, beta-blockers, and high blood pressure medications called calcium channel blockers. Alcohol, methamphetamines, cocaine, heroin, and ketamine may also negatively impact mitochondria.

7. **Sleep Deprivation:** Poor quality and quantity of sleep generate a wide array of downstream effects that damage the mitochondria. Lack of quality sleep leads to hormonal imbalances, including altered cortisol, insulin, growth hormone, and melatonin levels, all of which interact with the mitochondria. Additionally, sleep deprivation disrupts the expression of genes involved in the production of new mitochondria and replication of mitochondria. Like stress, sleep deprivation generates increased free radicals, both by activating cellular machinery that makes free radicals and by inhibiting the production of antioxidants.

8. **Environmental Toxins and Pollutants:** Many synthetic industrial chemicals that have entered our food supply, water, air, and consumer products over the last century are wreaking havoc on our mitochondria. A non-exhaustive list includes pesticides; polychlorinated biphenyls (PCBs); phthalates found in plastics and scented products; perfluoroalkyl and polyfluoroalkyl substances (PFASs) found in nonstick cookware, food packaging, and many other consumer products; bisphenol A (BPA) found in plastics and resins, dioxins, and others. Some natural substances, like heavy metals, have made their way into our environment and can directly impair the mitochondria as well. These include lead, mercury, and cadmium. In addition to these, cigarette smoke and vaping chemicals are some of the most potent toxins for our mitochondria and biology. Have you ever wondered why cigarettes are so terrible for our health? A key reason is that the chemicals in cigarette smoke (like cyanide, aldehyde, and benzene) directly cause Bad Energy: they impair mitochondrial function, mutate mitochondrial DNA, and cause mitochondrial structural changes (like mitochondrial swelling). Alcohol, too, can be considered a mitochondrial toxin and has been shown to change mitochondrial shape and function, damage mitochondrial DNA,

generate oxidative stress, and impair the generation of new mitochondria.

9. **Artificial Light and Circadian Disruption:** With the advent of portable digital devices, we are being exposed to constant sources of artificial blue light, which is now considered to be both a direct and indirect contributor to mitochondrial dysfunction. Exposure to intense light at unnatural times affects our circadian rhythms and the many metabolic pathways that are meant to be activated in specific daily cycles that are dictated by when our eyes (and therefore brains) are exposed to light. Compounding this, we now spend little time outdoors, depriving ourselves of viewing direct sunlight early in the morning, which is one of the best signals we can give our brains to reinforce our natural circadian rhythms.

10. **"Thermoneutrality":** A hallmark of modern industrial life is spending most of our time indoors at relatively consistent ambient temperatures, a concept we'll refer to as thermoneutrality. Interestingly, experiencing swings in temperature is great for mitochondrial function, as cold stimulates the body to generate more warmth by increasing mitochondrial activity and stimulates more ATP generation and use. Heat exposure has been shown to activate heat shock proteins (HSPs) within cells, which can protect mitochondria from damage and help to maintain their function. HSPs can also stimulate the production of new mitochondria and improve their efficiency in producing ATP.

Blood Sugar and Insulin

When mitochondria are damaged by the factors listed above, they are not able to do their job of converting food energy into cellular energy properly. They become inefficient machines, causing things to back up, which is a big problem.

Normally, fat and glucose breakdown products would be transported into the mitochondria to be processed into ATP and be done with. In ideal, healthy circumstances, our energy needs would roughly match our food intake, our mitochondria would not be damaged by the ten environmental factors outlined above, and the whole process would move along seamlessly.

But that's not what's happening. With the mitochondria not working properly, the conversion of fats and glucose to ATP becomes impaired, and these raw materials are stored as damaging fats inside the cell. Any cell that is not a fat cell that is filled with fats is a big problem, because the normal cellular activities we outlined earlier, like cell signaling and the transportation of items around the cell that allow for normal cellular functioning, get blocked. It's a traffic jam inside the cell caused by all this excess fat. One of the cell-signaling pathways that is blocked when a cell is filled with toxic fat is insulin signaling, which has a huge impact on the levels of blood sugar circulating in the body.

Under normal circumstances, when there is a surge of sugar in the bloodstream after eating and digesting a carbohydrate-rich meal, the hormone insulin is released from the pancreas and floats around the body, binding to insulin receptors on cells and signaling for those cells to bring glucose channels from the inside of the cell to the cell membrane to let the glucose flow inside. However, when a cell is filled with fat, this insulin signaling process is impaired; glucose channels don't get shuttled to the cell membrane, and glucose doesn't get let into the cell; it's blocked. This blocking, called insulin resistance, is a way the cell protects itself from being overly bombarded with too much energy from food (glucose). The cell "knows" that because of mitochondrial issues, it can't convert that raw material (glucose) to cellular energy, so it blocks the entry of glucose into the cell. Insulin resistance causes glucose to remain in excess in the bloodstream, where it causes a slew of problems.

That's not the end of the story. The body is very smart. It knows that excess blood sugar circulating around the bloodstream can cause problems, so it tries *extra* hard to encourage the cells to take it up. It does this by prompting the pancreas to produce much more insulin (leading to high insulin levels in the blood) to overcome the insulin signaling block. And, amazingly, this works—for a while. For years, the body can overcompensate for its insulin resistance just by pumping out excess insulin, bombarding the insulin receptors, and forcing glucose into cells. During this period of overcompensation, blood sugar levels can appear to be normal and healthy, when, in fact, severe dysfunction and insulin resistance are at play. Over time, the overwhelmed cell—filled with fat and dysfunctional mitochondria—just can't keep stuffing glucose into itself. This is when we start to see individuals have sharp rises in their blood sugar levels and difficulty controlling their levels.

And therein lies the root of blood sugar problems, such as prediabetes and type 2 diabetes, conditions that affect over 50 percent of adults and nearly 30 percent of children in the United States. It's a domino effect of mitochondrial dysfunction—caused by several environmental factors—which leads to a backup of glucose and fatty acids that convert to toxic fats that fill the cell, thereby blocking insulin signaling, leading to a cell that struggles to take in glucose from the bloodstream. Insulin resistance ultimately leads to a rise in our day-to-day levels of blood sugar.

Adding fuel to the fire, the rising blood sugar levels can independently stimulate the activation of the immune system and the generation of excess free radicals, thus contributing to a tornado of dysfunction in the cells and body. We've got mitochondrial dysfunction leading to inflammation and excess free radicals, and we've got high blood sugar doing more of the same. What's more, chronically elevated blood sugar floating around the bloodstream will lead to that excess sugar sticking to things—a process called glycation. Structures in the body that get glycated with sugar won't work properly and are considered foreign to the immune system, contributing even more to chronic inflammation.

A simple example of glycation causing dysfunction is in how it generates wrinkles. Excess blood sugar sticks to the most abundant protein in our skin, collagen. Normally, collagen gives our skin its structural integrity. Glycation causes collagen to contort in shape and "cross-link," leading to wrinkles and the appearance of premature aging. Much more serious and life-threatening effects of glycation can occur. For example, glycation can cause issues with the lining of our blood vessels and accelerate the process of vascular blockages called atherosclerosis, which lead to heart attacks, stroke, peripheral vascular disease, retinopathy, kidney disease, erectile dysfunction, and more.

About 74 percent of U.S. adults are overweight or obese, and 93.2 percent have metabolic dysfunction. These numbers sound high until you realize how many levers of modern society are stacked against our mitochondria and metabolism: too much sugar, too much stress, too much sitting, too much pollution, too many pills, too many pesticides, too many screens, too little sleep, and too little micronutrients. These trends—with trillions of dollars behind them—are causing epidemic levels of mitochondrial dysfunction and underpowered, sick, inflamed bodies.

The trifecta of cellular malfunction that is the root of virtually every symptom and disease plaguing modern Americans may not be the stuff of dinner table conversation. They may not be the most posted about topics on Instagram. But you need to know what they are—because when *you* know them, you get closer to understanding the root of the U.S. health care epidemic, more so than almost any doctor, and closer to helping yourself and your loved ones to heal, stay healthy, and be limitless during this precious lifetime. The trifecta of dysfunction inside our bodies that generates Bad Energy boils down to the following:

1. **Mitochondrial Dysfunction:** The cells can't make energy properly because they are overburdened with so much crap from the environment that their energy factories—the mitochondria—are overtaxed and damaged, leading to less ATP production and more fat stored inside cells, which blocks normal cellular functions.
2. **Chronic Inflammation:** Mitochondrial dysfunction and low cellular energy (ATP) production are perceived as a threat, so the body revs up a fighting response. This response becomes chronic because the perceived threat doesn't go away unless the environment changes.
3. **Oxidative Stress:** The cells create damaging, reactive waste in the form of free radicals while trying to process all the junk being thrown at them from the environment and from damaged mitochondria. These free radicals cause damage to cells, leading to dysfunction.

HOW TO MEASURE GOOD ENERGY

If you're like the many thousands of people with whom I have shared this information, you have probably come out of this dive into cellular biology with one pressing question: How on earth do I know if those invisible malfunctions are happening inside *me*?

It's a great question. And luckily, we have some good answers. Simple markers can show us "check engine" alerts. A most basic and accessible way to see if you have a reasonable level of metabolic health is by checking five markers that are almost always tested and tracked at your annual checkup: blood sugar, triglycerides, high-density lipoprotein (HDL) cholesterol, blood pressure, and waist circumference. When these markers fall into an optimal range, in the absence of medication—see Chapter 4 for exact specifications—you can deduce that your cellular energy production is doing OK. Typically, you will feel vibrant, healthy, and pain-free. These feelings, too, should tell you that your body has Good Energy, the foundation of general good health.

When several of those markers fall outside the optimal range, however, it's a different story. The markers are signposts to the opposite state: metabolic syndrome. Metabolic syndrome means cells are struggling to get their jobs done because of problems in their energy production system. Metabolic syndrome is clinically defined as having three or more of the following traits:

- Fasting glucose of 100 mg/dL or higher
- A waistline of more than 35 inches for women and 40 inches for men
- HDL cholesterol less than 40 mg/dL for men and 50 mg/dL for women
- Triglycerides of 150 mg/dL or higher
- Blood pressure of 130/85 mmHg or higher

The reason you want to know whether your markers have tipped into suboptimal states is that it gives you a surefire clue that the Bad Energy processes are happening inside the cells. And this needs to be corrected to prevent or reverse the innumerable problems that can result from an underpowered machine. You will learn much more about this in Part 2, where I will show you how—despite the monumental challenges your cells face on a daily basis—establishing (or reestablishing) proper functioning, improving your biomarkers, building (or rebuilding) better health, and recovering from (or preventing) the most common health issues and diseases of our time is something that every person can do.

We've been taught that disease is often random (or hereditary), and my definitive claim—that preventing some of the country's largest killers is within your control—probably sounds surprising. But when you dig into the scientific literature, you can see a phenomenal picture: People with Good Energy have a drastically lower risk of heart disease (#1 cause of death in the United States), many leading forms of cancer (#2 cause of death), stroke (#5 cause of death), Alzheimer's disease (#7 cause of death), type 2 diabetes (#8 cause of death), and liver disease (#10 cause of death). People with Good Energy will be much more likely to recover from pneumonia (#9 cause of death), COVID-19 (#3 cause of death), and chronic lower respiratory diseases (#6 cause of death). Studies show that 70 percent of people with heart disease and 80 percent of those with Alzheimer's have dysfunctional blood glucose levels.

Poor energy metabolism, which is in part represented by elevated glucose levels, is a target on your back for a slow and painful journey toward death, a shorter life, innumerable brain and body symptoms, and significantly higher costs. Even if you currently have more "minor" symptoms, such as fatigue, infertility, and foggy thinking, the evidence is clear: You can improve these issues by understanding the science of how your body processes energy, by treating food as the information to optimize this machine, and by utilizing some very simple behaviors in your daily life as high-level biochemical information your cells require to thrive. You can feel limitless, positive, sharp, powerful, and free.

But if you don't heed the warnings these "minor" conditions are trying to tell you, our Good Energy machinery will get worse over time, leading to more serious symptoms. This is why it is tragic that patients are told conditions like type 2 diabetes, heart disease, and obesity are totally separate conditions. They are all warning signs of Bad Energy and can be improved or reversed the same way.

Exiting the separatist, reductionist framework of medicine to take on unifying cellular perspectives of health and disease felt like a sea change to me. It probably feels that way as a patient as well. But now I feel like I have a solid gold key in hand that opens what seemed like an impenetrable lock. This key unlocks the possibility of your feeling and functioning better, even when you've gotten stuck in long-standing, challenging, or even defeating circumstances. This key holds a kind of superpower: one that can help all of us, young and old alike, avert chronic diseases and symptoms of the mind and body that have become tragically normalized today, and for people of shockingly young ages. It is not normal for 74 percent of the country to be overweight or obese, for fifty million people to have autoimmune diseases, or for 25 percent of young adults to have fatty liver disease. It is not normal for the leading cause of visits to the doctor to be vague feelings of "being tired."

You now have a powerful understanding of how nearly every common symptom of the Western world is connected and how one of the biggest misconceptions in medicine is that people in their twenties, thirties, and forties are "healthy"—simply because they're not overtly or egregiously sick or overweight. (In fact, data suggests that most Americans in this age group—regardless of weight—are not optimally healthy.) This superpower is priceless in a world where the deck is stacked against us (and all forms of life around us: plants, animals, and microorganisms alike), and where our animating life force is being systematically and dramatically dimmed.

To understand why exactly that is, we need to zoom out from looking at the interior of our cells to looking at something wide and far-reaching: the metabolic spectrum of disease.

To view the scientific references cited in this chapter, please visit us online at caseymeans.com/goodenergy.

CHAPTER 2

Bad Energy Is the Root of Disease

At thirty-six, Lucy was increasingly frustrated by a cluster of health issues impacting her well-being, confidence, and dreams for the future. In the previous year, she'd seen a dermatologist to treat her adult acne, a gastroenterologist to address her frequent bloating after meals, a psychiatrist for her low mood and anxiety, and her primary care physician for her insomnia. She and her husband had been trying for a baby for over two years to no avail, making regular visits to her OB-GYN for prescriptions to treat her polycystic ovary syndrome (PCOS). She was about to gear up for an expensive round of in vitro fertilization (IVF).

She was one of the first patients who sat across from me, looking for answers, in the private practice I established after leaving residency. Nothing had been working and she wanted to feel better, look better, and start a family. She looked eager and slightly nervous, sitting in a comfortable armchair in my plant-filled office, which intentionally looked more like a peaceful living room than a clinical space. She had seen on my website that I focused on addressing the root causes of illness rather than just treating isolated symptoms, and something in her knew that she wanted *that*.

By any statistical measure, Lucy was a typical American woman. After all, she had no flagrant "lethal" disease and wasn't at risk of being immediately hospitalized or dying. She didn't feel or look as good as she thought she could, but wasn't that the case for everyone? More than 19 percent of adult women take an antidepressant, and up to 26 percent of women experience PCOS. Lucy's conditions seemed so common that she always considered herself "healthy." But she had a nagging feeling that something wasn't quite right and that she could live a life with more ease, joy, and energy.

Over the course of a two-hour initial visit, Lucy and I began to peel back the onion. Fatigue, acne, gastrointestinal upset, depression, insomnia, and infertility seemed to Lucy and her doctors to be isolated issues. Noting Lucy's sense of defeat, I told her we would shift perspective and look at her body differently. Her varied conditions, though occurring in different parts of her body and having very different names, were more likely to be branches of the same tree. Our work was to figure out what that tree was and how to heal it.

In a routine doctor's appointment, Lucy would have said she "eats and sleeps well," and the conversation about lifestyle would have been over. But we dug deeper and found the following:

- **Sleep:** Her husband was going to bed later than she did, and their cat often jumped on the bed; both interrupted her sleep.
- **Food:** Her diet consisted of many refined and ultra-processed foods, like refined grain in tortillas, pita chips, and croutons, and added sugars in granola bars, baked goods, and drinks.
- **Movement:** She was doing yoga and going on weekend hikes, but these were discrete bouts; she was otherwise sedentary, working a desk job. She did no resistance training, and her body composition showed minimal muscle.
- **Stress:** She lacked community in a new city and felt somewhat lonely. She felt daily low-grade stress from her job as a software engineer, her parents' aging, and her lack of ability to conceive.
- **Toxins:** Her water was unfiltered, giving her a dose of chemicals and toxins throughout the day. Her personal care products and home care products contained several common toxins. She drank wine several nights per week.
- **Light:** She stared at blue light all day at her computer and then late into the night in front of the TV, while she finished emails. The light bulbs

in her house weren't helping, either. She spent most of her hours in her apartment, office, or favorite yoga studio, enjoying little time outdoors.

We created a plan that incorporated seeing food as medicine, optimizing sleep, reducing chronic stress, protecting her microbiome, reducing environmental toxins, and maximizing sunlight during the day.

Over the next six months, nearly every symptom melted away: her menstrual cycles normalized, the pain during her periods lightened significantly, her mood lifted, and her digestive function improved. She was able to taper off her medications, and—confident that her reproductive hormones were coming back into balance—she postponed her first IVF appointment. She hadn't simply started to feel better, more energized, and happier about herself today; she had also drastically reduced her chances of developing chronic illness in the future.

I saw similar turnarounds in patients who implemented consistent lifestyle changes in my practice. These changes were rooted in understanding three simple truths:

1. Most chronic symptoms and diseases afflicting modern bodies are connected by a shared root cause of cellular malfunction that often results in Bad Energy. *All* symptoms are the direct result of dysfunction in our cells; symptoms cannot arise out of thin air. And for most people in the United States, metabolic dysfunction is a key cause of their cellular dysfunction.

2. Chronic conditions linked to Bad Energy exist on a spectrum from not immediately life-threatening (e.g., erectile dysfunction, fatigue, infertility, gout, arthritis) to more urgently life-threatening (e.g., stroke, cancer, and heart disease).

3. "Mild" symptoms today should be seen as clues that more serious disease will likely follow.

The best way I can explain the interconnectivity of "small" and "big" diseases is by diving deeper into the story of my mother and me.

A "HEALTHY" BABY

When my mom was preparing to get pregnant in the 1980s, she had duly followed the nutritional advice of the time: copious grains, bread, crackers (we were told to eat six to eleven servings a day), and lots of low-fat snacks—since fats back then were to be eaten "sparingly." Sufficient healthy protein was, unsurprisingly, an afterthought, given its no-man's-land place in the confusing middle of the food pyramid. In her twenties and early thirties, my mom was known for despising vegetables, with her main veggie dish being broiled tomatoes with Parmesan on occasion. She never learned to cook in her youth and relied on takeout as a New Yorker in her twenties. She walked but wasn't a regular exerciser and was notorious for going to bed late. She smoked from her twenties to her fifties, stopping just for pregnancy.

Invisibly, metabolic abnormalities were going on in my mom that transferred to me in utero. You don't become an eleven-pound, nine-ounce baby for no reason. And having a large baby increases the risk of future metabolic problems for both mom and baby, including type 2 diabetes and obesity. This relationship is due to several mechanisms.

1. **Insulin Resistance:** Children born with macrosomia are often exposed to high levels of glucose in utero, which can cause insulin resistance in the child. This early exposure to high insulin levels can persist into adulthood, leading to an increased risk of developing type 2 diabetes and other metabolic problems.
2. **Fat Cell Number and Size:** Children born with macrosomia often have an increased quantity and size of fat cells, likely due to maternal fatty acids stimulating the conversion of fetal stem cells into fat cells. This can contribute to obesity and metabolic problems later in life.
3. **Inflammation:** Children born with macrosomia are often exposed to high levels of inflammation in utero, which can contribute to the development of metabolic problems as they age.

My mom's doctor insisted on a cesarean birth due to my size. But because I didn't pass through her vaginal canal, I didn't ingest the organisms from her microbiome that would have helped seed mine. Breastfeeding is more challenging for mothers after C-section, and my mother couldn't breastfeed. She was also told not to lift more than ten pounds while her C-section scar healed, and I was nearly twelve pounds, making breastfeeding additionally challenging. Given this, I didn't get the benefits of the healthy bacterial transfer and oligosaccharides that come with breast milk that shape the infant microbiome for life.

In early childhood, although we had many home-cooked, lovingly made meals as a family, I ate many standard children's foods: Reese's Puffs cereal, Lucky Charms, Dunkaroos, Utz Barbeque chips, Rice Krispies Treats, Goldfish, and Hostess CupCakes. The Bad Energy warning signs showed up quickly. When I was a toddler, my chronic ear infections and tonsillitis had my mom frequently running to the doctor, who prescribed antibiotics. I remember stories in my youth of her "living" at the pediatrician's office and being on a first-name basis with all the staff.

I now understand that those chronic infections likely were connected to a suboptimal immune system, which is in large part determined by our microbiome composition and the integrity of the lining of our gut (which houses 70 percent of our immune system). As I was a C-section-birthed, formula-fed baby who went on to eat processed foods and to frequently consume microbiome-destroying antibiotics, my gut function was likely a disaster (in the scientific literature, this "disaster" is referred to as a combination of "dysbiosis" and "intestinal permeability"), and it was contributing to a vicious cycle of worsening metabolic health, worsening cravings for processed food, and worsening immune function.

By the time I was just ten years old, my young body had packed on weight. I was 210 pounds before eighth grade. I experienced low-grade anxiety, painful menstrual cycles, acne along my jawline and back, semi-regular headaches, and recurrent tonsil infections in my early teen years. I didn't see these as red flags: they were customary rites of passage for American children, and doctors even called me "healthy." It seemed common to have cramps, intermittent headaches, zits, and strep throat here and there. While these might be common conditions in the modern world, I didn't understand that they all represented highly dysfunctional biology.

At age fourteen, at the end of my first year of high school, I became passionate and relentless about getting to a healthy weight, so I read a stack of nutrition books and cookbooks to learn how. I committed to a summer of health: I cooked all my meals and joined a gym and took the bus there every day, sweating on the elliptical machine and lifting weights while blasting a Backstreet Boys CD on my Walkman. I quickly and healthily lost all the extra weight over about six months. My other symptoms got quite a bit better, too. Though I couldn't have named it then, I probably reversed the insulin resistance and chronic inflammation that, since infancy, had been causing or aggravating my weight gain and other issues. Growing into a dedicated athlete and chef in my mid-teens, I kept many of my symptoms at bay.

"NORMAL" CHALLENGES IN MY TWENTIES AND THIRTIES

Ten years later, as a twenty-six-year-old freshly minted medical doctor and first-year surgical resident, I fell back into a matrix of cellular misery. The day I walked into the hospital as a bright and healthy surgical resident, my world shrank to a tunnel of chronic stress and adrenaline. My pager beeped around the clock, and the fluorescent lights of the hospital glared down at me during every moment of the day and night. I slept erratically during frequent night shifts, ate processed cafeteria food, got little exercise, imbibed caffeine constantly, and breathed stale air. I endured multiday stretches of zero sunlight, waking before dawn and leaving work after dark. My body was again an epicenter of Bad Energy, which cropped up almost instantly in multiple symptoms.

IBS

Irritable bowel syndrome (IBS) was the first sign that the cells in my intestine were dysfunctional and quite literally couldn't do their job. I didn't make a solid stool for almost two years. IBS can look like many different things, and for me it was painful lower abdominal gas coupled with watery diarrhea eight to ten times a day.

Strong evidence shows reduced mitochondrial activity and decreased energy production within the gut-lining cells in people with IBS. This reduced activity contributes to gut symptoms, such as abdominal pain and changes in bowel habits. As strange as the connection sounds, IBS is strongly linked to insulin resistance and problems with Bad Energy. If you have IBS, you are twice as likely to have metabolic syndrome and elevated triglycerides.

Insulin resistance can negatively affect the enteric (gut) nervous system, which some call our "second brain." The impact can alter gut motility, which is the coordinated contraction and relaxation of the muscles in the gut wall. Insulin resistance also alters gut barrier function, which is the ability of the gut lining to prevent the entry of harmful substances into the bloodstream. Altered gut barrier function can result in increased gut inflammation and sensitivity, leading to increased abdominal pain and other symptoms of IBS. What's more, chronic inflammation from a poor gut barrier can fuel metabolic issues throughout the body.

Acne

The acne cysts on my face and neck that erupted when I was a new doctor were clues that elevated glucose and insulin levels were driving hormonal changes. Studies have shown that individuals with acne have higher insulin levels than those without acne. High insulin levels are linked to increased production of male hormones that stimulate the production of skin oil, called sebum. When the skin's oil glands produce too much, sebum can mix with dead skin cells and clog hair follicles, creating an environment where bacteria can thrive. Multiple studies have found that a low-glycemic load (i.e., low sugar) or a low-carbohydrate diet can lead to significant reductions in acne.

People with acne have been shown to have a higher burden of oxidative stress and mitochondrial damage, both hallmarks of Bad Energy. Interestingly, over a dozen skin conditions are known to be downstream of oxidative stress and mitochondrial damage, including alopecia areata (a type of hair loss), atopic dermatitis (eczema), lichen planus, scleroderma, vitiligo, rosacea, sun damage, psoriasis, and many others. Dysfunction in various skin cell types can look like many different skin conditions and symptoms, and it appears that much of this dysfunction is driven by Bad Energy.

Depression

The onset of uncharacteristic depression during my surgical residency has a strong metabolic link. The brain is exquisitely sensitive to oxidative stress and inflammation and is one of the most energy-hungry organs of the body, using 20 percent of the body's total energy despite representing just 2 percent of the body's weight! As such, Bad Energy processes, like mitochondrial dysfunction, inflammation, and oxidative stress, are known to affect brain function and mood regulation—similar to how they impact gut function in IBS. My toxic work environment and residency lifestyle worked together to break the energy-producing pathways of my gut and brain.

The gut-brain axis refers to communication between the digestive and central nervous systems. This connection is vital in depression because the gut microbiome plays a significant role in making our neurotransmitters, which control our thoughts and feelings and regulate mood and behavior. Imbalances in these neurotransmitters contribute to depression. More than 90 percent of serotonin, the hormone that regulates mood and contentment, is made in the gut—*not* in the brain. Anything that disturbs gut function—like the Bad Energy physiology that leads to IBS—can strongly impact mental health. Unsurprisingly, IBS and depression have a strong link, with IBS sometimes even being called "depression of the gut." IBS, in fact, is often addressed with antidepressants.

Studies in animals and humans have also found that changes in the gut microbiome can influence the development of depression-like behaviors. Shifts toward unhealthy patterns in the gut microbiome are observed in individuals with depression. Microbiome transfer from depressed animals to healthy animals has been shown to quickly induce depression-like behaviors.

Problems with Bad Energy in our cells contribute to the pathophysiology of depression in several ways.

1. **Energy Production:** Mitochondrial dysfunction can lead to decreased energy production in the central nervous system, resulting in altered

neurotransmitter signaling, including the neurotransmitters that modulate mood, such as serotonin and norepinephrine.

2. **Inflammation:** Mitochondrial dysfunction can also lead to an increase in oxidative stress, which can trigger inflammation. Chronic inflammation has been linked to depression, and many studies have shown that individuals with depression have elevated levels of inflammatory markers.

3. **Neuronal Function:** Mitochondria are involved in several vital processes for neuronal function, including apoptosis (cell death), calcium regulation, and oxidative stress defense. Mitochondrial dysfunction can alter these processes and lead to neuronal dysfunction, contributing to depression.

4. **Stress Response:** The hypothalamic-pituitary-adrenal (HPA) axis, which regulates stress response, depends on proper mitochondrial function. Mitochondrial dysfunction can alter the regulation of the HPA axis and lead to altered stress response, which can contribute to depression.

Unstable blood sugar can derail the brain's cells, just as it can derail any other cell in the body. It can cause the brain's cells to promote the production of more stress hormones, creating an endless feedback loop of stress and dysfunction. Incredibly, our five primary metabolic biomarkers from Chapter 1 can tell us a lot about depression risk. One study showed that every additional 18 mg/dL of fasting glucose was associated with a 37 percent increased rate of developing depression. Additionally, for every one-unit increase in the triglyceride-to-HDL ratio, people had an 89 percent higher likelihood of developing depression. When I was describing my feelings of depression to my parents during my residency, I tearfully told them I felt as if my brain had rapidly gone from the full-color spectrum to black and white. My creativity, ability to synthesize concepts, and sharp memory were gone. A few times after thirty-hour call-shifts, I had the disturbing sense that it would be easier just *not to exist*. Through the lens of Bad Energy, this makes sense to me now: due to several changes in my lifestyle and stress levels as a new surgical resident, my brain cells likely did not have the power to provide me with the full spectrum of thought and emotion, nor the energy to want to keep going.

There have been several reported associations between metabolic syndrome biomarkers and suicidal ideation, a link that should be urgently investigated and addressed as rates of depression and suicide alarmingly rise, especially in young people.

Chronic Pain

Even the chronic neck pain I developed as a young surgeon was likely related to metabolic chaos. Research demonstrates how poor mitochondrial function and insulin resistance may play a role in the development of chronic pain. Oxidative stress and inflammation in the nerves and other tissues can lead to nerve damage and sensitization. Mitochondrial dysfunction can result in decreased production of neurotransmitters and other signaling molecules that regulate pain perception. Insulin resistance may also alter the metabolism of cells in the muscles and other tissues, leading to muscle wasting, joint degradation, and other pain-inducing changes. Likely, the manifestation of dysfunction within the energy-producing pathways of my cells was generating my pain, rather than the repetitive neck bending I'd originally attributed the pain to due to my long hours hunched over the operating room table. I was certainly not alone: an estimated 20 percent of U.S. adults suffer from chronic pain.

Sinus Infections and Migraines

While I ignored the root cause of my own health issues, the ENT department in which I worked also was ignoring what might be causing the head and neck issues in the patients who found themselves under our scalpels. Take sinusitis, the condition that plagued Sophia and thirty-one million other people in the United States. Doctors describe chronic sinusitis—characterized by facial pain and pressure, nasal congestion, headaches, postnasal drip, and green and yellow nasal discharge—as chronic inflammation of the tissue of the sinuses. But we never dig deeper: *What is causing that chronic inflammation?*

The higher a person's blood sugar, the higher the likelihood of their having sinusitis. The probability is 2.7 times higher if you have type 2 diabetes!

I recall my shock when I read an article on sinusitis in the *Journal of the American Medical Association* (*JAMA*). It showed a picture of the inflammatory pathways that increase in the nasal tissue in a person with sinusitis. Many of the inflammatory markers that are increased in the nasal tissue are the same ones that are elevated in people with heart disease, obesity, and type 2 diabetes. Staring at the figure in this journal in the bright light of my call room, I thought to myself, *Is it possible that the same fundamental problem with inflammatory overdrive is just showing up in different body parts as different symptoms?*

Migraine, like my patient Sarah had, also correlates closely to poor metabolic health. In the ENT otology clinic, we often saw this condition and had limited success in treating it. Sufferers of this debilitating neurological disease—about 12 percent of people in the United States—tend to have higher insulin levels and insulin resistance. A comprehensive review of fifty-six research articles identified links between migraine and poor metabolic health, pointing out that "migraine sufferers tend to have impaired insulin sensitivity." The review supports the "neuro-energetic" theory of migraine.

Additionally, evidence suggests that micronutrient deficiencies in key mitochondrial cofactors may also be a contributing factor of migraine. Research has suggested that migraines could be treated by restoring levels of vitamins B and D, magnesium, CoQ10, alpha lipoic acid, and L-carnitine. Vitamin B_{12}, for instance, is involved in the electron transport chain responsible for the final steps of ATP generation in the mitochondria, and studies have indicated that high doses of B_{12} can help prevent migraine. These micronutrients usually have fewer side effects than other drugs used to treat migraines, making them a promising option for relief, which can be obtained through a diet rich in these micronutrients, or supplementation.

Having high markers of oxidative stress, a key Bad Energy feature, is associated with a significantly higher risk of migraine in women, with some studies suggesting that migraine attacks are a symptomatic response to increased levels of oxidative stress. Less painful and more common tension-type headaches are also linked to high variability (excess peaks and crashes) in blood sugar.

Hearing Loss

The same story of metabolic ignorance in the ENT department unfolded for auditory problems and hearing loss, one of the most common issues that presented to our ENT clinic. We'd typically tell our patients that their auditory decline was inevitable, due to aging and loud concerts in their youth, and we would suggest interventions like hearing aids. Yet insulin resistance is a little-known link to hearing problems. If you have insulin resistance, you are more likely to lose hearing as you age because of poor energy production in the delicate hearing cells and blockage of the small blood vessels that supply the inner ear.

One study showed that insulin resistance is associated with age-related hearing loss, even when controlling for weight and age. The likely mechanism for this is that the auditory system requires high energy utilization for its complex signal processing. In the case of insulin resistance, glucose metabolism is disturbed, leading to decreased energy generation.

The impact of Bad Energy on hearing is not subtle: A study showed that the prevalence of high-frequency hearing impairment among subjects with elevated fasting glucose levels was 42 percent compared to 24 percent in those with normal fasting glucose. Moreover, insulin resistance is associated with high-frequency mild hearing impairment in the male population under seventy years of age, even before the onset of diabetes. These papers suggest that assessing early metabolic function and levels of insulin resistance is essential in the ENT clinic and counseling individuals on the potential warning signs is paramount.

Autoimmune Conditions

Even with rarer conditions such as autoimmune diseases, which occur when the body's immune system attacks its own tissues, research indicates a strong metabolic link. We addressed several autoimmune conditions in the ENT clinic, including Sjögren's syndrome, a condition leading to malfunction of the glands of the body, and Hashimoto's thyroiditis, a condition of immune infiltration of the thyroid gland that leads to low thyroid function. While I never learned in medical school to think through the lens of cellular metabolism and how it might generate autoimmunity, a growing body of literature shows that metabolic and autoimmune issues are tightly linked. Remember, after all, that a cell that can't make energy properly sends out danger signals, which can trigger the immune system to invade. People with autoimmune diseases have been shown to have 1.5 to 2.5 times the rate of insulin resistance and metabolic syndrome when compared to people without these conditions. Bad Energy can result in chronic inflammation and, at times, *auto*immunity.

Renowned researcher and physician Dr. Terry Wahls speculates that autoimmunity could be in part because of the body responding to the "cell danger response" (CDR), a biological reaction coordinated by the mitochondria that occurs because of perceived threats to the cell such as poor diet, injury, infection, and nutrient deprivation. The CDR activates a series of events that culminate in the release of ATP outside the cell. (Normally ATP should be inside the cell powering the cell's biologic processes.) The release of ATP outside the cell acts as a signal to other cells in the area, alerting them of the danger. Overstimulation of the CDR can lead to an increased risk of chronic diseases such as autoimmune disorders, cardiovascular disease, and cancer.

Research has shown that people with autoimmune diseases—like rheumatoid arthritis, lupus, psoriasis, inflammatory bowel disease (IBD), and multiple sclerosis (MS)—are more likely to develop metabolic disorders like obesity and type 2 diabetes. For people with rheumatoid arthritis, the risk of diabetes is up to 50 percent higher. People with lupus are nearly twice as likely to have metabolic syndrome. And studies have found that people with MS are nearly 2.5 times more likely to be insulin resistant, compared to those without MS. Plus, patients with MS and high fasting blood glucose levels experience more cognitive dysfunction. This link between metabolic problems and autoimmunity is likely due to chronic low-grade inflammation in the body, which disrupts insulin signaling and leads to insulin resistance, and the interrelated phenomenon of oxidative stress, which is both a cause and an effect of metabolic issues and triggers inflammation.

Unsurprisingly, autoimmune diseases have rapidly increased in the United States over the past few decades. According to the National Institute of Environmental Health Sciences, autoimmune diseases affect approximately fifty million people in the nation, around 20 percent of the population. Some studies estimate that the number of individuals with autoimmune diseases in the country has increased by 50 to 75 percent since the 1950s, with such conditions affecting significantly more women than men. Currently, 20 percent of the population lives with some of their body's cells attacking and trying to destroy others, a process that appears to be rooted, in part, in biological confusion related to modern dietary and lifestyle exposures. The skyrocketing rate of autoimmune disease is the most obvious example of the devastating results of biochemical fear. It represents the body's cells saying "WTF?" to our modern exposures and acting out.

Infertility

Beginning in my early thirties, I noticed some common discussions surrounding fertility and sex among my friend group. Many had trouble conceiving and some experienced miscarriage. There were also whispers over cocktails about partners having problems with sexual function, libido, and erections.

The PCOS that Lucy experienced was common and rapidly increasing among women in my age group. Today, it is the leading cause of female infertility. Though the problem of cysts growing on the ovaries may not seem connected to blood sugar and insulin issues, look again. A key driver of PCOS is high insulin, which stimulates the ovaries' theca cells to make more testosterone and disturbs the delicate hormonal balance of sex hormones and the menstrual cycle. The process impedes fertility in all sorts of ways. PCOS, which often appears alongside obesity and diabetes, is so tied in with metabolic health that a 2012 NIH panel proposed that the name of the disease be changed to "metabolic reproductive syndrome."

As metabolic issues have risen in prevalence, so has PCOS. A recent study out of China—which is facing a type 2 diabetes crisis like that of the United States—showed that PCOS has gone up 65 percent just in the past decade. Evidence suggests it is now affecting 20 percent of women worldwide. According to the Centers for Disease Control and Prevention (CDC), half of women with PCOS may eventually develop type 2 diabetes by the time they are forty years old. The prevalence of obesity in women with PCOS in the nation is 80 percent. Studies have shown that weight loss, diet and lifestyle changes, and medication can all play a role in improving insulin sensitivity and reducing symptoms of PCOS. Just twelve weeks of a vegetable-filled, low-glycemic diet can improve all key biomarkers of the condition.

Women with PCOS are frequently prescribed hormonal birth control pills or diabetes drugs, such as metformin, to overcompensate for hormone dysregulation or to regulate blood sugar. Sometimes women with PCOS use in vitro fertilization (IVF) in their attempts to conceive. The use of assisted reproductive technologies like IVF has steadily increased in the United States over the past four decades. In 2015, more than 182,000 assisted reproductive technology (ART) procedures were performed. But very few of the women who elect for these invasive procedures are told by their doctor the root causes of their infertility or how to reverse them. Nor are they told that people with blood sugar problems have *double* the miscarriage rate with assisted reproduction, and that "the higher percentage of sperm DNA damage because of oxidative stress seen in diabetic patients may be responsible for poor embryonic development and pregnancy outcomes." Increasing body mass index (BMI) also increases odds of miscarriage after ART, with risk starting to go up at a BMI of around 22.

The fertility crisis in America isn't confined to women. Sperm count has fallen precipitously this century—by more than 50 to 60 percent in forty years as of the last count—and metabolic dysfunction is one key reason. Low sperm count hits obese men particularly hard: they have an 81 percent higher chance of having *zero* sperm in their semen than men of normal weight. "Male factor" infertility contributes to up to 50 percent of infertility cases. This is directly related to metabolic issues, as fat tissue contains enzymes called aromatases that convert testosterone to estrogen and disrupt the delicate hormonal balance required for sperm production. Dr. Benjamin Bikman notes that fat tissue in men basically acts like a big ovary, causing low testosterone and higher estrogen.

Excess oxidative stress, a key (and preventable) hallmark of Bad Energy, damages sensitive sperm cell membranes, impairs healthy sperm development, and can fragment sperm DNA, causing reduced sperm quality and increased risk of miscarriage. Oxidative stress also directly decreases testosterone production. A 2023 research review states, "Evidence is mounting to support an association between elevated seminal reactive oxygen species [in the male reproductive tract] and recurrent pregnancy loss." The paper goes on to remind that oxidative stress is thought to be increased by "alcohol use, smoking, obesity, aging, psychological stress . . . medical comorbidities including diabetes and infection." Other causes include exposure to radiation, diets high in processed foods, certain medications, chronic sleep loss, pesticides, pollution, and many industrial chemicals.

What's more, sexual dysfunction is rising in men, with 52 percent of men over age forty having concerns, much of which is related to erectile dysfunction (ED). ED is generally rooted in metabolic disease, with reduced blood flow to capillaries and nerves of the penis being a key factor, driven by the impact of insulin resistance on forming arterial blockages (called atherosclerosis) and reduced blood vessel dilation. Metabolic and sexual health expert Dr. Sara Gottfried notes, "Erectile dysfunction is atherosclerosis of the penile artery until proven otherwise," and notes that ED is a neon sign that a man needs a metabolic evaluation. Additionally, glycation caused by high glucose levels impairs the health of penile tissues and blood vessels and also contributes to ED.

More than a few friends have shared that they were diagnosed with gestational diabetes when they were pregnant. The condition has risen 30 percent in the United States since just 2016. Others have shared sad stories of pregnancy loss, which—though seldom discussed—can also be a result, in part, of metabolic strain. Cases of miscarriage have increased 10 percent over the past ten years, with studies showing that metabolic dysfunction can be toxic to the placenta. Placental dysfunction (PD) can be more technically defined as a failure of the placenta to perform its normal functions, including nutrient and oxygen transport, waste removal, hormone synthesis, and immune regulation. Maternal metabolic issues, such as obesity and insulin resistance, can cause changes in the balance of hormones and growth factors involved in placental development and function. The more features of metabolic syndrome someone has (e.g., low HDL, high triglycerides, and elevated glucose), the higher the odds ratio of PD and fetal death, with an odds ratio of 7.7 for PD in women with three to four metabolic syndrome features. Metabolic imbalances can lead to alterations in placental angiogenesis (formation of new blood vessels) and blood flow, reducing oxygen and nutrient delivery to the fetus. Additionally, obesity and insulin resistance can cause oxidative stress in the placenta, resulting in oxidative damage to the tissues and PD.

Assessing the data holistically, it appears that modern diet and lifestyle are sterilizing the human population in part through Bad Energy.

Chronic Fatigue

Between 10 and 30 percent of all U.S. doctor visits are for symptoms of fatigue, making it the most common cause of medical appointments. And 67 percent of people in the United States experience regular fatigue at work, seventy million experience chronic sleep issues, and 90 percent consume caffeine daily. For postmenopausal women, the situation is much worse: recent research shows that 85.3 percent of postmenopausal women report symptoms of physical and mental exhaustion, compared with 46.5 percent of perimenopausal women and just 19.7 percent of premenopausal women.

I saw this up close when I was a resident. Most of us chalked our rampant chronic fatigue up to our institutionally enforced sleep deprivation. Some days, after being awake for thirty-six hours in the hospital on call, I would drive home from work and be unable to muster the energy to get out of my car to go up to my apartment for much-needed sleep. I would nap in my front seat till I could summon the will to move.

But even under less extreme conditions, we often accept fatigue and sleep issues as inevitable by-products of modern life. Reduced ATP production, unstable blood sugar levels, and hormonal imbalances—all hallmarks of metabolic dysfunction—contribute to persistent fatigue and dysregulated sleep. This causes a negative spiral because the lack of quality sleep contributes to increased mitochondrial dysfunction and fatigue. We've normalized this dynamic as almost inevitable, but it is often a warning sign of Bad Energy in our body.

BAD ENERGY AMONG CHILDREN: NORMALIZING UNPRECEDENTED TRENDS

Childhood Obesity and Fatty Liver Disease

The prevalence of childhood obesity has increased dramatically in the past fifty years, and this is just one face of Bad Energy in kids. According to data from the CDC, the rate of childhood obesity has more than tripled since the 1970s. During that decade, approximately 5 percent of children and adolescents ages six to nineteen years were considered to have obesity. By the late 2000s, this rate had increased to approximately 18 percent, and it's going up. Another face of Bad Energy is nonalcoholic fatty liver disease (NAFLD), now the most common liver disease in kids. The prevalence of NAFLD in children is rising sharply. The first case of NAFLD in children was reported in 1983, and now up to 20 percent of children have it (and up to 80 percent of obese children). For specific ethnic groups and sexes, this number is much higher. For instance, in Hispanic young men ages twenty-five to thirty, 42 percent have NAFLD. This prevalence should be close to zero. Similar trends have been observed in other countries around the world. Historically, fatty livers were found primarily in adults abusing alcohol, as alcohol disturbs several elements of lipid processing in cells, while also generating oxidative stress. But over the past thirty years, *non*alcoholic fatty liver disease has become the most common chronic liver disease in the world, increasing from 25 percent of the global population in 1990 to close to 40 percent by 2019. NAFLD is full-blown metabolic dysfunction in kids and adults, representing liver cells filling with fat, which worsens insulin resistance. Key contributors are processed foods, refined sugars, refined grains, sweet beverages, high-fructose corn syrup, fast food, low fiber and phytochemical intake, habitual eating close to bedtime, sedentary behavior, and oxidative stress. Liver transplants have gone up close to 50 percent in the past fifteen years, and while alcohol and hepatitis C used to be the leading causes, now NAFLD is taking the lead in women as the cause of liver failure and is a top cause for men. Fatty liver disease is now the most common cause of liver transplant in young adults in the United States. We are failing our children.

Brain Disorders Among Children

Children's brains don't escape from issues with Bad Energy. We are reaching epidemic levels of childhood mental illness, which is the dysfunction of these young brains. About 20 percent of all children will have an identified mental health condition in any given year. According to the CDC, by the time they reach age eighteen, 40 percent of all children will meet the criteria for mental health disorders! The prevalence has risen dramatically over the decades, with the increase going up sharply more recently. A new study in *JAMA Pediatrics* showed that the number of children ages three to seventeen years with an anxiety or depression diagnosis increased by 29 percent and 27 percent, respectively—all between 2016 and 2020.

During my years at Stanford and rotating at other hospitals, twenty children and young adults per year took their lives in the surrounding Santa Clara County. A report showed that 17 percent of Santa Clara high school students had seriously contemplated suicide. Suicide is now the second leading cause of death for young adults ages ten to thirty-four. According to the CDC, 25 percent of young adults contemplated suicide in 2020—a statistic I still can't wrap my head around. Among local leaders, there was little talk of whether metabolic factors—such as inflammatory food, lack of sleep, and chronic stress spurred by technology and academic pressure in the epicenter of Silicon Valley—could have contributed to these trends.

Cases of developmental conditions are also rising rapidly in youth, with autism and attention deficit hyperactivity disorder (ADHD) rates climbing yearly. A mother with obesity and diabetes has quadruple the risk of having a child with autism, and she has double the risk of having a child with ADHD. As our most energy-hungry organ, our brains are exquisitely sensitive to Bad Energy. A developing brain is particularly susceptible. In a rational health care environment, a key public health priority would be to support maternal and early childhood metabolic health as a high-leverage approach to support a thriving population.

Other Childhood Metabolic Conditions

Epidemic levels of obesity, liver dysfunction, and brain dysfunction demonstrate a cellular energy epidemic. And our children's small, not fully developed bodies are being set up to fail at an early age because our culture and daily lives have been co-opted by processed foods and the other factors that damage mitochondria and cellular energy production.

The following are just a sampling of health conditions that are increasing in children and are known to be related to poor cellular energy production, mitochondrial dysfunction, or oxidative stress: ADHD, autism spectrum disorder, type 2 diabetes, NAFLD, cardiomyopathy, depression, anxiety, high blood pressure, high cholesterol, IBD, asthma, atopic dermatitis, allergies, acne, psoriasis, eczema, schizophrenia, bipolar disorder, borderline personality disorder, and hidradenitis suppurativa (HS, a condition of painful inflammatory lumps under the skin).

Many friends who are parents have complained of having to take off work to take their kids to the doctor for recurrent throat, ear, and viral upper respiratory tract infections. Few, if any, understood that the way their kids' bodies were producing energy had a significant impact on the propensity for illness, given that just like the function of any other cell type, immune cell function is regulated by how well they can make and utilize energy.

Kids with metabolic dysfunction are at a significantly higher risk for infections—such as strep throat and ear infections—than kids without metabolic dysfunction or who are a healthy weight. For instance, one study found that the odds of having streptococcal pharyngitis were 1.5 times higher in children with obesity compared to those without. Another study found that children with obesity were 2.5 times more likely to experience middle ear infections than normal-weight children. The antibiotics we throw at these kids are in no way harmless. One of the most alarming research findings I've ever come across is that antibiotics in childhood increased the risk of mental health issues by an odds ratio of 1.44.

Destroying the microbiome with aggressive antibiotics impacts gut function, metabolic function, and chronic inflammation, and it sets up the conditions for Bad Energy and subsequent problems like mental illness. Unsurprisingly, a linear relationship exists between the number of antibiotics courses taken prenatally or in the first one to two years of life and having an increased BMI at ages four to five. Through the microbiome-gut-inflammation-metabolic lens, this relationship makes sense. We are creating a vicious cycle in kids, with poor immune function from Bad Energy leading to more infectious diseases, leading to more antibiotic use, and leading to worsened Bad Energy due to microbiome disruption.

It's this simple: kids' bodies, just like adult bodies, are made of cells that need energy to function. Our children are living in disastrous metabolic conditions, and their bodies are paying the price—while leaders in nutrition science (which is largely funded by food companies) and "health care" (whose research is largely funded by pharmaceutical companies to "manage" the rise of metabolic conditions) stand silent. Our society has failed to make meaningful preventive moves to counter the exploding epidemics of childhood chronic diseases. Not only are these conditions rooted in how diet and lifestyle are hurting our kids' mitochondria, but the conditions are also putting them squarely on the spectrum of metabolic diseases that will ultimately shorten their lives and decrease their quality of life. Our kids are entering a world where they will live fewer total years on average than their parents.

Despite these trends, our culture pushes a Bad Energy world onto kids who cannot protect themselves. Our culture has normalized giving one-year-olds packaged, ultra-processed foods like cake, Goldfish, rice puffs, juice, and french fries. We slather toxic, artificially scented lotions and shampoos all over their tiny bodies as soon as their first hospital bath. We damage their livers and antioxidant capacity with too much acetaminophen (Tylenol) at the first sign of fussiness or a cold. We blast their microbiomes with heavy-duty antibiotics at the first sign of a possible ear infection. And we interrupt their sleep for unconscionably early school times, then force them to sit at desks in school for six or more hours a day. We create terror and chronic stress in their bodies from social media and overall media exposure. The world kids live in is inflammatory and metabolically disastrous unless parents staunchly go against the tide of "normal" American culture. The irony is that so many parents wish that parenting were easier—fewer infections, less colic, easier behavioral patterns—without thinking through the lens of energy production in their children's bodies. We can do so much to make our lives and our kids' lives easier by controlling the controllable.

FIFTY AND BEYOND: THE RISE OF LIFE-THREATENING CHRONIC CONDITIONS

Many of us have watched as our parents develop chronic illnesses as they get older. To have a conversation with my group of friends without someone in the group sharing updates of their parents' declining health is unusual. The common conditions include high blood pressure, high cholesterol, heart disease, stroke, burgeoning dementia, arthritis, cancer, or upper respiratory conditions that have required hospitalization. In my time as a first-year resident, two coworkers' parents had debilitating strokes. As physicians, we are often the first call from our parents and elderly family members to seek advice or help regarding the recent health scare. These are all conditions rooted in Bad Energy.

Stroke

The relationship between high blood glucose and the risk of stroke is well established. A meta-analysis from 2014 found that people with type 2 diabetes have double the stroke risk compared to those without the condition. Another study found that people with prediabetic glucose levels (110 to 125 mg/dL) had a 60 percent higher stroke risk than those with normal glucose levels. More than 80 percent of acute stroke patients have a blood sugar problem, yet most of them are unaware of it. Insulin resistance leads directly to several problems with blood vessels that contribute to stroke, including excess clotting, reduced nitric oxide production (which dilates vessels), and increased atherosclerosis, the formation of blockages in arteries.

Dementia

Early-onset dementia and other devastating cognitive diseases are also charging through our population. Remember, the brain uses more energy and glucose than any other organ, so it is particularly vulnerable to the effects of Bad Energy and blood sugar variability. Evidence suggests that the impaired glucose uptake caused by insulin resistance may, over time, starve brain cell mitochondria of the energy they need to function properly, creating a state called *hypometabolism*, which research indicates is a potential cause of Alzheimer's disease.

Alzheimer's disease has been dubbed "type 3 diabetes" because of its higher prevalence among people with insulin resistance and impaired insulin sensitivity. In the United States, around 6.2 million adults ages sixty-five or older live with Alzheimer's disease, and this figure is predicted to more than double by 2050. The health care costs associated with Alzheimer's and other dementias in the United States were estimated to hit $355 billion in 2021. Add to that an estimated $250 billion worth of unpaid caregiving by patients' loved ones. With fifty million people living with dementia worldwide and ten million new cases expected each year, finding ways to prevent, treat, cure, or simply slow the devastating progression of dementia has become an urgent global challenge, particularly since medications for Alzheimer's are not effective and may even be harmful.

Fortunately, recent research in the top medical journal *The Lancet* shows that 40 percent of Alzheimer's cases are related to twelve modifiable risk factors (and therefore are likely preventable) and that we should be "ambitious about prevention" with Alzheimer's.

In a 2013 study, researchers tracked the blood glucose levels of more than two thousand adults for about seven years and found that higher blood sugar was associated with a greater risk of dementia, including Alzheimer's disease. This was true even among patients without diagnosed diabetes. However, independent research has confirmed that diabetes increases the risk for cognitive decline, and prediabetes is a risk factor for all types of dementia. Another observational study published in 2021 discovered that the earlier type 2 diabetes is diagnosed, the greater the risk of developing Alzheimer's disease.

Heart Disease

The heart is the organ that causes more deaths than any other part of the body in the Western world. Heart disease—across the spectrum of high blood pressure, high cholesterol, and coronary artery disease—is directly rooted in Bad Energy.

Back in 1979, the Framingham Heart Study, one of the longest-running and most important research studies in medical history, was one of the first to demonstrate that metabolic dysfunction—in the form of diabetes—is a risk factor for developing heart disease. Why? The usual suspects: high blood sugar leads to oxidative stress, and these cell-damaging free radicals lead to inflammation, which damages both large and small blood vessels by deteriorating their inner lining, known as the endothelium. In response to that damage, fatty deposits known as plaques build up inside your blood vessels, causing them to harden and narrow in the process of atherosclerosis. Eventually, the vessels can become so narrow that blood flow is blocked: the root of coronary artery disease. Heart disease leads to nearly seven hundred thousand deaths per year, and most of these cases involve some or all of the biomarkers from Chapter 1 being out of range.

A significant risk factor for heart disease is high blood pressure, which 50 percent of the population experiences. Inflammation, obesity, insulin resistance, high blood sugar, and oxidative stress all lead to strain on the blood vessel lining, which then results in decreased production by these cells of nitric oxide, a chemical that relaxes blood vessels. Insulin resistance and diabetes also directly affect the parts of the brain that set off this process, leading to dysfunction in how nitric oxide is synthesized and released. This all leads to arterial stiffness, increases in blood pressure, and an increased risk of heart disease. Additionally, dysfunctional vessel lining cells promote the improper accumulation of clots and plaques and ultimately lead to heart attacks. (Of note, these processes are nearly identical to those that lead to erectile dysfunction, caused by the narrowing and lack of dilatation of blood vessels in the penis.)

Respiratory Disease

The leading type of chronic respiratory disease is known as chronic obstructive pulmonary disease (COPD). It is a progressive inflammatory condition that causes damage to the lungs and makes breathing difficult. Sixteen percent of people newly diagnosed with COPD have type 2 diabetes, and an additional 19 percent will develop type 2 diabetes within ten years of a COPD diagnosis.

A key risk factor for COPD is smoking, which directly links this condition to mitochondrial dysfunction and the risk of type 2 diabetes. Cigarette smoke contains a multitude of toxic chemicals, including cyanide, which can directly damage the mitochondria within our cells. This damage to the mitochondria leads to decreased energy production, which in turn can lead to various health problems, including COPD, and a higher risk of developing diabetes. The toxic chemicals in cigarette smoke can also contribute to oxidative stress and inflammation in the body, exacerbating the negative impact on the mitochondria.

Multiple studies support the concept that improving blood glucose control leads to better outcomes for patients with chronic respiratory conditions. A 2019 analysis of over fifty-two hundred patient records showed that adults with type 2 diabetes who took metformin, a medication used to regulate blood sugar, were less likely to die from chronic lower respiratory diseases. Research suggests an antioxidant diet rich in fruits and vegetables can decrease COPD severity and lower risk, yet nutritional guidelines are not a part of standard treatment. Consumption of sugar-sweetened beverages is strongly linked to COPD risk (as well as the risk of pediatric and adult asthma and bronchitis). Research in the journal *Nutrients* reviewing the impact of diet on COPD states that "the magnitude of effect of diet on lung function is estimated to be comparable to that of chronic smoking." A healthy diet may quell inflammation and oxidative stress, potentially easing COPD severity.

Arthritis

One of the saddest things so many people experience when they age—aside from the development of life-threatening diseases—is that their bodies just don't feel as good or work as well as they used to. Even the aches, the pains, and the stiffness have a direct metabolic link. Leading orthopedic surgeons, such as Howard Luks, MD, have elucidated that arthritis may be more of a metabolic disease than a structural one. People with osteoarthritis have three times the risk of having cardiovascular disease and a 61 percent higher risk of having type 2 diabetes. Emerging research shows that even musculoskeletal pain, like arthritis, is downstream of Bad Energy processes, just like many of the other chronic cardiometabolic diseases.

One metabolic factor that has been linked to arthritis and musculoskeletal pain is chronic inflammation. Chronic inflammation can damage joint tissues and cause the release of pain-causing chemicals. Another metabolic factor that is important in the development of arthritis and musculoskeletal pain is chronic oxidative stress, which can lead to cellular damage and contribute to joint degeneration, while also slowing down the healing process and making recovery more difficult for the body.

Excess weight has been shown to increase the risk of developing osteoarthritis, which is the most common type of arthritis. A study conducted by the Arthritis Foundation found that for every pound of weight gained, the load on the knee joint increases by four pounds. This extra strain can lead to wear and tear on the joint and increase the risk of developing osteoarthritis. Additionally, obesity has been linked to a higher risk of developing knee osteoarthritis, with the risk increasing with an increasing BMI. A meta-analysis of seventeen studies found that for every one unit increase in BMI, the risk of knee osteoarthritis increased by 13 percent. Furthermore, obesity has been associated with increased pain and decreased physical function in individuals with knee osteoarthritis. Exercise is one of the best things an older person can do to minimize joint pain—likely, in part, because of how physical activity supports mitochondrial function. The medical establishment continues to see osteoarthritis as a nuisance often seen in patients with other cardiometabolic diseases, but we need to view arthritis as a warning sign of the brewing dysfunction inside our cells that can cause degeneration to all parts of the body, not just the joint tissues.

COVID-19

As I continued through my journey of discovering the metabolic links to common conditions in our country, around the bend came COVID-19. When the first news of this disease began circulating in early 2020, I had recently joined forces with my cofounders to launch Levels, a health technology company built to empower individuals to understand their metabolic health. The connections between Bad Energy and nearly every chronic disease and symptom were becoming crystal clear to those of us in metabolic research and medicine, and we couldn't avoid viewing the fast-moving viral phenomenon through metabolic glasses.

The COVID-19 crisis was one of the most dramatic and intense examples of conventional medicine's metabolic blind spot that I have ever seen. This acute disease cruelly ravaged the bodies of those who, often unknowingly, had a foundation of chronic conditions and diseases of Bad Energy caused primarily by diet and lifestyle. The connections were clear in scores of quality peer-reviewed papers. Experts around the world were trying to yell it from the rooftops. Yet the message did not get out. Societies worldwide lost so much by the missed opportunity to teach people about the proven connections between severity of illness and diet, exercise, and other modifiable factors.

In many studies on COVID-19 mortality, 80 to 100 percent of the people who died had other chronic health problems, of which the most common were metabolic issues, such as type 2 diabetes and high blood pressure. Other studies showed that patients with metabolic syndrome had a 77 percent increased risk of hospitalization and an 81 percent increased risk of death.

COVID-19 is not the first pathogen to biologically discriminate against people with diabetes. Bacterial infections and seasonal influenza both are much more morbid in people with diabetes, for reasons including the impairment of the acute immune response in the face of high blood sugar. In fact, people with diabetes are six times more likely to need hospitalization during influenza epidemics than those without the condition. High blood sugar negatively impacts immune function in many ways, including impairing the ability of immune cells to move through the body and get to the site of infection and engulf and destroy pathogens or infected cells. Additionally, antibodies may work less effectively when sugar is stuck to them through glycation. What's more, high blood sugar prompts immune cells to release excess pro-inflammatory cytokines, contributing to an exaggerated but dysfunctional immune response that yields unproductive collateral damage on body tissues.

THE CRUEL COST OF MISSING THE SIGNS

Early in our life, we accept conditions such as obesity, acne, fatigue, depression, infertility, high cholesterol, or prediabetes as common rites of passage for generally "healthy" adults as they get older.

This is the largest blind spot in medicine: these "small" conditions are invitations to become curious about the metabolic dysfunction brewing in our body. Bad Energy will almost certainly result in more serious conditions down the road if left unaddressed.

In my functional medicine practice, my patients with complex cases and serious diseases that have Bad Energy origins—like heart disease or cancer—had experienced one or more conditions on the metabolic spectrum years before.

In medicine, we call two or more conditions that tend to go together *comorbidities*—they happen comorbidly, meaning, we "happen to see them together." As doctors in training, we discover that people with diabetes often have comorbid high blood pressure and people with obesity often have comorbid depression. In medical school, the conclusion of these co-occurrences generally elicited a shrug and "Huh, interesting." On the hospital floor, the word *comorbidities* simply signaled, "If you see this disease, look for that one, too"—and then treat each one as you were trained, or send the patient to the appropriate specialist for what you didn't have the authority to treat. While arthritis and heart disease are comorbidities, very few orthopedists or cardiologists are deeply thinking about the causes of mitochondrial dysfunction, oxidative stress, and chronic inflammation in the cells of the patient in front of them and how to support getting those causative pathways back on track to improve *both* issues. Instead, they manage the symptoms and send the patient on their way, with their core physiology still a mess.

The pervasiveness of the word *comorbid* normalizes what should not be normal at all—clusters of serious conditions that are all branches of the same tree with the same root system. This normalization has, in a sense, reinforced our blind spots and has led to untold missed opportunities to help millions of people turn things around before their health gets worse and harder to heal. This is exactly what happened with my mom.

My mom did not know—nor did her doctors—that the extra fat on her body was a sign of cells that were overwhelmed and undersupported. My mom's metabolism rarely shifted into a fat-burning state, a state that will occur only if we don't overload the body with glucose and carbohydrates. She didn't know that her comorbidities—elevated glucose, dysregulated cholesterol, and high blood pressure—were *the definition* of metabolic dysfunction. They were telling a story and raising a warning that was ignored. Over time, her metabolism became more and more strained, losing its efficiency.

My mom tried so hard to get her health back on track. She stopped smoking. She hired a trainer. She joined a Curves gym. She read every book about nutrition that she could get her hands on and participated in several programs, including a medical weight-loss program through Stanford and WeightWatchers. She tried a whole-foods plant-based diet, and then tried a ketogenic diet through Virta Health. She tried and tried and tried. She felt discouraged with how many different ideologies there were, all of which claimed to be the silver bullet. But unfortunately, she didn't have the framework to look at her body through the lens of cellular energy production, she didn't have the resources to make sense of her biomarkers, and she didn't make a lot of progress. There were positive features to each of these endeavors, but since no plan focused all arrows *directly* toward the *right* problem of metabolic dysfunction, they didn't work and she didn't heal.

She was let down by the siloed medical system, which saw every health issue she faced as an isolated incident. She didn't have the support of practitioners who could teach her at each step that the large baby, the inability to lose weight, the high blood pressure and cholesterol, the prediabetes, and, ultimately, the pancreatic cancer were all branches of the same tree. Instead of offering synthesis and helping tie all the pieces together, her specialists actively held all the pieces apart.

The conditions that have affected me, my friends in middle age, our children, and our aging parents show that we are all starting to become entrenched on the Bad Energy spectrum. Our siloed approach to seeing these conditions as separate is fatally misguided. We don't have fifty different conditions to treat. Consistent pathways inside our bodies must be nurtured and healed: the function and quantity of mitochondria, the prevalence of chronic inflammation, the levels of oxidative stress, the health of our microbiome, and all the ways they interact.

We've lost our way, but we can change course quickly. Our cells have an incredible capacity for adaptability and regeneration. They are doing it all day, every day. Broken cellular functions can be repaired and restored quickly. This information applies to people of all ages. I have seen eighty-year-olds, eighteen-year-olds, and even eight-year-olds gain back their health, confidence, self-esteem, and happiness—all by starting with a foundation of protecting their cells' energy-making capacity. Becoming an empowered patient is possible, but breaking free from our current health care system requires a clear understanding of its incentives and shortcomings.

To view the scientific references cited in this chapter, please visit us online at caseymeans.com/goodenergy.

CHAPTER 3

Trust Yourself, Not Your Doctor

The most important thirteen days of my life came from ignoring a team of doctors.

Right after my mom's pancreatic cancer diagnosis, a medical team out of Stanford and Palo Alto Medical Foundation jumped to action, recommending a laundry list of surgeries and procedures—biopsies, blood transfusions, and a liver stent. In most cases, the patient would have agreed to these procedures, and the meeting would wrap up quickly. These recommendations were coming from some of the most prestigious institutions in the world, after all.

But based on my experience in medicine, I started asking questions.

I learned that these procedures had about a 33 percent chance of extending her life a few more months at most, a 33 percent chance of shortening her life span, and a 33 percent chance of not impacting her life span (yet keeping her away from the family). In all cases, the invasive route would mean that my mom would need to sit in a hospital room alone (because of COVID-19 protocols) and potentially longer if the surgery had complications (as they often do with immunocompromised cancer patients). Additionally, her cancer was causing her liver to fail by the day and her body to destroy its red blood cells, making the prognosis numbers even worse, potentially complicating her recommended procedures, and making her dependent on every-other-day multi-hour blood transfusions in the hospital, despite being so weak she could barely leave her bed. We were amid COVID lockdowns, and we also knew that she would be forced to check in for the hospital procedures alone and might not come out. My mom made it clear to the oncologist that she was not afraid of her rapidly impending death, but she wanted to minimize unnecessary pain or nausea in her final days. Despite the fact that she was clear, the system pushed the exact procedures that would yield pain and nausea and aggressively shamed our family for questioning the full-court press approach.

The doctor was not consciously trying to recommend a suboptimal procedure, but I knew the invasive route would generate hundreds of thousands of dollars for the hospital, and this doctor's pay was tied to booking these procedures.

I confirmed with the oncologist: "You are recommending an invasive diagnostic procedure that would under no scenario extend her life more than a couple of months and risk my mom dying alone in a hospital room? Even though we are certain that this is stage 4 pancreatic cancer based on the CA 19-9 blood test and CT scan, and that she has liver failure and almost no red blood cells left?"

"Yes, that is what we're recommending," the doctor replied.

With the family's full support, my mother chose to go without the confirmatory diagnostic procedure and to spend her final days at home with her family. The procedure was being recommended to alleviate the doctor's checklist, algorithm, chart note template, and billing codes—and decidedly *not* for my mom's benefit. At that moment, I felt sick for the families who navigate these decisions without the advocacy of a trusted support person who understands the incentives of the system and has the knowledge to ask difficult questions.

Rather than leaving my mom in the hospital, where she likely would never see or touch my brother, father, or me again, we drove back from Stanford to my parents' home in Half Moon Bay and spent her final days together.

On my mom's final day of consciousness, she woke up weak and started to lose control of her speech. Later in the day, in a burst of energy, she urged us to take her to the place where she would soon be buried—a rustic forest grove overlooking fields and ocean, just three minutes from her house. We quickly drove her there and took her in a wheelchair to the natural burial site. My mom expressed amazement at the beauty of the ocean view and the trees she would soon be buried under, and we hugged as a family. She asked my dad to kneel beside her in the wheelchair and cupped his face in her hands. She looked at him and talked about how magical their life was together. On this small patch of earth with the Pacific Ocean behind them, they exchanged silent looks that expressed emotion and gratitude for each other that are impossible to fully convey in words. The awe and connection they shared as they exchanged their final embrace will forever be my definition of the meaning of life.

"It's just . . . so perfect and beautiful," my mom burst out as she looked at her family embracing her at her final resting site.

Minutes later, she lost consciousness. Two days later, surrounded by her family holding hands around her, she died.

The final thirteen days I shared with my mom were the most meaningful of my life.

If we had taken the advice of the medical system, they wouldn't have happened.

THE INCENTIVE TO INTERVENE

During residency, one of my best friends was a cancer surgeon. During the meeting with my mom's doctors, words my friend spoke years before rang in my head: *If you walk through the doors of this surgical oncology department, you are going to get an operation, whether you need it or not.*

I remember speaking to this friend after work when she was visibly shaken after watching a patient encouraged to undergo a surgery that wasn't necessary. Frequently, she suggested patients with terminal cancer be put on palliative care (which prioritizes the patient's comfort and peace in their final days). The senior doctors generally shot this down. She told me her attending surgeon would "lose his mind" for suggesting anything other than surgery to a patient. If a patient said they wanted to decline a surgical intervention, the department leaders would ask them to sign "Against Medical Advice" (AMA) paperwork and be left with fewer resources to seek palliative care or less invasive treatment options.

A doctor-patient relationship is such a power imbalance: the patient is scared for their life and is not in a position to disagree when that doctor offers a perceived "cure" to solve diabetes or heart disease or depression or cancer.

Nobody gets into medicine to take advantage of patients to get rich. There are far easier ways to make money than four years of medical school, another three to nine years of residency and fellowship, an MCAT test, three USMLEs (United States Medical Licensing Examinations), and oral and written board examinations. Nearly every doctor I worked with dreamed as a child about curing disease and worked like crazy to become a doctor. They studied tirelessly to learn science, entered medical school with idealistic visions, and became the pride of their family. They entered residency with hundreds of thousands of dollars of student loan debt and initially saw the chronic sleep deprivation and verbal abuse by their superiors as integral parts of the experience—because "great achievement is born of great sacrifice."

But almost universally among doctors I have met, this idealism eventually turns to cynicism. My colleagues in residency talked often about questioning their sanity, of wondering whether this was all worth it. I spoke with successful surgeons who'd drafted their resignation letters dozens of times. Another had a recurring daydream of leaving everything behind and becoming a baker. Many of my supervising physicians were desperate to spend more time with their children. I witnessed more than one tearful breakdown in the operating room when surgical cases were delayed and led to yet another missed bedtime for their kids. Several had dealt with suicidal depression. I understood why doctors had the highest burnout and suicide rate of any profession.

Inevitably, these conversations led to an insight that I believe is whispered by doctors in every hospital in America: they feel trapped inside a broken system. For most, changing paths was unthinkable because of financial pressures and the fact that they'd tied their identities to the status of having "MD" at the end of their name.

These dedicated professionals are saddled with hundreds of thousands in debt and put into a system driven by one simple financial incentive:

Every institution that impacts your health makes more money when you are sick and less when you are healthy—from hospitals to pharma to medical schools, and even insurance companies.

This incentive has created a system that is demonstrably hurting patients.

Imagine you were an intelligent alien who was transported from outer space to the United States and saw the health landscape: more than 75 percent of deaths and 80 percent of costs are driven by obesity, diabetes, heart disease, and other *preventable* and *reversible* metabolic conditions we have today. Now imagine you asked that alien to allocate $4 trillion—the amount we spend on health care annually—to fix the problem. Never in a million years would that alien say that we should wait for everyone to get sick and then write prescriptions and perform procedures that don't reverse the underlying reasons they're sick. But that is what we are doing today because it generates recurring revenue for the largest industry in the country.

TRUST THE SYSTEM ON ACUTE ISSUES, IGNORE IT ON CHRONIC

Most health care books give recommendations and end with a disclaimer to "consult your doctor."

I have a different conclusion: when it comes to preventing and managing chronic disease, you should *not* trust the medical system. This might sound pessimistic or even frightening, but understanding the incentives of our medical system and why it does not deserve our benefit of the doubt is the first step to becoming an empowered patient.

In the last twenty years of her life, my mom had what many would consider the best medical care in the world. She frequently visited the Mayo Clinic for preventive tests and routinely visited doctors at Stanford Hospital. And yet despite faithfully going through their revolving doors, year after year, her cells never healed. Her doctors turned little knobs on her biomarkers with a slew of medications, but those drugs did not help her heal the disarray in her cells. Like almost any chronic disease, pancreatic cancer is largely preventable by implementing the lifelong Good Energy habits in this book. But nobody at these preeminent medical institutions gave her strong recommendations on improving how her cells fundamentally functioned. The only aggressive, assertive interventions they espoused were ones they recommended when she was flagrantly and lethally sick.

I hear you asking these questions: Hasn't our system produced medical miracles over the past hundred years? Hasn't life expectancy almost doubled during that time? Medicine is complicated—why should we question a system that has worked so well?

Life expectancy has increased primarily because of sanitation practices and infectious disease mitigation measures; because of emergency surgery techniques for acute and life-threatening conditions, like an inflamed appendix or trauma; and because of antibiotics to reverse life-threatening infections. In short, almost every "health miracle" we can point to is a cure for an acute issue (i.e., a problem that would kill you imminently if left unresolved). Economically, acute conditions aren't great in our modern system, because the patient is quickly cured and no longer a customer.

Starting in the 1960s, the medical system has taken the trust engendered by these acute innovations and used it to ask patients not to question its authority on chronic diseases (which can last a lifetime and thus are more profitable).

But the medicalization of chronic disease in the past fifty years has been an abject failure. Today, we've siloed diseases and have a treatment for everything:

- High cholesterol? See a cardiologist for a statin.
- High fasting glucose? See an endocrinologist for metformin.
- ADHD? See a neurologist for Adderall.
- Depressed? See a psychiatrist for a selective serotonin reuptake inhibitor (SSRI).
- Can't sleep? See a sleep specialist for Ambien.
- Pain? See a pain specialist for an opioid.
- PCOS? See an OB-GYN for clomiphene.
- Erectile dysfunction? See a urologist for Viagra.
- Overweight? See an obesity specialist for Wegovy.
- Sinus infections? See an ENT for an antibiotic or surgery.

But what nobody talks about—what I think many doctors don't even realize—is that the rates of all these conditions are going *up* at the exact time we are spending trillions of dollars to "treat them."

In the face of these unprecedented trends happening to our brains and bodies across our life span—which all have metabolic dysfunction as a root—we are told to "trust the science." This obviously doesn't make sense. We have been gaslighted to not ask questions over the past fifty years at the exact time chronic disease rates have exploded.

Our intervention-based medical system is by design. One of the most cited doctors in medical school classes is Dr. William Stewart Halsted, a Johns Hopkins founding physician in the early 1900s who created the concept of residency. To Halsted, medical education was "a superhuman initiation into a superhuman profession that emphasized heroism, self-denial, diligence, and tirelessness."

In Halsted's view, there was no more important or higher calling in a hospital than a surgeon cutting into a patient's body and ridding them of disease. Aggressive medical interventions were heroic—necessarily barbaric and aggressive—to inflict short-term pain on the patient for long-term gain. To achieve the honor of becoming a surgeon, a Darwinian system that ensured only the best and brightest attained this privilege was necessary. He would engage in multiday surgical benders with residents to test and weed out students.

During this time, John D. Rockefeller—realizing he could use by-products from his oil production to create pharmaceuticals—heavily funded medical schools throughout the United States to teach a curriculum based on the intervention-first Halsted model. An employee of Rockefeller's was tasked to create the Flexner Report, which outlined a vision for medical education that prioritized interventions and stigmatized nutritional, traditional, and holistic remedies. Congress affirmed the Flexner Report in 1910 to establish that any credentialed medical institution in the United States had to follow the Halsted/Rockefeller intervention-based model.

Initially, I agreed with Dr. Halsted's mindset. When I applied for surgical residency, I was eager to "solve" problems by simply cutting them out. I believed that becoming a doctor, particularly a surgeon, is a privilege, and there should be a rigorous process to ensure that only the best make it. As a young resident, I judged people who complained about the grueling schedule.

I didn't learn in medical school that Dr. Halsted suffered from a lifelong addiction to cocaine and morphine. He would embark on multiday drug-fueled marathons in the surgical wards and then experience psychotic breakdowns where he would be confined to home for days or weeks. He often couldn't perform surgeries because his hands were shaking vigorously from sleep deprivation and cocaine. But the Flexner Report—and the Halsted/Rockefeller intervention-based brand of medicine—has not been changed by Congress since 1910 and continues to define U.S. medicine.

The truth: we should consider listening to the medical system if we have an acute issue like a life-threatening infection or broken bone. But when it comes to the chronic conditions that plague our lives, we should question almost every institution regarding nutrition or chronic disease advice. All you need to do is follow the money and incentives.

BIAS FOR ACTION

During my undergraduate years, the dean of Stanford Medical School was Dr. Philip Pizzo, a pain specialist appointed in 2011 to lead a government-supported Institute of Medicine panel to make recommendations on treating chronic pain in America. Nine of the nineteen people he appointed to the panel had direct ties to opioid manufacturers. At the same time he was appointed to the panel, Dr. Pizzo secured a $3 million donation to the school from Pfizer, one of the largest opioid makers. The committee recommended lenient opioid guidelines that have contributed to the crisis of addiction we are seeing today.

Between 2012 and 2019, NIH grants went to at least eight thousand researchers with "significant" financial conflicts of interest, many with pharma companies. Over $188 million in conflicts were reported.

Deans of leading institutions have taken millions of dollars in direct payments from pharmaceutical companies.

At the start of my residency, the Affordable Care Act (ACA) was passed and all doctors had to get up to speed on the Merit-Based Incentive Payment System (MIPS), a new program under the Quality Payment Program (QPP), where a physician would now receive substantial adjustments to payments from Medicare if they met specific quality-of-care criteria. One would think that "quality" and "merit" in medicine would mean that *the patient was actually getting better.* But when I dug deep through the MIPS website to find the specific quality metrics for each specialty, I was shocked to see that these quality criteria were primarily based on whether doctors prescribed drugs regularly or did more interventions. Yes, a government incentive program focused less on actual patient outcomes (i.e., Did the patient get healthier?) and more on whether doctors prescribed long-term pharmaceuticals. For instance, there are four quality metrics under the domain of "Effective Clinical Care" for asthma, and none references the improvement or resolution of asthma; rather, doctors report on metrics like "percentage of patients aged five through sixty-four years with a diagnosis of persistent asthma who were prescribed long-term control medication." This is consistent across hundreds of metrics for a multitude of conditions. Only later did I learn that pharma spends three times more on lobbying than the oil industry, and pharma has heavily influenced virtually every piece of health care legislation and guideline I operated under.

I heard doctors frequently talk about their variable pay being based on relative values units (RVUs)—a measure of their productivity in generating profitable billing codes. Many hospitals incentivize doctors to increase their RVUs. Doing something like performing bariatric surgery on someone is awarded significantly more RVU points than counseling a patient with obesity to eat healthily. Even in hospitals that don't explicitly tie RVUs to pay, the administration almost always expects a doctor to hit a minimum number of RVUs in a year. The metric is also used to assess promotions. RVUs are an explicit gauge of the economic value a doctor is driving to the hospital. Maximizing RVUs is an overarching concern for hospital administrators and doctors who work within them. This makes sense. Interventions, measured by RVUs, are how hospitals make money. This incentive leads doctors not to ask questions about root-cause solutions when a surgical case lands in their department. And it leads doctors to recommend surgery more than they should. From early in my residency, I was counseled by faculty physicians to learn to bill properly, because as a surgeon "you eat what you kill," a disturbing euphemism meaning that you get paid more if you do more and bill more.

Whenever I asked why we were performing surgery or suggested a potential dietary intervention (for people like my migraine patient Sarah), doctors with seniority reprimanded me with comments like "We didn't become surgeons to give dietary advice." Even if it means that terminal patients are brutally traumatized and separated from family during their remaining time, doctors are indoctrinated to do whatever it takes to keep patients alive, even if it's about squeezing out a few more days of life in the ICU.

Billing is based on completing and coding an interventional action rather than addressing why people get sick. Measuring and reimbursing an act (such as prescribing a pill, conducting surgery, running an MRI) can be coded, while a multifactorial physiological outcome that improves patients' health (reversing diabetes, preventing cancer, reducing inflammation or oxidative stress) cannot be.

Because revenue depends on the billing codes used, hospitals are incentivized to conduct as many procedures and have as many quick patient visits as possible to maximize reimbursements. If you come to the hospital with a broken arm, the hospital will make more money if they prescribe a narcotic to you in addition to treating your arm. The more you do, the more you get paid, no matter what the outcome for the patient.

In residency, I sat by a sign in the ENT workroom that read FUCK CANCER!—presumably to motivate the poor souls already terrified and weakened by the disease running through their bodies. At Stanford Medicine, I saw powerful, wealthy cancer patients laud their oncology team for helping them wage war on their disease and confidently tell their families, between exams, that they had the "best doctors in the world" on their side. Obviously, there are benefits for patients to get psychologically motivated to beat a disease, and there is nothing wrong with having enthusiasm for your medical team. But I couldn't help but start wondering where these motivational slogans were in the decades prior when these patients inevitably demonstrated symptoms like diabetes, mild dementia, and hypertension. Cancer is often a *preventable* disease, but the fervor to "fight" comes only after the damage has been largely done.

The truth is that the caliber of your doctor matters very little after a cancer diagnosis. They will prescribe you the same thing as every other doctor, conduct the same chemotherapy procedures with the same machines, and perform the same surgery to roughly the same standards, all based on National Comprehensive Cancer Network (NCCN) guidelines (which are dripping with conflicts of interest). Saying "You have the best medical team" after a cancer diagnosis is like saying you have the best mechanic after totaling your car.

After my mother's death, I spoke with one of her oncologists on the phone. I leveled with her—doctor to doctor, woman to woman—and expressed my frustration that she'd recommended procedures we both knew would take my mom away from her family in her final days without meaningfully improving her life span. I felt empathy, knowing she'd gotten into medicine to help people, but she was so deep in the system, she couldn't conceive of a different way.

THE BIGGEST LIE IN HEALTH CARE

The most blatant and deadly example of the intervention-based incentives of our medical system is that medical leaders are absolutely silent on the things that are actually making us sick: food and lifestyle.

If the surgeon general, the dean of Stanford Medical School, and the head of the NIH gave a press conference on the steps of Congress tomorrow saying we should have an urgent national effort to cut sugar consumption among children, I believe sugar consumption would go down. People in the United States generally listen to medical leaders. Smoking plummeted when the Surgeon General's Report on Smoking was released, and we changed our diet to more carbs and sugar (to disastrous effect) when the Food Pyramid was released in the 1990s.

But instead, our medical leaders are silent on the true causes of our nearly universal metabolic epidemic.

They don't sound the alarm that U.S. teenagers are so sedentary and eating such poor food that 77 percent of twenty-one-year-olds aren't physically fit enough to join the military.

They aren't calling out media companies like Viacom (Nickelodeon) that spend millions on lobbying the FTC *not* to regulate food ads to kids. Fast-food companies alone spent $5 billion to target kids in 2019, with 99 percent of the ads highlighting unhealthy options that are against the USDA's guidance.

They aren't demanding later start times for schools, even when we have a scientific consensus that sleep patterns of teenagers differ significantly from those of other age groups and the current early start of school disrupts normal brain development.

They aren't decrying that 40 percent of funding for the Academy of Nutrition and Dietetics comes from the food industry. These financial conflicts have led the largest and most influential dietician group to endorse mini cans of Coke as healthy, to publicly attack the idea that sugar causes obesity, and to lobby against sugar taxes.

They aren't expressing outrage that 10 percent of SNAP (Supplemental Nutrition Assistance Program, a nutrition program 15 percent of the country relies on) funds are spent on sugar-sweetened beverages, representing billions of taxpayer dollars being funneled directly to companies like Coca-Cola and PepsiCo (which also benefit from taxpayer-funded Farm Bills that subsidize the high-fructose corn syrup that goes into their disease-generating drinks).

They aren't calling for medical organizations to reject donations from ultra-processed food companies, which have donated millions of dollars to medical groups such as the American Academy of Pediatrics (which takes money from formula companies like Abbott and Mead Johnson) and the American Diabetes Association (which has received money from the likes of Coke and Cadbury).

They aren't calling for tighter regulation on the more than eighty thousand synthetic chemicals filling our food, water, air, soil, homes, and personal care products, of which less than 1 percent have been adequately tested for human safety, but for which many are known to be hormonal and mitochondrial disruptors linked to diabetes, obesity, infertility, and cancer.

They aren't calling for a stop to the billions in agricultural subsidies that generate the components of processed food: Eighty percent of American Farm Bill subsidies go to corn, grains, and soy oil. Amazingly, tobacco receives four times more government subsidies (2 percent) than all fruits and vegetables combined (0.45 percent).

Obesity doctors and pediatricians are not calling to lower the recommended added sugar for children to zero; they are saying obesity is a "brain disease" and that the government should subsidize bariatric surgeries and pharmaceutical injections to manage it.

Cardiologists are not screaming from the rooftops for an urgent national effort to reduce processed food to curb America's number one killer, heart disease.

The American Diabetes Association (ADA) is not declaring a War on Sugar. They have in fact accepted millions from processed food companies like Coke and put the ADA logo on products from brands such as Cadbury chocolate, Kool-Aid, Crystal Light, Jell-O, SnackWell's, Cool Whip, and Raisin Bran.

Our medical leaders aren't protesting the USDA's decision to blatantly ignore its scientific advisory board's recommendation to lower added sugar from 10 to 6 percent of total calories in the recent food guidelines. They aren't calling for the reversal of the USDA's decision to broker a deal with Kraft to offer ultra-processed Lunchables in schools and to relax regulations around whole foods in cafeterias while being able to offer more processed foods.

We would expect institutions like the NIH, medical schools, and the American Medical Association (the group representing doctors) to be ringing alarm bells about why so many patients are getting sick: diet and other metabolic habits. We would expect them to use their respected voices to be calling aggressively for changes to our food system and launching a national effort to decrease sedentary lifestyles. But these critical institutions of medicine have stayed silent and profited as more patients have gotten sick.

Often I would hear in medical training that patients are "lazy" and that they will inevitably eat bad food and make bad decisions. This pessimistic view of patients is endemic in medicine. Looking around, I do not see people in the United States systematically trying to be obese and metabolically unhealthy or trying to live tortured lives and miss critical milestones of their kids and grandkids. No. Patients are being crushed by the devil's bargain between the $6 trillion food industry (which wants to make food cheap and addictive) and the $4 trillion health care industry (which profits off interventions on sick patients and stays silent about the reasons they're getting sick).

This is not a conspiracy but a statement of hard economic reality that every patient should clearly understand. Your doctor—and the entire system they work within—directly and unequivocally benefits from your continued suffering, symptoms, and sickness. Your doctor also likely doesn't understand the role they play in this medical industrial billing complex or the economic and political puppet strings controlling their educational curriculum, the research literature around nutrition, and their decision-making.

The incentives of our medical and food systems pressure patients to not ask questions. These incentives also lead to the biggest lie in health care: that the reasons we are getting sicker, fatter, more depressed, and more infertile are complicated.

The reasons are not complicated; they all tie to Good Energy habits.

I deeply respect doctors, but I want to be very clear on something: at every hospital in the United States, many doctors are doing the wrong things, pushing pills and interventions when an ultra-aggressive stance on diet and behavior would do far more for the patient in front of them. Suicide and burnout rates are astronomical in health care, with approximately four hundred doctors per year killing themselves. (That's equivalent to about four medical school graduating classes just dropping dead every year by their own hand.) Doctors have twice the rate of suicide as the general population. Based on my own experience with depression as a young surgeon, I think a contributor to this phenomenon is an insidious spiritual crisis about the efficacy of our work and a sense of being trapped in a system that is not working but seems too big to change or escape.

SAVING YOURSELF

It might not sound like it, but the theme of this chapter is optimism. We are amid a modern health crisis. The good news is that our system can be fixed, and the crisis can end.

Just 120 years ago, starvation, malnutrition, and early death were the norm. Tuberculosis and pneumonia were leading causes of death. Life expectancy in the United States was around age forty-seven. Back then, 30 percent of all U.S. deaths occurred in children under five years of age, compared to just 1.4 percent in 1999. If you transported someone living in those times to the present day, they'd be in utter shock as they tried to process society's advancements. There is no question that our system can produce positive results when focused on the right problem.

U.S. hospitals today are filled with some of the world's most dedicated, intelligent, and hardworking professionals. But they are operating in a system that has lost its way, one that now makes money when patients are sick and loses money when they are healthy.

The modern medical system has systematically, overwhelmingly, and unequivocally let us down in preventing and reversing chronic disease. In fact, if you pull out deaths from the top eight infectious diseases (which were decreased by antibiotics) from historical data, life expectancy rates haven't improved much in the past 120 years—despite, of course, the fact that health care is the largest and fastest-growing industry in the United States—with the vast majority of health care dollars going to chronic disease care.

We will all grow old before the system changes itself. But a bottoms-up revolution is happening where patients are better equipped today to take charge of their metabolic health. Let's dive into specific ways to implement Good Energy principles to feel better today and prevent disease tomorrow.

To view the scientific references cited in this chapter, please visit us online at caseymeans.com/goodenergy.

PART 2

CREATING GOOD ENERGY

CHAPTER 4

Your Body Has the Answers

How to Read Your Blood Tests and Get Actionable Insights from Wearables

Emily did what every pregnant woman in the United States does at twenty-four weeks of pregnancy: she walked into a doctor's office, drank a concoction of 50 grams of glucose dissolved in water and artificial colorings (an oral glucose tolerance test, or OGTT), waited an hour, and took a blood sugar test to see if she had gestational diabetes. She was told her blood glucose level didn't indicate the condition and she was "in the clear."

Emily had a personal affinity for data and had gotten access to a continuous glucose monitor (CGM), which she was wearing on her arm when she went in for her OGTT. Given this, she was able to personally obtain dozens of glucose data points over the several hours before and after her test and see a much more dynamic picture of her blood sugar than the single data point from the lab. The CGM results showed a very different story than what her doctor told her: she actually had high glucose levels (well in the gestational diabetes range), even hours after drinking the glucose drink. "I walked away thinking that I didn't trust that lab anymore—or the hospital mixed up my results," said Emily.

Without that CGM data, Emily would have left her doctor's office not knowing about her underlying condition and the risks it could have for her child and herself. According to the journal *Diabetes Care*, 20 percent of women with gestational diabetes will remain undiagnosed, even with universal screening. Failure to manage the condition can lead to insulin resistance in the fetus and set the stage for the high risk of lifelong metabolic issues. As we saw in the case of my mother, metabolic dysfunction often first shows signs in the mother during pregnancy, providing a warning signal to get blood glucose levels in a healthy range to avoid additional (and increasingly serious) related conditions.

Managing the condition "was a fun challenge . . . with the CGM," said Emily. During pregnancy, she launched an exploration to protect herself and her child. "Data shows that glucose levels and type 2 diabetes may play a role in Alzheimer's development," she added. "So I started to think, *Wow, I have a child, and I need to start thinking about protecting my brain long term.*"

She continued, "Before wearing a CGM, my body was a mystery to me. I wasn't connecting what I was doing to how I was feeling. Now it's *Oh, if I'm feeling tired or stressed, how have I been eating in the past twenty-four hours?* because I usually see the answer there. It's funny because, as women, we're always told to lose weight and be thin and look better. Once I wore the glucose monitor, my mindset shifted to *Actually, I'm eating food to take care of my body and protect it long term.* Food stopped being an enemy and started being a tool for my health."

Getting insight into how food impacts our health to empower people to make decisions is a good thing; that seems obvious. But most expecting mothers—and most patients in general—don't get nearly as much insight into their bodies as Emily did with a CGM.

Today, we understand more about how our cars, finances, and computers work at any given moment than we do about the function of our own bodies. We jump through hoops to get a basic once-a-year sense of our metabolic health. In twenty-two U.S. states, patients still don't legally own their own medical records; instead, doctors and hospitals do.

If we lack access to tests that show us how food directly affects our biology, the health care system prevents us from understanding our health trajectory and whether our choices are leading to good outcomes. Instead, we have industry-funded movements aimed to convince us that there is "no such thing as bad foods." Such perverse campaigns have spread among the public health and nutrition ecosystem.

Most of us have had the disappointing experience of going to the doctor to review our lab work only to have them tell us one of two things:

1. "Everything looks fine! You're good to go." *Even when you definitely don't feel fine.*
2. "This result is a little off. We're going to put you on this medication." *Without talking in depth about why or what you can do about it.*

The truth is that most doctors don't understand how to interpret the lab results in a meaningful way. Sure, doctors can order a potassium infusion if potassium is low, prescribe a statin if LDL cholesterol is elevated, and prescribe an antibiotic if the white blood cell count is above 11,000. But push a little deeper into how labs are interconnected or what the constellation of labs and biomarkers says about the underlying cellular physiology in your body, and you're likely to get a blank stare. Physicians are trained to follow rules with lab interpretation rather than to step back and read the integrated tea leaves of what it all means. And in more than 93 percent of U.S. adults, the tea leaves read "Bad Energy."

Fortunately, we're entering a new era of medicine. Doctors no longer need to serve as the middlemen for interpreting lab results. This new era will benefit patients profoundly. Levels CEO Sam Corcos calls this concept "bio-observability"—the ability to observe your own biology through technologies like wearables, continuous monitors, and direct-to-consumer (DTC) lab testing. Let me be clear: bio-observability is one of the most disruptive trends our health care industry faces. You should *not* blindly trust your doctor and you should *not* blindly trust me. You should trust your own body. Your body can "speak" to you through accessible testing and real-time data from wearable sensors that help you understand how individual symptoms are connected to overall metabolic health.

We are living in an exciting time where we have the potential to live the longest, healthiest lives in human history, but this will require optimization. *You* are the primary person in charge of understanding your body.

You may have been indoctrinated to think you're not capable of understanding your body, to distrust common sense, and to outsource your health agency. This stops now. A movement exists of people demanding to understand and own their health data so they can use it to live healthier lives. The time is now to join this movement to learn more about the signals coming from your body. For the remainder of this book, let's dive into how to use symptoms, blood tests, and real-time biosensors to see inside your body and determine the success of the Good Energy plan.

SYMPTOMS ARE A GIFT: HOW DO YOU FEEL?

So many patients I've seen in my practice tell me that they "feel fine" and are "healthy." But when we dig into a detailed symptom questionnaire, we find they have ten or more discrete symptoms or conditions, which their previous doctors have chalked up to "normal." These symptoms often include neck pain, seasonal sinus infections or recurrent colds, eczema, itchy ear canals, lower-back pain, acne, headaches, bloating, reflux, chronic cough, a little anxiety, trouble falling asleep, low energy, and PMS symptoms like cramps and moodiness.

None of this is normal. You can and should feel incredible—mentally and physically—most of the time. We have so normalized what Dr. Mark Hyman refers to as "FLC" (feel like crap) syndrome that many of us can't even imagine what it could feel like to be symptom-free. Every one of the handful of symptoms I just listed is a sign from the body that the cells are not getting what they need and could be improved by minimizing oxidative stress, mitochondrial dysfunction, and chronic inflammation with food and lifestyle changes.

Taking stock of baseline symptoms is a simple, critical step in enhanced bio-observability. I urge you to take the symptom questionnaire on my website (caseymeans.com/goodenergy), adapted from the Institute for Functional Medicine, and see what has been affecting you over the past thirty days.

We are told that symptoms are things to fear and immediately treat. But they are a gift. Think of your cells as thirty-seven trillion infants in your care. Like infants, the cells can't communicate with words, so symptoms are their way of wailing to get your attention to have their needs met.

Every time a symptom crops up, I ask, *What is my body trying to tell me?* If my neck pain starts acting up, I always look at how my sleep and stress levels have been. If I have anxiety, I think about whether I've been exercising and how much alcohol I had that week. If a pimple pops up out of the blue, I ponder whether sneaky sugar crept into a recent restaurant meal I ate. If I have a headache, I think back on my hydration over the day. If I have PMS symptoms, I think about all the factors that may have affected my hormones differently that month, like fiber intake, alcohol, stress, and sleep.

Another important way our body speaks to us is through our biomarkers.

HOW TO ANALYZE A STANDARD BLOOD TEST

Triglycerides, fasting glucose, "good" cholesterol, "bad" cholesterol—we have all nodded as the doctors quickly glossed over our test results, but very few of us have any idea what these numbers mean. These numbers have limitations: they are a single snapshot when our body is highly dynamic. But they can still give powerful clues to metabolic health and cellular energy management when interpreted together properly.

The question you're trying to answer with standard blood tests is whether you are part of the 6.8 percent of people in the United States who meet the normal criteria for the five basic metabolic biomarkers without medication, and therefore are a step in the right direction to having Good Energy. To answer this question, you will need to obtain your lab results and vital signs from your most recent annual physical and get a measuring tape. Among your life's top priorities should be making it into that 6.8 percent. If you don't achieve that goal, you'll almost certainly experience more conditions like depression, acne, headaches, and deadly chronic diseases in life. If you're a woman, you'll be more likely to pass metabolic dysfunction on to your child in utero, be infertile, have a miscarriage, experience worse menopausal symptoms, and develop Alzheimer's. We have normalized an environment where 70 percent of the nation's population will have an overt chronic disease soon. That doesn't have to be you.

I am a huge believer in personal choice and individual freedoms—and for people to eat or do things that are unhealthy if they choose to. But we should all at least *know* where we are on the spectrum of Good (or Bad) Energy so we can make informed decisions. Scientific research on behavior change has shown that patients who have access to their own health data have significantly better outcomes. I believe that if a patient with a high triglyceride-HDL ratio clearly understands that this biomarker makes them 89 percent more likely to have depression, they would be more likely to follow a diet and lifestyle plan to optimize their metabolism.

To be empowered about our health, we must understand the five basic metabolic biomarkers that generally come at no cost during our annual physical.

Triglycerides: Am I Overwhelming My Cells with Glucose?

When we consume more sugar and carbohydrates than our liver mito-chondria can handle, the excess glucose is converted into triglycerides and shipped out into the bloodstream to be stored in tissues and muscles in a process called *de novo lipogenesis* (de novo = new, lipo = fat, genesis = to make).

Evolutionarily, this process makes sense. Triglycerides are a form of fat that can be used for energy when humans are fasting (which they were of-ten forced to do in the feast-or-famine cycles of premodern life) or exerting themselves. But in our modern society—where we are constantly fed and largely sedentary—these triglycerides pile up in the bloodstream.

Insulin resistance causes overburdened fat cells throughout the body to break down fat (via *lipolysis*), which sends more fat back to the liver for tri-glyceride production. Unfortunately, liver cells filled with fat don't work properly and block insulin signaling, exacerbating insulin resistance in a vicious cycle occurring in most U.S. bodies today.

In terms of what raises triglyceride levels, the simple message is that high triglycerides are almost certainly a warning sign that you are eating too much sugar, refined carbs, and/or alcohol, and probably not engaging in enough physical activity. You need to reduce the amount of carbs that are overwhelming your liver and turning into fat. This means cutting out the soda, sugar-sweetened beverages, juices, added sugar of any kind, candy, products with refined grains (breads, pasta, crackers, tortillas, chips, cookies, pastries, cakes, cereals, etc.), and other high glycemic foods. And you need to increase your daily movement to burn the excess fuel.

Excess alcohol consumption has a negative impact on triglyceride levels due to its impact on liver function, with triglyceride levels going up as alcohol consumption goes up (which will likely be even worse if the drink has any added sugar, mixes, or juices in it). Additionally, when alcohol is consumed with a meal containing fat (specifically saturated fat), it may worsen post-meal triglyceride levels by impairing the activity of lipoprotein lipase, an enzyme that normally clears triglycerides. Aside from increased triglycerides as alcohol consumption goes up, alcohol also depletes antioxidant resources in the cells and generates reactive oxygen species, both of which contribute to poor metabolic health.

RANGES:
- The triglyceride range that's considered "normal" by standard criteria: <150 mg/dL
- Optimal range: <80 mg/dL

That the normal range for triglycerides is anything under 150 mg/dL is a travesty. The range should be much lower. The research shows that the probability of a cardiovascular event (i.e., heart attack and stroke) is 50 percent less in people with triglycerides under 81 mg/dL versus in people with levels between 110 and 153 mg/dL. (Yet doctors tell both groups they are in the "normal" range.) Levels above 153 mg/dL sharply drive up the risk.

In my own case, my triglyceride levels on two very different diets—one a high-carb, low-fat vegan diet and the other a more omnivorous, higher fat, moderately low-carb diet—were both 47 mg/dL. Why did both diets keep triglycerides low? Neither diet overwhelmed my cells with too much energy to process, because both focused on unprocessed, whole foods that cued my complex satiety mechanisms to signal me not to overeat. If you pair dietary strategies with comprehensive Good Energy habits (such as sleep, stress management, toxin avoidance, exercise, etc.), your whole metabolic system will churn through excess energy substrates from food and maintain mitochondrial health. And you'll be set up for healthier triglyceride levels.

High-Density Lipoprotein (HDL) Cholesterol

When we talk about cholesterol in lab testing, it's a misnomer. Cholesterol and triglycerides can't travel around the body by themselves, because these two fatty substances can't dissolve in the blood (which is mostly water). Instead, they are packaged together inside a sphere made of molecules that *can* dissolve in water, and this sphere is covered in protein markers (like shipping labels) that allow cells to recognize and interact with it, so the sphere can drop off its fat and cholesterol cargo. The specific proteins on the surface, along with the ratio of cholesterol and fat inside the sphere, determine whether it's considered a high-density lipoprotein cholesterol (HDL-C) particle, a low-density lipoprotein cholesterol (LDL-C) particle, or other types.

HDL is often referred to as "good" because it helps remove cholesterol from the blood vessels and carries it back to the liver for processing and elimination from the body. This process of reverse cholesterol transport can help prevent the buildup of plaque in the arteries and reduce the risk of heart disease and stroke. Therefore, high levels of HDL in the bloodstream are considered beneficial for cardiovascular health.

Meanwhile, LDL (low-density lipoprotein) is often referred to as "bad" cholesterol because it can deposit cholesterol in the walls of the arteries, leading to the formation of plaque. This process, known as atherosclerosis, can narrow the arteries and increase the risk of heart disease and stroke.

High levels of HDL have been associated with a lower risk of heart disease and stroke, while low levels of HDL have been linked to an increased risk of these conditions. In fact, HDL is often used as a predictor of cardiovascular risk, along with other factors such as blood pressure, smoking, and age. Additionally, HDL has anti-inflammatory and antioxidant properties, which can help protect against the development of atherosclerosis. For inflammatory cells to cause problems in the blood vessels, they need to first bind to the vessel walls; HDL helps decrease this ability for inflammatory cells to adhere. More research is coming out daily about the nuances of HDL, with more attention being paid to the subtypes of this larger class of molecules. But HDL is generally associated with better metabolic health, and HDL is one of the only lab tests you want to be high rather than low.

RANGES:
- Range considered "normal" by standard criteria: >40 mg/dL for men and >50 mg/dL for women
- Optimal range: There is a U-shaped relationship between HDL levels and development of diseases, with both low and very high levels being associated with increased risk. The sweet spot for lowest risk appears to be about 50 to 90 mg/dL, although sources vary.

Fasting Glucose

Fasting glucose measures your blood sugar levels unaffected by a recent meal and should be tested after not eating or drinking any calories for eight hours. We learned why this is important in earlier chapters: a high fasting glucose level is a sign of insulin resistance blocking glucose from getting into our cells. We also learned that the body initially overcompensates for this insulin block by producing more insulin, which can work for a while in "pushing" the cell to let glucose in. Because of this overcompensation, fasting glucose levels can look normal for a long period while insulin resistance is developing full force.

Unfortunately, though, you won't know if insulin resistance is brewing unless you test fasting insulin, which is—catastrophically—not a standard lab test in the United States, despite being cheap and easy. A study from *The Lancet* showed that insulin resistance can be picked up more than a decade before fasting glucose hits the diabetic range, meaning that we are knowingly missing a huge window of opportunity to intervene. More on this later in the chapter.

With that said, if your glucose is rising, it's a big warning sign of problems with how your cells are functioning and a clue that Bad Energy processes—like mitochondrial dysfunction, oxidative stress, and chronic inflammation—are at play and that issues inside your cells are preventing the normal transmission of the insulin signal.

RANGES:
- Range considered "normal" by standard criteria: <100 mg/dL
- Optimal range: 70–85 mg/dL

We call blood sugar less than 100 mg/dL "normal." That's another travesty. As Dr. Robert Lustig says, "Once the fasting glucose rises over 100 mg/dL (signifying prediabetes), metabolic syndrome is in full force, and there are no options for prevention anymore; now you're in full-fledged treatment mode. But in fact, a fasting blood glucose of 90 mg/dL is already questionable."

> **The Six Stages of Diabesity According to Dr. Mark Hyman**
> "There are six stages of diabesity [diabetes + obesity, aka insulin resistance]. The first stage of insulin resistance is high spiking levels of insulin 30 minutes, one hour, and two hours after the introduction of a sugar load. Your blood sugar may stay completely normal in these time frames. The second stage is elevated levels of fasting insulin with a perfectly normal blood sugar level while fasting and after a glucose challenge test. The third stage is the elevation of blood sugar and insulin after a sugar load at 30 minutes, one hour, or two hours. The fourth stage is an elevation of your fasting blood sugar level higher than 90 or 100 mg/dl and elevation of fasting insulin. As you can see, by the time fasting blood sugar is higher than 90 or 100 mg/dl, this is far down the progression of insulin resistance." —Dr. Mark Hyman

Blood Pressure

High blood pressure is the most common preventable risk factor for cardiovascular diseases, such as heart disease, heart failure, stroke, heart attack, arrhythmias, chronic kidney disease, dementia, and arterial blockages in the extremities. High blood pressure is the largest contributor to death and disability in the entire world. It exerts its ill effects on the body by damaging blood vessels and contributing to stiffness and blockages in the vascular system that can cut off critical blood flow in subtle ways over long periods of time.

Blood pressure is directly related to insulin resistance. Interestingly, one of the many functions of insulin is to stimulate nitric oxide, which is the chemical that dilates vessels and is released from cells of the blood vessel wall. In insulin-resistant bodies, this process is impaired, leading to less dilation of vessels. Bad Energy processes make this worse: increased inflammation leads to high blood pressure by downregulating nitric oxide synthase (the protein enzyme that makes nitric oxide), and oxidative stress induces hypertension by causing damage to blood vessel walls and decreasing nitric oxide.

RANGES:
- Range considered "normal" by standard criteria: <120 systolic and <80 diastolic mmHg
- Optimal range: Same as "normal"

Waist Circumference

Waist circumference matters because it is a marker of fat in and around your abdominal organs. Excess fat here is a sign of excess energy being deposited in places it is not supposed to be. Fat can be stored in the body's following three compartments, and each carries a different level of risk for metabolic dysfunction:

- *Subcutaneous fat* is the fat under the skin that you can pinch with your fingers. This fat is not considered to be dangerous and more of it is not associated with increased mortality.
- *Visceral fat* is fat coating the organs in the abdomen. Think of it as a blanket of fat on top of your liver, intestines, and spleen. This fat is dangerous, promotes chronic inflammation, and increases the risk of disease and early death.

- *Ectopic fat* is fat *inside* the cells of various organs like the liver, heart, and muscle. This fat is extremely dangerous, blocks insulin receptor signaling, and increases the risk of disease and early death.

Visceral fat and ectopic fat are strongly associated with insulin resistance and metabolic abnormalities. Visceral fat is unique in that it acts as a hormone-secreting organ, secreting pro-inflammatory chemicals that recruit inflammatory cells. This stew of inflammation causes fat to leak into the bloodstream (lipolysis), block insulin signaling, and drive insulin resistance. Ectopic fat directly blocks the cells' normal internal activities, like insulin signaling.

Waist circumference is a useful—albeit rudimentary—indicator of the level of visceral fat, which expands our midlines. This is measured just above the top of your hip bone, at about the level of your belly button. The amount of visceral fat helps predict metabolic dysfunction, regardless of whether someone is normal weight or obese. We can measure visceral fat in more precise ways, including via imaging studies, such as dual X-ray absorptiometry (DEXA) scans. But knowing your waist circumference is a great place to start.

RANGES:
- Range considered "normal" by standard criteria: <102 cm (40 inches) for men and <88 cm (35 inches) for women
- Optimal range: The International Diabetes Federation has proposed tighter cut points of <80 cm (31.5 inches) for women and <90 cm (35 inches) for men of the following ethnicities: South Asian, Chinese, Japanese, and South and Central Americans. For those of European, Sub-Saharan African, Middle Eastern, and Eastern Mediterranean origin, the cut points are <94 cm (37 inches) in men and <80 cm (31.5 inches) in women.

Triglyceride-to-HDL Ratio
After assessing each of these five biomarkers, there is one more step: calculate your triglyceride-to-HDL ratio to better understand insulin sensitivity.

Simply divide your triglycerides by your HDL. Interestingly, studies have shown that this value correlates well with underlying insulin resistance. So even if you are unable to access a fasting insulin test, the triglyceride-to-HDL ratio can give you a general sense of where you're at.

According to Dr. Mark Hyman, "the triglyceride-to-HDL ratio is the best way to check for insulin resistance other than the insulin response test. According to a paper published in *Circulation*, the most powerful test to predict your risk of a heart attack is the ratio of your triglycerides to HDL. If the ratio is high, your risk for a heart attack increases sixteen-fold—or 1,600 percent! This is because triglycerides go up and HDL (or 'good cholesterol') goes down with diabesity."

Dr. Robert Lustig agrees: "The triglyceride-to-HDL ratio is the best biomarker of cardiovascular disease and the best surrogate marker of insulin resistance and metabolic syndrome." In children, higher triglyceride-to-HDL is significantly correlated with mean insulin, waist circumferences, and insulin resistance. In adults, the ratio has shown a positive association with insulin resistance across normal weight and overweight people and significantly tracks with insulin levels, insulin sensitivity, and prediabetes.

Perplexingly, the triglyceride-to-HDL ratio is not a metric used in standard clinical practice. If you remember one thing from this chapter, remember this: you need to know your insulin sensitivity. It can give you lifesaving clues about early dysfunction and Bad Energy brewing in your body, and is best assessed by a fasting insulin test, discussed below. Right now, this is not a standard test offered to you at your annual physical. I implore you to find a way to get a fasting insulin test or to calculate your triglyceride-to-HDL ratio every year. Do this for your children, as well. And take the steps outlined in the following chapters to ensure it does not start creeping up.

RANGES:
- Range considered "normal" by standard criteria: none specified in standard criteria
- Optimal range: Anything above a ratio of 3 is strongly suggestive of insulin resistance. You want to shoot for less than 1.5, although lower is better. I recommend aiming for less than 1.

My HDL cholesterol is 92 mg/dL and triglycerides are 47 mg/dL, making my ratio 0.51.

SIX FURTHER TESTS

The blood tests we've covered so far should come standard (and generally for free) on your annual physical and give you a decent picture on whether Bad Energy is brewing in your body.

Below are the six most important additional tests that are relatively inexpensive and can be run at almost any standard lab to give an expanded view of your metabolic and overall health. These tests should be completed at least yearly. Confirm that these six tests are on your annual physical or order them as additional tests if not.

Fasting Insulin and Calculation of HOMA-IR
Fasting insulin is the most valuable lab test you can get.

An elevated fasting insulin is a red alarm that your cells are under siege and Bad Energy is at play. It tells you that cells in your body are likely filling up with toxic excess fat, blocking the insulin signal, disavowing glucose from entering the cell, and forcing your pancreas to oversecrete insulin to try to overcompensate for this dysfunctional block. Elevated fasting insulin also tells you that inflammation may be directly blocking the transmission of the insulin signal from the outside to the inside of the cell. Ask your doctor for a fasting insulin test on your next lab draw. From the fasting insulin along with a fasting glucose test, you can calculate your HOMA-IR (homeostatic model assessment for insulin resistance)—one of the most standard measures of insulin resistance in research. To calculate, search "HOMA-IR" on MDCalc (a medical calculator tool) and input your lab values.

Most likely your doctor will push back and say, "Oh, your blood sugar is fine. You don't need an insulin test" or "You're a healthy weight. You don't need an insulin test" or "This test varies day to day, so it won't be reliable." Do not accept any of this.

Dozens, if not hundreds of papers show the clinical utility of understanding the degree of insulin resistance, even in people without diabetes who are a healthy weight. If your doctor pushes back on this test, I recommend providing the following quote from *The Lancet*, a premier medical journal that your doctor will be aware of (Note: "hyperglycemic" means "high glucose"):

> [There are] marked changes in the HOMA 2 scores in the patients that progress to the overt hyperglycaemic stage of type 2 diabetes up to 15 years before diabetes diagnosis by glycaemic parameters, which remained mostly in the normal range during this anterior period of time. . . .
>
> Excessive pancreatic ß-cell function is characterised by hyperinsulinaemia . . . as this organ attempts to overcome the body's increasing insulin resistance, characterising subclinical diabetes within the non-diabetic glycaemic range. At this hyperglycaemic insulin-resistant stage, hyperglycaemic insulin-resistant individuals already present with an increased risk of diabetic comorbidities long before overt diabetes develops.

Translation: You can develop insulin resistance up to fifteen years before you can diagnose type 2 diabetes based on testing glucose. Any level of insulin resistance means your cells are overburdened, you are dealing with Bad Energy processes in the cells, and you will be at a higher risk for developing innumerable symptoms and diseases associated with metabolic dysfunction (see Chapter 2).

HOMA-IR is a calculation that considers your insulin level for a given fasting glucose level. Two people might have the exact same fasting glucose level, but the more insulin-resistant person will be producing much more insulin to keep the glucose at that level (to overcome the insulin block). The following example illustrates why knowing your HOMA-IR is crucial.

Person A has a fasting glucose of 85 mg/dL and an insulin level of 2 mIU/L.

> Person B has the same fasting glucose of 85 mg/dL and an insulin level of 30 mIU/L.
>
> Person B's body is having to churn out significantly more insulin to keep fasting glucose at 85 mg/dL, representing that person B is extremely insulin resistant.
>
> Person A has a HOMA-IR of 0.4 (extremely good, very insulin sensitive).
>
> Person B has a HOMA-IR of 6.3 (very insulin resistant) and will likely develop many more diseases and symptoms and die earlier.
>
> However, doctors rarely test fasting insulin. Both people have normal fasting glucose levels, so their doctors will tell them they are both totally in the clear.

Recent research shows that in children with obesity, elevated fasting insulin levels and HOMA-IR are highly predictive of future blood sugar diseases, whereas fasting glucose levels and hemoglobin A1c were not predictive.

RANGES (FASTING INSULIN):
- No standardized range for "normal," but according to some sources, <25 mIU/L
- Optimal range: fasting insulin 2 to 5 mIU/L. Above 10 mIU/L is concerning, and above 15 mIU/L is significantly elevated.

RANGES (HOMA-IR):
- Less than 2.0, but lower is better

Brand-new research has shown that when a young, healthy adult is on the high end of "normal" for fasting glucose, waist circumference, and fasting insulin, they have a five times higher risk for a future major cardiovascular event. The absolute tragedy of our current health care system is that a doctor will tell this young person they are fine and normal.

High-Sensitivity CRP (hsCRP)

When you have inflammation, hsCRP, a protein primarily made by the liver, rises in blood concentration. This test is one of the most common and easy-to-access measures of inflammation. It is often elevated in people with metabolic dysfunction. Think obesity, heart disease, type 2 diabetes, leaky gut, Alzheimer's disease, and sleep disorders like obstructive sleep apnea. The marker can also rise during infection. You definitely want to know your level of inflammation every year—given how strong the relationship is between insulin resistance, oxidative stress, chronic inflammation, mitochondrial dysfunction, the cell danger response (CDR), and the development of nearly every chronic disease and symptom facing people in the United States today.

RANGES:

- Range considered "normal" by standard criteria: The CDC and American Heart Association recommend the following ranges:
  - Low risk: <1.0 mg/L
  - Average risk: 1.0 to 3.0 mg/L
  - High risk: >3.0 mg/L
- Optimal range: <0.3 mg/L. This level is one you want as low as possible, and certainly below the "low-risk" range indicated by the CDC. A study of nearly thirty thousand individuals showed that very low hsCRP (<0.36 mg/L) was associated with the least risk of cardiovascular events, such as heart attack and stroke, and the risk steadily increased from there. Even a range of 0.36 to 0.64 mg/L conferred higher risk than <0.36 mg/L, and by the time one reached 0.64 to 1.0 mg/L, the relative risk was 2.6 for a cardiovascular event.

Chronic inflammation is one of the three key hallmarks of Bad Energy. If it's not low, take stock of which Good Energy pillars outlined in the following chapters may be driving a state of "threat" in the body, and address it.

Hemoglobin A1c (HbA1c)

HbA1c (often referred to as just A1c) measures the percentage of hemoglobin in your body that has sugar stuck to it via glycation. HbA1c is one of the three main screening tests for type 2 diabetes (along with fasting glucose and an oral glucose tolerance test). Hemoglobin is the molecule in all red blood cells that carries oxygen. If more glucose is floating around in the bloodstream, it has a higher chance of bumping into hemoglobin and bonding with it. This bonding will increase the percentage of glycated hemoglobin, which can be translated into an approximation of average glucose levels.

Red blood cells float around in the bloodstream for around 90 to 120 days before the spleen clears them out. So HbA1c represents a longer-term estimate of average blood sugar levels over a few months. But many factors can affect HbA1c, like red blood cell life span (which can be related to genetics and ethnicity), anemia, kidney disease, an enlarged spleen, and more. Therefore, we should use an HbA1c test as just one tool among many to understand metabolic status.

RANGES:

- Range considered "normal" by standard criteria: <5.7 percent
- Optimal range: Research suggests that the lowest risk range for HbA1c is 5.0 to 5.4 percent.

Uric Acid

Uric acid is a metabolic by-product of the breakdown of fructose and purine-rich foods, which include animal proteins (especially red meat, seafood, and organs) and alcohol (especially beer). When we overwhelm the body with too much fructose too quickly (like when we chug a soda laden with high-fructose corn syrup), uric acid levels quickly rise, creating several problems. Excess uric acid generates oxidative stress that disturbs mitochondrial function, shunting things that should go to cellular energy (ATP) production toward fat instead. Then, as fat builds up in the cells, particularly in the liver cells, it worsens insulin resistance. Uric acid also generates systemic inflammation by stimulating the release of inflammatory chemicals (cytokines) and increases blood pressure by inactivating nitric oxide, which normally relaxes blood vessels.

When uric acid levels are high, it can crystallize in our joints, leading to gout, an extremely painful inflammatory condition that, unsurprisingly, is associated with a 71 percent higher likelihood of having type 2 diabetes (in women), a 78 percent higher risk of kidney disease, a 42 percent increased risk of depression, and a twice as high risk of sleep apnea and heart attack. Hopefully, the relationship between these varied conditions no longer seems perplexing: they are each organ-specific expressions of the same underlying physiology of Bad Energy.

RANGES:
- Range considered "normal" by standard criteria: usually around 1.5 to 6 mg/dL for women and 2.5 to 6 mg/dL for men
- Optimal range: Research suggests that keeping uric acid <5 mg/dL for men and 2 to 4 mg/dL for women is associated with the lowest development of cardiometabolic diseases.

Liver Enzymes: Aspartate Transaminase (AST), Alanine Transaminase (ALT), and Gamma-Glutamyl Transferase (GGT)

AST and ALT are proteins made in liver cells that can be released into circulation when liver cells die or become damaged. One of the key ways that liver cells can become dysfunctional is via insulin resistance. So elevated AST and ALT are associated with increased risk of fatty liver and metabolic disease.

GGT is a protein made throughout the body. But it is especially concentrated in the liver. It is a unique marker in that it is one of the few tests that can offer a hint of oxidative stress, one of the three key processes underlying Bad Energy, which is notoriously hard to test for directly. Because GGT's role is to metabolize the protein glutathione, a key antioxidant our bodies make that neutralizes free radicals, levels will increase in the face of more oxidative burden and glutathione activity. Given the relationship between oxidative stress and metabolic dysfunction, high GGT is significantly associated with increased risk of type 2 diabetes, cardiovascular disease, cancer, liver disease, and premature death.

The liver could not be more important to our overall metabolism and our ability to make Good Energy. It is the first site of nutrient delivery from the intestines after we eat and it determines how the body will process and use energy. The liver is a master balancer of blood sugar levels by having the skills to break down glucose, store glucose, and make glucose from other substrates, like fat. It creates bile to help break down food in the gut, so we can absorb critical micro- and macronutrients necessary for metabolism and mitochondrial function. It packages and exports fats and cholesterol to other parts of the body for storage or use. It also receives fats and cholesterol from the bloodstream to process them. As we've learned, when the liver becomes overburdened and damaged, it will store fat inside its cells, creating fatty liver disease—a toxic and preventable process now affecting close to 50 percent of U.S. adults. Modern life is decimating this key metabolic organ.

Interestingly, when insulin is released from the pancreas, it doesn't immediately enter the general circulation. It goes straight to the liver through a special vein: the portal vein. So if the liver becomes insulin resistant, the pancreas receives direct feedback to make more insulin, generating damaging hyperinsulinemia and the vicious cycle of Bad Energy. I cannot overstate how much we want a pristine, healthy, optimally functioning liver for all aspects of health. The strategies in the next chapters will help you achieve that. You may have never thought about how your liver health can directly contribute to heart disease, Alzheimer's, PMS, erectile dysfunction, or infertility, but it can. The liver is a master orchestrator of metabolism, hormone processing, detoxification, digestion, and cellular energy production across the whole body.

RANGES:

- Range considered "normal" by standard criteria: the Mayo Clinic states that normal ALT is 7 to 55 U/L, AST is 8 to 48 U/L, and GGT is 8 to 61 U/L.

- Optimal range: Research suggests that all-cause mortality starkly increases when AST and ALT levels rise above about 17 U/L. For GGT, lowest risk for men is about <25 U/L and women <14 to 20 U/L. Some sources recommend <8 U/L. Sources vary, but these are good targets to aim for.

Vitamin D

Vitamin D is a hormone made when we expose our skin to sunlight. Vitamin D serves dozens of critical biological functions related to calcium and phosphate levels, insulin secretion, immune function and cytokine regulation, cell death, and vascular growth pathways, among others.

Many proteins made inside cells get released into circulation to act elsewhere in the body. These proteins include insulin, neurotransmitters, inflammatory cytokines, antibodies, and others. They require calcium as an activating signal for their release, and vitamin D highly regulates calcium levels.

Healthy vitamin D levels not only improve insulin sensitivity but also improve the function of the pancreatic cells that make insulin. Vitamin D also manages the healthy regulation of the immune system, while low vitamin D levels can stimulate the master inflammatory gene NF-𝜘B, increase pro-inflammatory cytokine levels, and cause the overproduction of immune cells. Simply put, low vitamin D signals a chronic "pro-threat" to the body, which we've learned is antithetical to Good Energy. Various aspects of the pro-inflammatory state can directly impair insulin signaling and reduce glucose channel expression in the cell. Vitamin D supplementation has been shown to decrease fasting glucose levels and decrease the incidence of type 2 diabetes.

RANGES:

- Range considered "normal" by standard criteria: the NIH recommends levels from 20 to 50 ng/mL.
- Optimal range: research suggests that vitamin D levels from 40 to 60 ng/mL are associated with the lowest all-cause mortality. Vitamin D toxicity is generally not observed until levels are much higher.

GOING FURTHER

There are deeper layers of lab testing that can give you an even more nuanced picture. Options include looking at expanded cholesterol panels, thyroid hormones, sex hormones, kidney function, and micronutrient levels. At my functional medicine clinic, I often tested over one hundred biomarkers in patients. To receive full blood work to target where Bad Energy is brewing in your body and a specific plan of how to reverse it, I recommend searching the functional medicine doctor database (https://www .ifm.org/find-a-practitioner/) or utilizing Function Health (a telehealth service that tests over one hundred biomarkers from all body systems for a very affordable price, with detailed interpretations and optimal ranges for each test).

What About Total Cholesterol and Low-Density Lipoprotein Cholesterol (LDL-C)?

On a standard cholesterol panel, you'll see Total Cholesterol and LDL-C as part of your results. While these are given a lot of weight in the health care conversation, they are nuanced to interpret. Below is a primer on Total Cholesterol and LDL-C from Dr. Robert Lustig, professor emeritus of endocrinology at the University of California, San Francisco, as paraphrased from his book *Metabolical*:

When you get a total cholesterol result, throw it in the garbage. It means absolutely nothing. Anyone who tells you that "my cholesterol level is high" doesn't know what they are talking about. You need to know what kind of cholesterol you're talking about. . . .

LDL-C has a checkered history. There is no doubt that LDL-C levels correlate with heart disease risk in large populations, and you do need to know your LDL-C. But, the medical profession places way too much significance on this test, and they do that because we have a drug for it. . . . The hazard risk for high LDL-C and heart disease is 1.3 (high LDL-C leads to 30 percent higher risk of having a heart attack in your lifetime), but there is something that is much more concerning: high triglycerides. High triglyceride levels confer a hazard risk of 1.8 for heart attack.

The takeaway of the Framingham Heart Study was that if you had very high LDL-C, you were more likely to suffer a heart attack. But when the data were analyzed, unless LDL-C was very high (over 200 mg/dL), it wasn't a risk factor. Those with an LDL-C less than 70 mg/dL develop relatively little heart disease. But for the rest of the population, LDL-C is not a great predictor of who will suffer a heart attack. More people are suffering heart attacks with lower LDL-Cs than before, because the standard test of cholesterol assumes all the LDL-C particles are the same.

There are two different types of LDL-Cs, but the lipid profile test measures them together. The majority (80 percent) of circulating LDL-C species are called large buoyant, or type A LDL-C, which are increased by dietary fat consumption. This is the species reduced by eating low-fat or taking statins. However, large buoyant LDL-C are cardiovascularly neutral— meaning it's not the particle driving the accumulation of plaque in the arteries leading to heart disease. There's a second, less common (only 20 percent) LDL-C species called small dense LDL-C (sdLDL-C) or type B LDL-C, and it is predictive of risk for heart attack. The problem is that statins will lower your LDL-C because they are lowering the type A LDL-C, which is 80 percent of the total; but they're not doing anything to the type B LDL-C, which is the problematic particle.

If you have a high LDL-C level, your provider is likely to tell you to eat a low-fat diet. Similar to statins, while your LDL will go down, it's only affecting the large buoyant LDL and not the small dense LDL, which is the actual problem. Small dense LDL rise because they are responsive to dietary refined carbohydrates (i.e., fiberless food) and especially sugar consumption.

According to Dr. Mark Hyman, "more than 50 percent of people who show up in the emergency room with heart attacks have normal cholesterol. But they have small cholesterol particles (sdLDL-C), which are caused by insulin resistance. What causes these small dangerous cholesterol particles? It is the sugar and refined carbohydrates in our diet. Insulin resistance causes these small cholesterol particles to form, and taking statins won't fix the problem."

To better understand your level of disease-promoting cholesterol, ask your doctor for an NMR Lipoprotein Fractionation test, which tells you about your amounts of type A and type B LDL-C, and also may report oxidized LDL (oxLDL), a marker of LDL-C particles damaged by oxidation and prone to stoke inflammation. An additional test that may be more useful than LDL-C to understand the total amount of disease-causing cholesterol particles in the body is apolipoprotein B-100 (ApoB). ApoB is the protein that wraps around specific cholesterol particles to help them dissolve in the blood, and uniquely, it is present on the forms of cholesterol particles in the blood that are known to be *atherogenic,* or promote blocked vessels and causative of heart disease. These include several interrelated cholesterol particles, including LDL-C, very-low-density lipoprotein (VLDL-C), intermediate-density lipoprotein (IDL-C), and lipoprotein(a)—also called Lp(a). Because ApoB measures the total number of *disease-promoting* cholesterol particles in the blood, it may be a more accurate marker of heart disease risk than LDL-C alone. This is not a test that is ordered in standard practice and must be requested or ordered through a specialty service, like Function Health, and optimal ranges have not been established.

Ranges (LDL-C):

- Range considered "normal" by standard criteria (from Cleveland Clinic):
  - Less than 70 mg/dL for those with heart or blood vessel disease and for other patients at very high risk of heart disease (those with metabolic syndrome)

- Less than 100 mg/dL for high-risk patients (for example, some patients who have diabetes or multiple heart disease risk factors)
- Less than 130 mg/dL otherwise
- Optimal range: According to Dr. Robert Lustig in his book *Metabolical*, "If LDL-C is below 100 mg/dL, the small dense fraction can't be high enough to be harmful. If it's over 300 mg/dL, you might have the rare genetic disease familial hypercholesterolemia (FH) and you can't clear LDL-C, and you need a statin. If it's between 100 and 300 mg/dL, then you need to look at the triglyceride level. If the triglyceride level is above 150 mg/dL, that's metabolic syndrome until proven otherwise."

Also look at the LDL-C value in the context of triglyceride-to-HDL ratio, as this ratio is a helpful biomarker for risk of cardiovascular disease and the presence of insulin resistance.

REAL-TIME TOOLS

Levels cofounder Josh Clemente is an aerospace engineer who developed life support systems for SpaceX before conceiving of and starting Levels. He observed that when we build rockets, we put over ten thousand sensors on them to understand the functioning of all parts of the spacecraft and to enable prediction of mechanical dysfunction and systems failure *before* it happens. You really don't want a rocket to break down in the middle of space. Yet with human health, we adhere to an opposite paradigm: we *wait* for the human body to develop fulminant systems failure, which shows up as symptoms and meeting diagnostic thresholds for disease-specific biomarkers. And only then do we recommend sensors or more frequent testing to address the problems. Almost the entirety of what is plaguing U.S. adults today is largely preventable chronic illnesses. What if we treated humans like rockets, equipping them with sensors *before* systems fail, to understand where dysfunction is arising so we can address it?

If you notice on your wearable device that your resting heart rate is slowly rising and has bumped from 55 bpm (beats per minute) to over 70 bpm over a few months, you need to dig into why. Have you been more sedentary? If you notice on a CGM that your waking glucose is slowly creeping up from about 75 mg/dL to 90 mg/dL, you need to address what might be causing it before it gets worse: Is it the ultra-processed foods? Recent work stress? Too little sleep? We're just beginning to be able to answer these questions for ourselves. But this ability will change health care forever, transforming it from a reactive sick care system to a true health empowerment system.

The following are the most impactful real-time biomarkers you can measure today to make actionable decisions.

Continuous Glucose Monitoring

I believe CGM is the most powerful technology for generating the data and awareness to rectify our Bad Energy crisis in the Western world. A CGM is a biosensor that can alert us to early dysfunction, coach us on how to eat and live in a way that promotes Good Energy in our unique bodies, and promote accountability. My belief in the potential of this technology to reduce global metabolic suffering is why I cofounded Levels, which enables access to CGMs and software to understand and interpret the data.

A CGM is a small plastic disc worn on the arm that automatically tests your blood sugar roughly every ten minutes, twenty-four hours a day. And it sends that information to your smartphone. As opposed to just having a single yearly snapshot of glucose—like a fasting glucose test in a lab—a continuous glucose monitor tells you exactly how your body is responding in real time to every action you take, like eating breakfast, exercising, walking, getting a poor night's sleep, or experiencing stress. These factors can change glucose levels almost immediately. In working to prevent the metabolic issues that 93.2 percent of people in the United States are facing, rather than just one data point, I'd rather have up to 35,040 painless data points per year to drive personalized decision-making.

Wearing a CGM as part of a journey to understand and optimize health provides seven main benefits:

1. **Improve Glycemic Variability:** Glucose levels should be generally stable and rise only slightly after meals. High variability in glucose levels can damage tissues and lead to heart disease, diabetes, and metabolic dysfunction. A study from Stanford found that even among people considered healthy by standard glucose ranges, 25 percent of them showed severe glucose variability based on CGM data, and the percentage of time spent in severe variability patterns correlated with worse metabolic markers.

2. **Reduce Cravings and Anxiety:** High glucose spikes lead to bigger glucose crashes, which can lead to cravings, fatigue, and anxiety. Recent CGM research showed that glucose dips—or reactive hypoglycemia— after meals can predict how hungry people would be later in the day, how soon they would eat again, and how much they would eat at the next meal. And bigger crashes led to eating more calories in a twenty-four-hour period. CGMs can teach you how to avoid reactive hypoglycemia by keeping blood sugar more stable and avoiding sharp spikes.

3. **Learn Your Reaction to Individual Foods and Meals:** Different individuals respond differently to the same food (in terms of blood sugar rise), depending on factors such as microbiome composition, sleep, recent meals, and body type. Simply reading carb content or looking at a food's glycemic index is not sufficient to help you find a diet and lifestyle that allows you to maintain stable glucose. Chronic overnutrition is a key cause of Bad Energy that overwhelms our cells and causes oxidative stress, inflammation, mitochondrial dysfunction, glycation, and insulin resistance. CGMs can be useful in showing you the exact impact of a meal on your blood glucose levels. An extra-large spike after a meal is a clear sign that the meal had too much refined grain or refined sugar and is creating a big stress of food energy for your cells to deal with.

4. **Learn to Use Strategies to Stabilize Glucose:** Balancing meals with enough fiber, protein, and fat; eating meals earlier in the day and avoiding late-night meals; walking after meals; and not eating while stressed are

some strategies that can help keep glucose stable. A CGM can help you experiment with different stabilizing strategies.

5. **Train the Body to Be Metabolically Flexible:** Burning fat produces ketones, which have health benefits. But if the body is constantly getting fed glucose—the body's preferential source of food energy to convert to ATP—it's not going to prioritize burning fat. By learning to keep blood sugar levels low and healthy through diet and lifestyle, we increase the opportunity for our body to tap into fat stores for energy, which improves metabolic flexibility (an indicator of better health).

6. **Catch Metabolic Dysfunction Earlier:** Fasting glucose can remain low despite increasing insulin resistance as the body pumps out excess insulin to overcompensate for an insulin block. By viewing a continuous glucose curve on CGM, we can see more subtle clues indicating early dysfunction, like how high our post-meal glucose levels are and how long glucose spikes take to come down to normal.

7. **Motivate Behavior Change:** Seeing real-time glucose data and the impact of meals and activities on glucose levels can motivate behavior change and encourage healthier choices, which can lead to better overall health outcomes.

What data can a continuous glucose monitor tell you?

1. **Morning Glucose:** After a poor night's sleep or a late-night dessert, morning glucose can be elevated. Ideally, morning glucose should be 70 to 85 mg/dL, the level associated with a lower risk of future cardiometabolic disease.

2. **Dawn Effect:** This refers to a rise in glucose driven by the growth hormone and cortisol release that happens naturally before we wake up. As people become more insulin resistant, they tend to have a larger magnitude of this effect. Their body becomes less efficient at clearing the morning glucose rise. Research has found that only 8.9 percent of people without diabetes have a dawn effect, while it is present in 30

percent of people with prediabetes and 52 percent of people with new type 2 diabetes. Presence of the dawn effect is indicative of poor glucose control in people with diabetes. Definitions of the dawn effect vary, but this study defined it as a 20 mg/dL rise. If you note a pronounced dawn effect, you could have brewing insulin resistance.

3. **Post-Meal Glucose (Postprandial Glucose):** Immense learning comes from understanding how different foods, meals, and ingredient combinations affect your blood sugar in the one to two hours after you eat. Post-meal spikes are a contributor to glycemic variability. We want to minimize spikes because they are associated with worse health outcomes. Aiming for a post-meal glucose level of less than 115 mg/dL, with not more than a 30 mg/dL increase from premeal levels, is likely more optimal than standard ranges (which recommend keeping blood sugar below 140 mg/dL). This lower post-meal goal also correlates with the average peak postprandial glucose levels seen in healthy populations wearing CGMs and is supported by extensive expert opinion. In your first week of using a CGM, I recommend eating your normal diet to get a baseline and note any interesting observations. For instance, you might realize that when you eat eggs, avocado, and an orange for breakfast, you have a much lower spike than when you eat breakfast cereal and skim milk or a doughnut and latte. In this case, the protein and fat from eggs and avocado likely offset the glucose impact from the orange. In contrast, cereal and pastries tend to be high in quickly absorbed refined carbs.

4. **Area Under the Curve (AUC):** AUC reflects both the height of the spike and how long the glucose stays elevated after a meal. Generally, people with normal glucose tolerance should return to baseline glucose levels within one to two hours after a meal, while those with prediabetes or type 2 diabetes may see their glucose stay elevated for longer.

5. **Reactive Hypoglycemia:** These post-meal crashes are usually the result of your blood sugar spiking and then crashing below normal levels after a meal. If you find that your blood sugars are going high and then

dropping below their baseline, try balancing future meals better by doing the following:

- Reduce any refined grains and sugars.
- Pair carbs with more fiber, protein, and healthy fat sources.

6. **Impact of Stress on Glucose:** One of my highest glucose spikes ever was after an argument with my brother (my coauthor!). We hear examples of this all the time from Levels members: stress alone can raise glucose levels, regardless of your diet. The reason is that a key stress hormone, cortisol, signals our liver to break down stored glucose and release it into the bloodstream to fuel the muscles, anticipating a threat that we'll need energy to physically move away from. In the modern world, however, the "threats"—like arguments, emails, honking, and the alerts on our phones—that cue our stress pathways rarely require our muscles to be active. As such, that mobilized glucose sits in our bloodstream, causing more harm than good. CGM can be a powerful tool in teaching us how stress impacts our metabolic health and motivates us to address acute stress in healthy ways, like deep breathing.

7. **Impact of Exercise on Glucose:** CGMs are a powerful feedback tool on how exercise impacts your metabolic health. For instance, you might learn and internalize that a ten-minute walk or thirty squats right after a meal significantly lowers your post-meal glucose rise. Similarly, you might notice that after two to three months of consistent daily movement, all your CGM metrics are improving.

8. **Impact of Sleep on Glucose Levels:** Just one night of reducing sleep to four hours can plummet insulin sensitivity by 25 percent in healthy people. What's more, poor sleep efficiency (meaning the time awake tossing and turning as a percentage of the whole night's sleep), later bedtimes, and deviating from one's usual sleep pattern all lead to higher glucose responses to breakfast the next morning. CGM can offer subtle clues about how sleep is affecting your body's ability to clear glucose from the bloodstream. Almost nothing has motivated me to prioritize sleep

quality, quantity, and consistency more than CGM biofeedback. Seeing how skimping on sleep hurts you in real time is incredibly valuable.

9. **Glucose During Sleep:** Late-night high-carbohydrate meals can cause high variability through the night because of our relative insulin resistance when melatonin levels are high (more on this in Chapter 7). And during REM sleep, glucose levels can naturally drop. Add late-night alcohol into the equation, and this can lead to lower glucose levels by blocking the liver's ability to synthesize and produce glucose (something the liver does in the background to make sure blood levels don't drop too low). Simply put, glucose during sleep can be all over the place, and knowing this can help you troubleshoot sleep problems that may be related to glucose patterns.

10. **Average Glucose:** Your twenty-four-hour mean or average glucose level is not a standard metric used in medical practice, but given the increasing use of CGM, I anticipate it will likely become more recognized. Average glucose takes into account fasting glucose, nighttime glucose, and magnitude of glycemic variability and can be a crude measurement of how much glucose your bloodstream is exposed to every day. In a study of a young, healthy population, mean glucose was 89 mg/dL with a standard deviation of 6.2 mg/dL.

11. **Long-term Trends in Glucose:** If you wear a CGM always or just a few times a year, you can view long-term trends in glucose that can help you see the trajectory of your metabolic health. One thing you can be certain of: if you are able to track your blood sugar and keep it in a low and healthy range over the course of your lifetime, you will never have to walk into the doctor's office and get a bomb dropped on you about a diagnosis of type 2 diabetes, which develops gradually over years and decades. You will know exactly where you stand, and that is powerful.

Food Journaling

To understand your body, you must know what is going into it. A food journal is a powerful tool for accountability, making sure that you are getting in what you need to optimize Good Energy, and keeping out what hurts these processes. In my practice, I will not see new patients unless they agree to temporarily keep a food journal. I can't counsel them if I don't know what two to three pounds of molecular information are going into their bodies every day. (Imagine a patient taking two to three pounds of medications every day but not telling the doctor what they're taking.)

What's more, research has shown that people on diets who keep food journals lose twice as much weight as those who don't. A Kaiser Permanente study, involving 1,685 patients, looked at the efficacy of a twenty-week weight-loss program. The number of food records the participants kept per week was one of the key statistically significant variables predicting weight loss. We have seen similar preliminary correlations in the Levels dataset: Levels members who input more food logs have a more significant reduction in body mass index while using CGM.

Several food-logging apps can be helpful, including MacroFactor, MyFitnessPal, and logging within a continuous glucose monitoring app like Levels. But just as effective might be using a paper journal or a note in your phone. Every Saturday I review my food logs from the week with my nutrition coach to understand where I was on track and where I could have made healthier choices.

Sleep Data

As we'll learn in Chapter 7, all-cause mortality and risk of type 2 diabetes are higher in both people who get too little sleep (less than seven hours) and those who get too much sleep (more than nine hours) per night.

Use a wearable sleep and step tracker (examples are listed on page 280) to understand your average *quantity* of sleep per night, with the goal of aiming for about seven to eight hours. Note which days—if any—tend to be outliers for you. Then reflect on why. Research has shown that people significantly overestimate the amount they sleep when their self-reports are compared to their wearable sleep data. Research shows that people who are actually sleeping five hours per night overestimate their sleep by eighty minutes on average. Imagine that: you *think* you are getting close to seven hours of sleep per night (optimal), when you are actually sleeping an amount that puts you at a high risk for a range of metabolic issues. Wearables can help us really see where we're falling short on critical health behaviors like sleep.

To get maximal benefits, use your sleep tracker to assess quality of sleep as well, including how many awakenings you experience per night and how much deep and restorative sleep you get. Actionable, evidence-based steps can help you improve sleep quality, like minimizing alcohol and reducing blue light before bedtime. Understanding your patterns can uncover specific—and simple—areas to focus on to improve Good Energy. Sleep consistency—the regularity of your sleep and wake times—is the third pillar of sleep to track with a wearable. Having a set sleep schedule is a key factor in optimal health.

Activity Data

Movement is one of the best things you can do to improve mitochondrial health and churn through excess food energy substrates. Step count is a great proxy metric to show you how much you're moving. Certainly, steps aren't the only form of exercise that's important, but we do know that low-grade activity that occurs more frequently and regularly throughout the day is extremely important for cellular health and glucose control, even more so than chunking all your physical activity in one discrete block and sitting for the rest of the day (a pattern most Americans adopt).

I'll explain the science of the Good Energy benefits of movement in Chapter 8. But a preview of why it's so important is that exercise stimulates glucose channels to come from inside the cell to the cell membrane to allow glucose to travel from the bloodstream into the cell to be processed for energy for the muscle. Exercise also increases mitochondrial function, mitochondrial quantity, and antioxidant proteins in the mitochondria to protect it from oxidative stress. More movement means we have an increased quantity and quality of high-resiliency energy-producing machines in our cells to work through all our energy substrates, reducing the likelihood that the foods we consume will end up shunted to toxic intracellular fat that leads to insulin resistance.

Use a wearable step and sleep tracker (examples listed on page 280) to understand your average steps per day, with a goal of getting a bare minimum of 7,000 steps per day, and ultimately working up to 10,000 steps per day. Researchers are still debating whether step count matters. I hope to put this debate to rest.

In a study of 2,110 adults followed for almost eleven years, published in the premier medical journal *JAMA*, adults who got at least 7,000 steps per day had a 50 to 70 percent lower risk of dying during the follow-up period than those getting fewer than 7,000 steps per day. Other studies have shown similar findings: data from 6,355 men and women followed for an average of ten years showed that those who walked 8,000 to 12,000 steps per day had a 50 to 65 percent lower risk of death than those who took fewer than 4,000 steps per day.

Aside from step count, you also want to understand the number of your active hours per day, meaning hours where you were up and moving more than about 250 steps. If you sit all day but get 10,000 steps over the course of one hour by going for a run, that's less health promoting than if you space out those steps over every hour of the day (more on this in Chapter 8). Wearables can help alert you to times of the day when you tend to be more sedentary and ping you to get up.

Research shows large discrepancies between how much we think we're moving and how much we are. For instance, in a study of 215 participants, the self-reported amount of moderate to vigorous physical activity was 160 minutes per week, while wearable data over the same period showed that these people were actually performing moderate to vigorous physical activity only 24 minutes per week. Wearable data provides us clarity about how much we really are moving.

Number of Cardiovascular Minutes per Day and Week

Research strongly suggests that a minimum of 150 minutes of moderate aerobic activity per week is crucial for cardiometabolic health (and is as effective as antidepressant medication for mood), which translates into about 30 minutes, five days a week. Wearables that track heart rate can help you know if you are getting this amount per week.

Heart Rate Variability (HRV)

Heart rate variability is a metric that indicates how much variability in time there is between each heartbeat. HRV is a biomarker that can help us understand the trends in our stress and strain levels, which we know impact our cells' ability to produce energy effectively. Counterintuitively, *more* variability in the time between each heartbeat is indicative of better health status and outcomes. Under times of more stress and strain on the body, the cardiovascular system will act like a metronome with regularity in the time between each heartbeat. In a more relaxed, rested, and recovery state, the whole system is more "elastic" and the time between each heartbeat will vary slightly. For instance, one beat might be 859 milliseconds, the next 763 milliseconds, the next 793 milliseconds, and so forth. So if your heart rate is 60 beats per minute, it doesn't mean that each beat is exactly one second; in fact, it's better if they're not.

A high HRV reflects the ability of the nervous system to adapt effectively, and low HRV can indicate strain, fatigue, overtraining, or chronic disease. Low HRV has been associated with physical inactivity, immune dysfunction, high blood pressure, diabetes, cardiovascular disease, depression, decreased social engagement, decreased psychological resilience in the face of stressors, decreased cancer survival, and infertility, among many other conditions that we learned are related to Bad Energy in Chapter 2. What's more, a drop in HRV can predict the onset of COVID-19 before PCR testing is positive.

The interrelationship between HRV and how our cells make energy is complex, multidirectional, and not fully understood, but this is how I see it: Cells that are subjected to the daily insults that result in Bad Energy (chronic overnutrition, sleep deprivation, chronic psychological or excess physical stress without time to recover, toxins, etc.) will send out distress signals and can activate the "stress" arm of the autonomic nervous system, which is the sympathetic nervous system. All of these insults indicate that the body is under threat and needs to be at the ready to "fight" the battle, even when there isn't one. When Bad Energy manifests in our body and we develop insulin resistance, we know that it can reduce nitric oxide activity and decrease the ability of the vascular system to dilate and adapt, which will exacerbate a cycle of having a rigid vascular system and low HRV. Nitric oxide also directly stimulates the relaxation arm of the nervous system, which is the parasympathetic nervous system, and specifically the vagus nerve (which regulates relaxation). Ideally, we want a balance between the two arms of the autonomic nervous system, with the ability to gear up when there is a threat and the ability to relax in times of safety. Low HRV indicates that the gas pedal of stress and strain is too high, and the body—particularly the vascular system—cannot relax.

You can monitor HRV via a wearable device and see trends over time. HRV is very individual and lacks a universal optimal range. You might naturally be a lot lower or higher than the people around you. What matters most is determining what lifestyle factors seem to bump or crash your personal HRV levels compared to your baseline, so you can make lifestyle adjustments to raise HRV. Whoop, an innovative wearable that tracks HRV, fitness, and sleep, has discovered that several factors are associated with increasing HRV over time:

- Giving the body time to recover after intense athletic training.
- Staying hydrated.
- Avoiding alcohol: just one night of drinking can decrease HRV for up to five days.
- Getting consistent and adequate quality sleep.
- Maintaining a consistent eating schedule.
- Eating a healthy diet.
- Avoiding eating within three to four hours of bedtime.
- Getting cold exposure: exposing the body to cold temperatures for brief periods of time (like cold showers and ice baths) stimulates the parasympathetic nervous system.
- Writing in a gratitude journal. This also impacts HRV. Focusing on abundance and thankfulness is a calming signal to the body.

Resting Heart Rate

Resting heart rate is the number of times the heart beats per minute when a person is at rest. It is considered an essential metric to evaluate overall health and fitness. A lower resting heart rate indicates that the heart is efficiently pumping blood and is less stressed. Research has shown that having a lower resting heart rate can improve overall life span and metabolic health. A higher resting heart rate is associated with an increased risk of heart disease, type 2 diabetes, and all-cause mortality. Studies also suggest that resting heart rate can be lowered by consistent exercise. Someone with a resting heart rate of more than 80 bpm (considered in the middle of the "normal" range of 60 to 100 bpm by Harvard, Mayo Clinic, and the American Heart Association) has a 2.91 times higher risk of having type 2 diabetes than someone with a heart rate of less than 60 bpm. In a meta-analysis of over one million people, all-cause mortality and cardiovascular mortality increased linearly and significantly for any resting heart rate above 45 bpm.

THE REPLACEMENT OF THE DOCTOR'S OFFICE

We are entering the era of bio-observability: more readily available blood tests and real-time sensors filtered through AI analysis to give us a highly personalized understanding of our bodies and a personalized plan to meet each body's needs with daily choices. This can't be crystallized in a fifteen-minute doctor's visit. We should all welcome more technology in the interpretation of our biomarkers.

Now that we know how to measure Good Energy, let's jump into the specific mindset shifts and steps we can take to optimize it.

Recap: Recommended Ranges

Below are recommended optimal ranges for key metabolic blood tests. Falling outside of these ranges is an indicator that you could have brewing dysfunction. The remainder of Part 2 and the plan in Part 3 will give specific steps to increase Good Energy and improve these biomarkers:

- Triglycerides:
  - Less than 80 mg/dL

- HDL:
  - 50 to 90 mg/dL
- Fasting Glucose:
  - 70 to 85 mg/dL
- Blood Pressure:
  - Less than 120 systolic and less than 80 diastolic mmHg
- Waist Circumference:
  - <80 cm (31.5 inches) for women and <90 cm (35 inches) for men (South Asian, Chinese, Japanese, and South and Central Americans)
  - <80 cm (31.5 inches) for women and <94 cm (37 inches) for men (European, Sub-Saharan African, Middle Eastern, and Eastern Mediterranean)
- Triglyceride-to-HDL Ratio:
  - Below 1.5. Above 3 is a clear sign of metabolic dysfunction.
- Fasting Insulin:
  - From 2 to 5 mIU/L. Above 10 mIU/L is concerning and above 15 mIU/L is significantly elevated.
- HOMA-IR:
  - Less than 2.0
- High-Sensitivity CRP (hsCRP):
  - Less than 0.3 mg/dL
- Hemoglobin A1c:
  - From 5.0 to 5.4 percent
- Uric Acid:
  - Less than 5 mg/dL for men, and from 2 to 4 mg/dL for women
- Liver Enzymes: aspartate transaminase (AST), alanine transaminase (ALT), and gamma-glutamyl transferase (GGT)
  - AST and ALT levels of 17 U/L or less. For GGT, lowest risk for men is less than 25 U/L and women from 14 to 20 U/L. Sources vary slightly, but these are good targets to aim for.
- Vitamin D
  - 40 to 60 ng/mL
- Recommended real-time metrics to track:
  - Glucose (continuous glucose monitor)

- Food (food journal or app)
- Sleep (quantity, quality, consistency)
- Activity (steps, number of active minutes per day and week with elevated heart rate)
- Resting heart rate and heart rate variability

To view the scientific references cited in this chapter, please visit us online at caseymeans.com/goodenergy.

CHAPTER 5

The Six Principles of Good Energy Eating

"Let me talk to your fucking manager," one patient screamed at me during my fourth year of residency. He was irate that I wouldn't prescribe him a refill of opioid pain medication, despite the fact that several weeks had passed since his surgery. He was well-versed that patient satisfaction surveys dictated physician performance ratings. These tools also determined physician compensation—even though patient satisfaction is often at odds with patient well-being. On several occasions, patients called the clinic repeatedly and threatened to leave bad reviews if I did not write an opioid prescription.

How weak that someone can be so blinded by their addiction to make them act like this, I used to think. But then I learned that most opioid addictions result from a legal prescription and often overdose deaths occur when addicts are forced to buy drugs off the street loaded with unknown poison. About eighty thousand people died of opioid overdoses in the United States in 2022, many of whom started taking opioids by getting their prescription from a doctor.

We have another, more hidden addiction crisis, in which highly addictive substances are being pushed on every person in the United States from birth, and these substances are causing well over one million deaths per year. These substances are ultra-processed foods.

The NIH defines addiction as "a chronic, relapsing disorder characterized by compulsive drug seeking and use despite adverse consequences," which is obviously what is happening when it comes to modern industrial food. We have no other way to explain how people in the nation are going against their evolutionary impulses to such a systematic degree—which is exactly what's happening when 30 percent of teenagers have prediabetes and nearly 80 percent of adults are overweight or obese. We have a compulsive collective food addiction. We are eating ourselves to death.

The solution to this crisis is very simple—promote unprocessed whole foods and discourage ultra-processed industrial foods. Yet we are in a state of confusion about what the right diet is—about 59 percent of people report that conflicting information about nutrition makes them doubt their choices.

Organic, plant-based, natural, non-GMO, fair trade, sustainable, cruelty-free, hormone-free, regenerative, gluten-free, free-range, pasture-raised, conventional—we have innumerable terms we need to sort through when selecting food.

We need to stop falling into traps of dietary philosophies and start breaking food into its individual parts and analyzing whether those parts are good or bad for our cells. Food is nothing more than a set of molecular components, and whether those components meet our cells' needs largely determines health. When we see someone who is addicted to opioids or alcohol, it is easy to identify the cause of the problem. But when it comes to food, we have trouble analyzing individual components that are helping our cells or harming them, because we don't think of food in this framework of molecular components.

Let's take an extreme, simple example:

- A glass of water is good and will help hydrate you.
- A glass of water mixed with arsenic is bad and will kill you.

In the example above, we can easily see the water with arsenic as two separate parts, one that can help (water) and one that will kill you (arsenic). But we don't think about this when it comes to most food. Let's take a less obvious case of a "burger," which could be made from several different things despite looking the same:

- Beef from a cow raised on an industrial farm in a concentrated animal feeding operation (CAFO), eating an all-grain diet
- Beef from a cow raised outside, free to roam in a pasture, eating exclusively pesticide-free grass
- Beef alternatives, like Beyond Burger or Impossible Burger

The molecular makeups of these three versions of burgers are *highly* different. A cow has evolved over millennia eating grass, which delivers anti-inflammatory omega-3 fatty acids to its body. Grain-fed beef contains five times fewer omega-3 fats and significantly more inflammatory omega-6 fats than grass-fed beef. In terms of micronutrient content, grass-fed beef is generally higher in vitamin A, vitamin E, and beta-carotene, which are all critical for maintaining metabolic and immune function.

The two main ingredients of Beyond Burger are pea protein and canola oil. Canola oil is high in omega-6 fats, making Beyond Burger more inflammatory than grass-fed beef. Additional ingredients include natural flavors (a misnomer, as natural flavors can be highly processed and contain chemical additives) and methylcellulose, a main ingredient in laxatives manufactured by heating wood in acidic solutions to extract and purify cellulose. Clearly, these three different versions of burger deliver vastly different molecular information to the cells.

Food empowerment involves seeing beyond the labels of food and into how the parts build functional cellular health. For instance, you could see broccoli as simply a green veggie. Or you could see it more accurately as an ecosystem of molecular components that can support many of the hallmarks of Good Energy by quelling oxidative stress, chronic inflammation, and mitochondrial dysfunction. The high fiber content of broccoli feeds your gut bacteria and lining, minimizing leaky gut and chronic inflammation and helping to produce mitochondria-optimizing chemicals like short-chain fatty acids (SCFAs). Its vitamin C protects your mitochondria from oxidative stress. Vitamin K decreases mitochondrial dysfunction by serving as a mitochondrial electron carrier. And folate serves as a lock-and-key cofactor in the mitochondrial proteins that generate ATP. Broccoli also contains numerous antioxidants that protect your cells from oxidative damage. All these substances turn the knobs on the key processes of Good Energy. You don't need to know all these scientific terms, but it is *vital* to start thinking of food as molecular information that dictates our day-to-day and long-term function, and Chapter 6 will get into the details.

Here is a hopeful message: daily, we make hundreds of micro-decisions about food that can change our genetic and physiologic "fate."

Like any doctor, I would end appointments by giving patients vague dietary advice such as "eat more fruits and veggies" and then writing a pharmaceutical prescription. But in training, doctors are told that nutrition is a soft topic that "isn't evidence based." You will rarely find specific nutrition recommendations in the *official* treatment guidelines for any given condition; for example, within the hundreds of cumulative pages of guidelines for migraine, sinusitis, COVID-19, and prostate cancer treatment, you won't find a *single* mention of specific dietary patterns to adopt, despite hundreds of scientific papers showing benefits of dietary interventions for these conditions. Interventions like prescribing a pill or performing surgery are seen as "heroic," while nutritional interventions are seen as fuzzy and wimpy. We ignore that natural foods have over five thousand known phytochemicals alone—each of which is a small molecule that impacts health: the definition of medicine.

The pounds of molecular information we put into our bodies daily impact our health. Every thought you have and feeling you feel comes from food. Inside your mother's body, you were 3D printed out of food, and every item you ingest continues to print the next iteration of yourself. Bodies, neurotransmitters, hormones, nerves, and mitochondria are all made, exclusively and necessarily, from what you (or your mom) put in your (or their) mouth; we don't arise from thin air, we arise from food.

So often, doctors and patients are taught that genes are our destiny—but that's not true. Our genes don't determine most health outcomes. What we eat and how we live impact our gene expression and cellular biology, determining our outcomes. Food chemicals go into your body and act as signaling molecules. They can directly increase or decrease gene expression, change DNA folding, and activate key cell-signaling pathways, like those controlling whether your cells produce Good Energy.

What we put into our bodies is the most critical decision for our health and happiness. To learn why food is our most potent weapon against chronic disease, I had to learn the principles for myself long after becoming a doctor.

PRINCIPLE I: FOOD DETERMINES THE STRUCTURE AND FUNCTION OF OUR CELLS AND MICROBIOME

Our bodies are built entirely of food. Eating is the process of transforming and assimilating matter from the external world into our own form. Every day, food breaks down into different types of "bricks" in our gut, and then those bricks get absorbed into our bloodstream to be used to continually rebuild the next iteration of our body. When we provide the body with the right "bricks," we build the right structures, and we get health. Below are five examples of how food acts as a structural element in cells, as a functional messenger, and as a shaper of the microbiome and what it produces.

Food as Structure: Dietary Fats in Our Cell Membranes

Cell membranes are the structural layer around cells. They are made of a fatty layer studded with cholesterol molecules (which make the membrane malleable) and proteins (which serve as receptors, anchors, and channels). Our modern industrial diets have fundamentally changed the structure of our cell membranes, which are a key functional unit of our cells, housing the cell receptors, channels, enzymes, and anchors that kick off innumerable cell-signaling activities. Healthy membranes are critical for all aspects of health because they are the gatekeepers of every material and signal that goes into the cell. Both omega-3 and omega-6 fats are necessary for optimal biological function, but we want them to be balanced, because omega-3 fats are anti-inflammatory and promote membrane elasticity, and omega-6 fats promote inflammation. With the advent of ultra-processed, industrialized foods—loaded with high concentrations of omega-6 fats from processed vegetable and seed oils—our dietary intake of omega-6 fats relative to omega-3 fats skyrocketed, radically changing our cell membrane structure and function. Adjusting dietary intake of omega-3s and omega-6s can change the membrane ratio in as little as three days, as cell membranes turn over rapidly.

Food is a message from the external world that can directly activate and inhibit genetic pathways deep inside your body. More than just being the *structural* bricks, food also is a *signaling* molecule that directs key functions in cells and the overall body, including how our genes are expressed. It can act like a hormone at hormone receptors and can directly create or alleviate oxidative stress. It can change the function of protein enzymes by serving as cofactors for chemical reactions, like a key in a lock that turns on machines in the cell that make ATP or do other jobs.

Eating spices like turmeric (which directly minimize chronic inflammation) or cruciferous vegetables (which directly minimize oxidative stress) are two examples of ways that food can functionally signal for Good Energy.

Food as a Functional Message: Minimizing Oxidative Stress

Isothiocyanates are molecules from cruciferous vegetables, such as broccoli or brussels sprouts, which help combat oxidative stress, one of the key Bad Energy processes. Normally, if excess oxidative stress is present, the cell increases gene expression of antioxidant molecules by sending a protein called Nrf2 into the nucleus to bind to the genome and increase the expression of antioxidant genes. When it's not doing this function, Nrf2 is inactivated by staying bound to a protein called Keap-1. Isothiocyanates from cruciferous vegetables act by binding to Keap-1, causing it to release Nrf2 to go to the nucleus and promote antioxidant gene expression—which supports Good Energy by minimizing damaging oxidative stress. Isothiocyanate from food acts to functionally activate key genes involved in Good Energy.

Food as a Functional Message: Inhibiting Inflammation

Curcumin, which gives turmeric its yellow color, acts similarly to isothiocyanates, but instead of increasing antioxidant genes, it *blocks* pro-inflammatory genes. Normally, a protein lives in the cell called NF-$\varkappa$B, which, upon interacting with the DNA, leads to the expression of an array of genes involved in inflammatory signaling. Overactivation of NF-$\varkappa$B—occurring from excess oxidative stress, processed foods, sleep deprivation, and psychological stress—leads to chronic inflammation, which can damage the body and directly promote insulin resistance. When unstimulated, NF-$\varkappa$B is bound to IkB proteins and inactivated (like how Keap-1 inactivates Nrf2). IkB proteins are themselves inactivated when another set of proteins, called IkB kinases, tags IkB with a molecule called phosphate. So when IkB kinases are activated, they inactivate IkB, and NF-$\varkappa$B is free to go to the nucleus and exert its pro-inflammatory effects. In the cell, curcumin suppresses IkB kinase, thereby keeping IkB bound to NF-$\varkappa$B, deactivating it. Curcumin therefore functionally inactivates pro-inflammatory genetic activity in the cell, supporting Good Energy.

Food Also Defines the Composition of Our Microbiome

Our microbiome is the trillions of bacteria cells that make up the second body living inside our body. It determines our metabolic health, mood, and longevity. In a sense, the microbiome is like our soul: it's invisible, lives inside of us, and determines the quality and quantity of our life and what we think and do. And it's immortal, because after we die, it breaks down our body and persists. A big part of the purpose of eating is to feed this well-intentioned beast so that it serves us by converting the food we eat into various chemicals that control our thoughts and bodies. Mistreat or misfeed the microbiome, and our life will suffer in unbelievable ways: depression, obesity, autoimmune disease, cancer, sleep disturbances, and more. Care for the microbiome, and *poof*: our life magically becomes easier.

Fiber, probiotic-rich foods, and polyphenol-rich plant foods all feed and support microbiome health, allowing for a robust gut lining (which minimizes chronic inflammation) and for the microbiome to generate metabolism-supporting chemicals like SCFA. You can think of your microbiome as a magical transformer of food to medicine.

Food Determines Whether the Microbiome Generates Mitochondria-Boosting Urolithin A

When certain gut bacteria in our microbiome encounter plant compounds called ellagic acid and ellagitannin—which are found in pomegranates, some berries, and certain nuts—they convert it into a class of compounds called urolithins, of which urolithin A is a common one. These are absorbed and then travel throughout the bloodstream. When urolithin A enters cells throughout the body, it acts to improve Good Energy through several mechanisms. The first is by acting as an antioxidant, and the second is by stimulating the critical process of *mitophagy*, a mitochondrial quality-control mechanism that allows for degradation of damaged and superfluous mitochondria.

In serving structural, functional, and microbiome-supporting roles in the body, foods need to be chosen wisely to yield health and Good Energy. This brings us to principle 2.

PRINCIPLE 2: EATING IS THE PROCESS OF MATCHING CELLULAR NEEDS WITH ORAL INPUTS

Any diet that sufficiently generates optimal cellular function, eliminates chronic symptoms, and leads to optimal biomarkers is the right diet for you.

Let's think about what food is from your cells' perspective: the inside of your body is warm, wet, and dark. Most of your thirty-seven trillion cells live in moist darkness within you, just waiting for the signals and information on what to do and when in order to give you a good life. Cells obviously can't see, hear, or smell. They only have receptors and channels on their membranes that allow them to receive inputs by patiently waiting for nutrients to float by that they can take up and use to do their work.

If what floats by is the needed structural and functional information to do their work, your cells (and therefore you) will be healthy.

If the right information isn't floating by, they'll get confused. If dangerous signals float by, they'll get damaged. In desperation, they will try to build the structures they need to build or do the work they need with this shoddy material—but it will go poorly, like a builder constructing a house out of low-quality or insufficient bricks. Everything you eat determines what your cells will blindly interact with and what will determine their fate.

Eating is a matching problem: Matching the food inputs with the cells' needs produces health. If we don't properly match inputs with needs or if we put in damaging substances that the body shouldn't be exposed to, we get symptoms and disease.

We eat an astonishing seventy metric tons of food in our lifetimes. Food constantly rebuilds our rapidly dying and regenerating bodies. We turn over our skin cells entirely every six weeks or so, and our gut lining turns over almost every week. Everything is rebuilt from food. Unfortunately, several factors have led to the majority of that seventy metric tons being either useless or harmful to our body's constant turnover process and baseline functioning. No wonder so many of us are sick or don't feel good.

The first is that industrial agriculture practices—like monocropping, tilling, pesticides, and factory farming of animals—lead to vastly fewer nutrients in our food. A fruit or vegetable you eat today has up to 40 percent fewer minerals, vitamins, and less protein than the same food would have had seventy years ago.

The second is that our food is being transported over large distances, causing degradation and damage to nutrients. The average distance that produce travels from farm to plate in the United States is approximately fifteen hundred miles. During this journey, some fruits and vegetables can lose up to 77 percent of their vitamin C content, a critical micronutrient for ATP production in the mitochondria and antioxidant activity in the cell. You may have thought that "eating local" or shopping from farmers' markets is frivolous, but it is actually a critical step to ensure you are getting maximal helpful molecular information in the bites you take to build and instruct your body.

The third is that most of our U.S. calorie consumption is ultra-processed foods, stripped of their nutrition. About 60 percent or more of the calories adults in the nation consume is ultra-processed garbage. You're looking at just a fraction of that seventy tons meeting the cells' functional needs.

No wonder we are insatiable as a culture and eating ourselves into early graves. We are not getting what we need from the nutrient-depleted industrial material we eat, so the deep wisdom of our bodies and microbiomes pushes us to consume more.

Eating most of your food from high-quality, unprocessed sources is crucial. When you eat ultra-processed foods, where key nutrients have been stripped from the whole-food form, you immediately slash the possibility of your cells getting what they need. When you eat whole, unprocessed foods, you have a much better chance of giving your cells the good stuff. And if you eat food grown in healthy, thriving soil that hasn't been tarnished by pesticides, your food will have the highest likelihood of being filled with the necessary molecules to get your cells what they need to thrive and the least amount of damaging stuff that hurts them. Hunger will effortlessly subside because your cells' needs are met.

Interestingly, the "matching problem" of eating for the cells' needs is dynamic and can change day to day and in different phases of life. For instance, during the second half of the menstrual cycle (the post-ovulation luteal phase), women tend to be more insulin resistant due to relatively high progesterone levels, which can induce oxidative stress in the mitochondria by promoting the generation of hydrogen peroxide (a free radical). Ramping up antioxidant food support during the second half of the menstrual cycle, as well as minimizing high-glycemic foods that could exacerbate insulin resistance–induced glycemic fluctuations, is a dynamic food intervention. During the luteal phase, I tend to focus on antioxidant-rich berries, cruciferous vegetables, and spices like cardamom and turmeric, and I emphasize low-glycemic foods, like leafy greens, nuts, seeds, fish, eggs, and pasture-raised meats.

A second example of the shifting needs of the cells is how several micronutrients, including zinc and magnesium (both of which are necessary for over three hundred chemical reactions in the body), can become depleted during times of psychological stress. Researchers theorize several possible reasons as to why this occurs, including increased metabolic demands, higher excretion of micronutrients, or greater utilization of antioxidant micronutrients when stress increases. Given this, supporting the body with additional micronutrients during periods of increased psychological stress could emerge as an intervention to minimize the cellular dysfunction and increased illness that is known to accompany chronic stress.

Bites are opportunities, and you don't want to waste any. You want every bite you take to communicate with your cells about what you expect them to do, which brings us to the next principle.

PRINCIPLE 3: FOOD IS HOW YOU COMMUNICATE WITH YOUR CELLS

Think of your consciousness and free will as a military general. Your cells are the troops defending the integrity and safety of your life. Foods are the messages the general chooses to send to motivate and tell the troops what to do. The general's ability to survive—as well as the troops' survival—depends on the quality and clarity of the messages. We must speak clearly and correctly if we want to survive.

In an optimal state, food sends our cells clear messages about what our body needs to do to thrive. Specific food choices and food behaviors can tell your body different things, such as the following:

- Omega-3 fatty acids (in, e.g., salmon, sardines, chia seeds, walnuts) to immune cells: *Put down your defenses. Things are safe now.*
- Cruciferous vegetables (in, e.g., cauliflower, cabbage, brussels sprouts, and kale) to the DNA: *It's a tough time and we must produce more defenses.*
- Leucine (an essential amino acid found in, e.g., beef, pork, yogurt, lentils, and almonds) to the muscles: *It's time to build. Let's go.*
- Magnesium (found in, e.g., pumpkin seeds, chia seeds, beans, leafy greens, and avocados) to neurons: *Relax!*
- Fiber to the microbiome: *I love you.*
- Intermittent fasting: *We need to clean things up.*

- Synthetic herbicides and pesticides to healthy bacteria in the gut: *It's time to die.*

Example of Clear Communication with the Body: Thylakoids Regulating Hunger

You may recall from high school biology that chloroplasts are the parts of plants that generate energy from the sun. Inside chloroplasts, green discs called thylakoids are the workhorses of this process, and you'll consume them if you eat any unprocessed green vegetables. When thylakoids enter the gut, they block the activity of the hormone lipase, which is released from the pancreas to digest fat. Inhibiting lipase slows fat breakdown and increases a sense of fullness. Thylakoids also suppress hunger by stimulating two hormones that promote satiety: cholecystokinin (CCK) and glucagon-like peptide 1 (GLP-1). These are both significantly increased when high thylakoid levels are present in meals. People eating thylakoids have a profoundly decreased urge for sweets. Thylakoids represent a way of sending your body the communication that you have eaten enough. They are found in high levels in raw spinach, kale, parsley, arugula, broccoli, and spirulina.

When I make a smoothie in the morning, loaded with a dozen organic ingredients, I'm thinking through exactly what conversation I want to have with my body that day: safety, strength, satiety, and resilience.

Like any relationship, communicating poorly can lead to confusion and problems.

PRINCIPLE 4: EXTREME FOOD CRAVINGS ARE FEEDBACK FROM YOUR CELLS THAT YOU'RE GIVING MIXED MESSAGES

The genesis of cravings is complex, involving over a dozen hormones, several brain regions, and the microbiome. But a fundamental way to think about it is that cravings—meaning a hedonistic desire for a specific food—are a sign that you have confused your cells through your diet. You can overcome cravings by communicating clearly to your body through food choices.

Many patients and people I talk with about changing their diet understandably feel like they just can't give up what they crave.

"It's just too hard."

"I just can't stop eating this stuff!"

"I'd rather cut five years off my life than give up X [insert highly addictive food]!" Sadly, I've heard this last one dozens of times.

A key point in understanding how to overcome cravings and create a sense of total freedom with food is this: if your body is pushing you to acquire specific foods (cravings), that is a signal that your human cells' or your microbiome cells' biological needs are not being met, and they are employing their tools—like hunger hormone secretion—to get you to aggressively seek food with the chance that you'll eat something that scratches their fundamental itch. You can think of yourself and your behavior as a robot acting at the will of your cells and microbiome.

We are eating ourselves into a state of Bad Energy because the food we eat is tapping into addictive pathways rather than meeting our needs or checking our bodies' boxes. We learned in Chapter 1 that "chronic overnutrition"—a.k.a. overeating—is a key root of why we're straining our mitochondria and generating intracellular fat buildup and insulin resistance. We can't *will* ourselves to avoid chronically overeating. Our drives are too strong, and our microbiome's signals are too powerful. The best chance against chronic overnutrition is eating real, unprocessed food. When you do this, you tap into the body's exquisitely sensitive regulatory mechanisms, which will stop you from eating more than you need. When eating real, unprocessed foods, you also experience more pleasure and stop wanting the other stuff—effortlessly. I spent much of my childhood and surgical training controlled by cravings to the point where I would not leave the house without a stash of sweet treats in my bag, especially Hershey's Kisses or Reese's Peanut Butter Cups. Learning to simply load my body with more unprocessed foods wiped away these cravings, which once felt part of my identity.

When I think about the worst examples of food that confuse our cells,

I think about fructose. Liquid fructose came onto the scene in the 1970s and completely changed the relationship between humans and sugar, increasing our consumption of added fructose intake from 6 grams a day (from fruits) to 33 grams per day—a fivefold increase in this substance. When fructose enters the body in high quantities, it depletes ATP levels in the cell, leading to less available cellular energy. It also generates uric acid as a by-product in its metabolism, which causes mitochondrial oxidative stress and mitochondrial dysfunction. To the cell, this rapid depletion in ATP and lower cellular energy signals starvation and induces intense appetite and food-seeking behaviors for more sugar in hopes of raising ATP levels in the cell. Simultaneously, to counteract the perceived starvation, uric acid–induced mitochondrial dysfunction leads to the sugar being stored as fat. Fructose says to the cells (and therefore the body): *You are starving and preparing for winter. Eat as much as you possibly can and store it!*

Many animals aim to store as much fat as possible before winter's low food supply. They gorge themselves with ripe, fructose-rich fruit. The short-lived spike in fructose consumption during autumn drives foraging (food-seeking) behaviors and even increases violence and aggression. For the animal, this time of gorging on fruit is a life-or-death situation, and an influx of fructose turns on this survival switch that changes metabolism and behavior. The survival switch concept is from Dr. Rick Johnson, author of *Nature Wants Us to Be Fat*. But now that ultra-concentrated high-fructose corn syrup is available 24-7, our survival switch has been used against us to turn us into aggressive food-seeking addicts, preparing for a hibernation that never comes.

Food companies have also mastered the science of glucose spikes to make food more addictive. Research has shown that intense cravings often happen after a blood sugar spike followed by a crash (reactive hypoglycemia), which we learned about in Chapter 4. When you load your body with sugar, like after eating refined carbohydrate foods or foods with added sugar, the body releases a surge of insulin to help take all this glucose out of the bloodstream. What can result from the surge is a stark crash in blood sugar, with levels often dipping below the premeal baseline. This time of post-spike low blood sugar—or hypoglycemia—has been shown to be the time when people often crave a high-carbohydrate snack, and the average post-meal glucose dip relative to baseline can even predict an increase in hunger at two to three hours post-meal and a greater caloric intake at the next meal and in the twenty-four-hour period following. The choice of blood sugar–spiking (and crashing) foods puts the body into a confused panic, seeking food to stabilize itself. We can prevent this cycle by avoiding skyrocketing glucose via simple blood sugar–stabilizing strategies (explained in the next chapter). Interestingly, when wearing a CGM, many people who believe they or their kids suffer from "hypoglycemia" actually find that the real problem is that they are *spiking* their blood sugar too high, which is then followed by a reactive hypoglycemic crash. The solution, therefore, is to stabilize the blood sugar, learn how to eat to avoid big spikes, and become more metabolically flexible.

In a fascinating study on hunger led by Dr. Kevin Hall, published in *Cell* in 2021, researchers put twenty participants with stable weight in an inpatient facility at the NIH for an entire month. There, they ate only food delivered to them by the research team. They could not leave. For the first two weeks, participants were able to eat unlimited quantities of ultra-processed, industrially manufactured foods. This diet consisted of common American staples, including Cheerios, croissants, Yoplait yogurt, blueberry muffins, margarine, packaged beef ravioli, diet lemonade, oatmeal raisin cookies, white bread, store-bought gravy, canned corn, low-fat chocolate milk, deli turkey, tortillas, Heinz pickle relish, Hellmann's mayonnaise, shortbread cookies, Fig Newtons, orange juice, Tater Tots, french fries, cheeseburgers with American cheese, Heinz ketchup, turkey bacon, English muffins, chicken nuggets, hoagie rolls, crackers, hot dogs, burritos, tortilla chips, and so on.

In the second two weeks, participants were able to eat unlimited quantities of unprocessed foods, like fresh egg scrambles and omelets, steamed and roasted vegetables, rice, nuts, fruits, oatmeal with berries and raw almonds, salads with chicken, apples, homemade dressing, sweet potato hash, unsweetened Greek yogurt with fruit, shrimp, salmon, chicken breast, beef roast, and baked sweet potatoes.

The researchers weighed every morsel of food left behind on the plates, so they knew the precise amount each participant had eaten. Amazingly, the participants ate over 500 *fewer* calories per day in the two weeks of consuming unlimited unprocessed foods, adding up to around 7,000 fewer calories in just two weeks. The participants lost two pounds on average during the unprocessed food period and gained two pounds during the ultra-processed food period. And, unsurprisingly, satiety hormones were significantly different between the two periods, with the unprocessed foods yielding higher satiety hormone levels and lower hunger hormones. So in the same bodies, two different food signals (unprocessed versus ultra-processed) gave very different messages: one that confused the body into thinking it needed more food than it did and one that satisfied it completely. Clearly, ultra-processed food intake drives weight gain and overeating, but it took locking up individuals in a prisonlike setting at the NIH to prove that ultra-processed foods make you hungrier, make you eat more, and make you gain weight.

In *The End of Craving*, Mark Schatzker makes the case that our insatiable desire for food stems from a unique feature of processed food called "variable reward." The body—which prepares itself for digestion from the time of looking at and tasting a food by predicting what nutrition will hit the GI tract—can never be sure what nutrition is coming in with unnatural ultra-processed foods. To the body, ultra-processed food is a nutrition gamble. One day it's Coke Zero, the next it's the full-sugar Coke, but they taste the same, and as with gambling, variable reward drives us to keep seeking by triggering our key motivation pathway: dopamine. Ultra-processed foods confuse our body's ability to accurately predict nutritional inputs and therefore drive us to keep seeking. In contrast, eating unprocessed foods at fairly stable times lets the system run smoothly.

The food industry uses the science of cravings to make food more addictive, rigorously studying how specific combinations of ultra-processed foods get consumers to their "bliss point" of pleasure, driving them to want more. We are being naive if we don't plainly realize that our food is weaponized to confuse our bodies at a sophisticated level. Over twenty-one million people in the United States depend on the food industry for employment, and that industry is built to grow, and growth means more cravings and addiction to processed foods.

The beauty of eating unprocessed, whole foods is that you have the best chance of getting a diverse array of nutrients that check the human cells' and microbiome cells' boxes and therefore diminish cravings. If you do this, the cravings will stop, the hedonistic desire for food will stop, and it will feel effortless to enjoy and love food that helps you.

The best advice I can give anyone in transforming their health is to find a way—*any* way—to stick with totally unprocessed, organic food for just a month or two. By the end of this time, I can guarantee that your preferences and cravings will have changed.

PRINCIPLE 5: IGNORE DIET PHILOSOPHIES AND FOCUS ON UNPROCESSED FOOD

Diet controversy is a charade.

I personally know brilliant, hardworking, highly educated people who believe polar opposite ideologies about nutrition. One group feels that a low-fat, high-carb diet is the only diet that yields Good Energy, and another feels that a high-fat, low-carb diet is the best way. Both have data that show that these diets reduce liver fat (a key marker of insulin sensitivity), lower weight, lower triglycerides, improve insulin sensitivity, and lower inflammation. And both are right. And in between is the Mediterranean diet, which also has masses of literature to support a more omnivorous approach. All these diets can "work" for good health because *all* emphasize primarily unprocessed, whole foods to give the cells what they need to function and cue satiety mechanisms so that we don't overeat.

Countless Instagram and blog posts from vegan health professionals blast the carnivores for ruining the planet. And the vitriol from the ketogenic and animal-based crowd toward the vegans is some of the cruelest stuff I've seen on the internet. Both are wrong in their attacks and right in their dietary choices. I know vegan and carnivore elite athletes, both of whom are absolutely thriving with low insulin levels, low glucose, low triglycerides, and low visceral fat.

I am so grateful that I have had a foot in both worlds. I know that both movements have merit and are championed by science-focused, mission-driven people. And I'm not being wishy-washy. The reality is that eating unprocessed, clean, natural foods—in a pattern that keeps you energized, symptom-free, and with optimal biomarkers—is the right diet for you.

How can different whole-food dietary patterns "work" for Good Energy? Chronic overnutrition and mitochondrial dysfunction are what clog up the cell with fat and lead to Bad Energy. In the absence of chronic overnutrition, the cell will work through the substrates it has available to it, whether it be glucose or fat, or a mix of both. If you're eating unprocessed, nutrient-dense food from healthy soil, your satiety mechanisms work exquisitely (like every other animal species that *doesn't* get metabolic disease because they *don't* eat ultra-processed foods) and you likely won't overconsume. Therefore, your body processes the energy it needs and the cell doesn't fill itself with fat and doesn't become insulin resistant.

We need to get over dietary labels and just start thinking of food as molecular information. The key is understanding what molecular information is in the food, how much is getting absorbed, and whether the cells are "happy" as a result.

It's important to realize that the body is remarkably capable of getting to similar outcomes with different inputs through redundant mechanisms— that is, you could be eating a sustainably sourced, unprocessed plant-based diet *or* an animal-based diet and still get the same molecular information for your cell. Here's how you can get several key nutrients to your cells from very different dietary sources.

Multiple Ways for Cells to Get What They Need from Food: Butyrate, EPA/DHA, and Vitamin C

Butyrate

Butyrate is a key signaling molecule in the body that serves as a positive regulator of mitochondrial function. Higher levels of butyrate are correlated with reducing depression and obesity risk, two states that are tied to mitochondrial dysfunction. Butyrate is an SCFA produced when bacteria ferment fiber in the gut, which is then absorbed by the gut lining cells and enters circulation. Butyrate production is a key reason why high-fiber diets are touted to be so beneficial. Often, ketogenic diets are theorized to be problematic partly because they lack fiber. However, people on a low-fiber ketogenic diet still can reap the benefits of butyrate by making it *themselves* in their own cells, bypassing the microbiome. When the body is starved of carbohydrates, the liver will make a chemical called beta-hydroxybutyrate, a chemical almost identical to the butyrate formed by gut bacteria with the addition of one oxygen atom, yielding a different pathway to give your cells the same Good Energy benefit. On a diet high in fiber, you may make about 50 grams of butyrate per day from the bacteria in the gut. On a ketogenic diet, you make a similar amount or more. Throughout human evolution, cultures have thrived on over 100 grams of fiber a day from foraging (like the modern hunter-gatherer Hadza tribe in Tanzania) while others ate a mostly animal-based diet of milk and meat and consumed little fiber (like the Maasai tribe in Kenya). I predict that the people in both cultures had sufficient butyrate in their cells, albeit through two different physiologic pathways.

EPA/DHA

One of the reasons people eschew a vegan diet is because it can lack the key omega-3s eicosapentaenoic acid (EPA) and docosahexaenoic acid (DHA), which are largely found in animal foods (although they are also found in algae). Omega-3s serve profound metabolic roles in both signaling in the mitochondria and minimizing chronic inflammation. The predominant omega-3 found in plants is alpha-linolenic acid (ALA), which must go through a several-step conversion process to become the biologically critical EPA and DHA. Many people, as a key criticism of plant-based diets, cite this conversion pathway as "inefficient." But we must dig deeper and look at biology before making these judgments. Three cellular protein machines (enzymes)—delta-6-desaturase, elongase, and delta-5-desaturase—process ALA to make EPA and DHA. And these enzymes require several micronutrients to function properly, including B_2, B_3, B_5, B_6, B_7, vitamin C, zinc, and magnesium. In the United States, 92 percent of people are deficient in at least one critical micronutrient, likely because of our ultra-processed diet, poor soil, and poor gut health. So if you're deficient in these micronutrients, you will likely not convert ALA to EPA/DHA efficiently, and if you are replete with these micronutrients, you will. What's more, omega-6 fats also use these *same* enzymes to convert to their downstream versions. The conversion occurs in several steps, going from linolenic acid to arachidonic acid (a downstream omega-3 that generates pro-inflammatory chemicals). So if you are like a typical American who is eating twenty times more omega-6 fats than we have historically—because you're consuming processed vegetable oils and processed foods—you are also going to stunt your ability to convert ALA to EPA and DHA by blocking access to these enzymes.

A thoughtful approach to vastly different diets can yield the positive outcomes you want, illustrating why we have healthy, uninflamed people who fall into different diet camps: one that's whole foods plant-based (WFPB) and one that's more animal-based.

Vitamin C

Vitamin C is a critical micronutrient that serves the purpose, among many other functions, of reducing oxidative stress in the cell. Vegans get vitamin C from numerous colorful plants, including bell peppers, tomatoes, and citrus fruits. More carnivorous people get it from eating organ meats, specifically liver, one of the only animal sources of vitamin C. Both do just fine.

Focus on cell biology over diet dogma. Put all your energy into finding and eating unprocessed foods grown in healthy soil. Your health will vastly improve. It actually *is* that simple.

With that said, *knowing* the principles of healthy eating and actually *living* them out day to day are two different things, which brings us to Principle 6.

PRINCIPLE 6: MINDFUL EATING—FINDING AWE IN FOOD

If adhering to an organic, unprocessed diet as a human in the twenty-first century were easy, we'd all be eating clean healthy food all the time.

Instead, it takes conscious daily work to go against the tide of normal culture to make consistently healthy food decisions. I tap into a sense of awe and wonder about food that lets me appreciate its impact on my life and inspires me to make the healthiest choices possible. The following are some of the things I reflect on as I tap into my appreciation for the miraculous interaction between food and my body:

I reflect that all the energy stored in the cellular bonds of the plants I'm eating was originally a packet of photon energy that started in the sun, traveled through space, and then was absorbed by a plant's chloroplast, transformed into glucose, and taken up by an animal that I might eat. Chloroplasts in plants are remarkably like the mitochondria in humans, which ultimately convert that glucose formed in plants from the sun into ATP that I can use to power my life and my ability to think and love. And when I eventually die and go back to the earth—hopefully in a natural burial like my mother's, where my body is put directly in the soil to be decomposed by worms, fungi, and bacteria and reenter the greater ecosystem— my body's material building blocks will help grow new plants that will convert more of the sun's energy into glucose in an infinite loop of mystical transformation.

I reflect that the mitochondria that process energy from food to animate our tissues are inherited entirely from our mothers, passed down through millennia in an endless progression of nesting dolls along a matrilineal line. The mitochondria from the sperm essentially melt upon fertilization with an egg, while our mother's mitochondria persist and create all the energy we need to do *everything*.

I reflect on how mitochondria historically started out as bacteria that were engulfed by more complex cells and worked together to create a more powerful entity. When I think about my mother in quiet moments, I visualize that unbroken lineage over millions of years and of my mother's cellular engines living through me in this spectacular way. She—and every woman before her in our lineage—are living through me as I type these words. I do not want to hurt that gift through my food choices. Modern life is an assault on our mitochondria, which means it's an assault on our ancestors and our mothers, an assault on the creative, generative force of the feminine in all of us, and an assault on our animating life force. It's an assault on the miraculous flow of cosmic energy from the sun, through the soil and plants, through bacteria in my gut, through my cells' mitochondria to create the energy that sparks my consciousness and the statistical near impossibility of *me*. Out of respect for all of this, I must push back. And I do that through what food I choose to buy, cook, and eat.

I reflect on the fact that a teaspoon of healthy soil has more living organisms in it than there are people on the planet, and all those little bacteria, nematodes, and fungi are working around the clock to alchemize air, water, sunlight, soil, and seed into everything humans need to survive and be happy. I think about how we have murdered our soil's life force with pesticides and industrial agriculture, but how there is an incredible, hopeful movement of regenerative farming advocates fighting to bring this life back because our lives—and the biodiversity that allows for our lives—depend on it.

I reflect on the nature of the gut. In one frame of reference, the gut is just a tube of tissue. In another frame of reference, it's the interface between the cosmos (i.e., everything in the universe) and "ourselves." As with all relationships, poor boundaries lead to toxic outcomes. No boundary—physical or psychological—is more important than your gut lining. I've worked on personal boundaries a lot in therapy, and I am convinced that healthy emotional boundaries—such as being clear and vocal about what you will and will not let into your life—are what make relationships functional. Your gut lining is a boundary between you and everything else in the universe that is poised to inundate and overwhelm your biology and generate unrelenting inflammation. Healing and strengthening your gut lining with food—therefore creating and strengthening this critical boundary and reducing intestinal permeability or "leaky gut"—allows you to be selective about what you want to take in from the universe on a material level. You can choose what serves you.

I reflect on the fact that many of the problems in society—including violence, mental illness, developmental issues, and pain—start in humans, and humans are made by cells that become dysfunctional largely because of oxidative stress, mitochondrial dysfunction, and chronic inflammation.

How miraculous that food can directly combat those things. We can't have a healthy society without well-functioning humans. We can't have well-functioning humans without well-functioning cells. And we can't have well-functioning cells with mitochondrial dysfunction, oxidative stress, chronic inflammation, and cellular and hormone disruption from toxic chemicals in our food. We combat those things through nutrient-dense, unprocessed foods grown in living, thriving soil. Many of us are addicted to processed food but have had trouble mustering the strength to quit because we don't really know what awaits us on the other side. What awaits us is a maximally positive experience of our one life.

Pausing before eating to think about these concepts, expressing gratitude for my food before I start, and eating slowly are ways I reinforce these concepts. From a place of awe and appreciation for the magic of food, I find it vastly easier to make healthier choices. And with that, the obvious next question is: What should we and shouldn't we eat?

Recap: The Six Principles of Good Energy Eating

Principle 1: Food Determines the Structure of Our Cells and Microbiome

Principle 2: Eating Is the Process of Matching Cellular Needs with Oral Inputs

Principle 3: Food Is How You Communicate with Your Cells

Principle 4: Extreme Food Cravings Are Feedback from Your Cells That You're Giving Mixed Messages

Principle 5: Ignore Diet Philosophies and Focus on Unprocessed Food

Principle 6: Find Awe in Food

To view the scientific references cited in this chapter, please visit us online at caseymeans.com/goodenergy.

CHAPTER **6**

Creating a Good Energy Meal

———

At Stanford Medical School, I didn't take a single dedicated nutrition course. In fact, 80 percent of medical schools to this day do not require their students to take a nutrition class, despite food-driven diseases decimating our population.

I saw occasional references to nutrition research, but the main messages were that "nutrition is complicated" and findings often contradict themselves. For example, some studies have shown that red meat causes heart disease, while other studies have shown that it prevents heart disease. Some studies have shown that sugar causes obesity, while others have shown that it doesn't. And some studies have shown that low-carb diets are best, while others have shown that low-fat diets are preferred.

Only after leaving medicine did I learn that so many of these studies were funded by food companies, which spend eleven times more on nutrition research than the NIH. Unsurprisingly, this money slants findings: 82 percent of independently funded studies show harm from sugar-sweetened beverages, but 93 percent of industry-sponsored studies reflect no harm. When food companies fund research, the studies are six times more likely to have a favorable result about the food in question.

Policymakers use this highly compromised research. It dictates food guidelines, school lunches, and food subsidy decisions. About 95 percent of the academics on the USDA panel that created the 2020 Dietary Guidelines for Americans had conflicts of interest with food companies. The food industry's influence on studies has led the current guidelines to say that 10 percent of a child's diet can come from *added refined* sugar, which should be unequivocally zero percent.

In 2022, one of the nation's preeminent nutrition studies (jointly funded by the NIH, the Gerald J. and Dorothy R. Friedman School of Nutrition Science and Policy at Tufts, and processed food companies) reported that Lucky Charms ranks as far healthier to consume than whole foods like lamb or ground beef. And seventy brand-name cereals from General Mills, Kellogg's, and Post were ranked twice as high as eggs. This would be funny if the stated goal of the study wasn't to impact "marketing to children."

No animals in the wild suffer from widespread metabolic conditions, nor did humans as little as seventy-five years ago. Somehow, animals left to their own devices—not confused by the advice of "experts"—figure it out. According to PubMed, 45,668 peer-reviewed nutrition studies were conducted between 2020 and 2022.

I believe the United States would be a healthier, happier, more prosperous place if we replaced all those studies with these simple guidelines that will transform anyone's health. Eat the following:

- Organic (ideally regenerative) unrefined or minimally refined fruits
- Organic (ideally regenerative) unrefined or minimally refined vegetables
- Organic (ideally regenerative) unrefined or minimally refined nuts and seeds
- Organic (ideally regenerative) unrefined or minimally refined legumes and beans
- Pasture-raised, organic, 100 percent grass-fed meats and organs, including elk, venison, bison, lamb, beef, pork, goat
- Pasture-raised, organic, 100 percent foraging poultry and eggs
- Pasture-raised, organic, 100 percent grass-fed, ideally A2-strain dairy products like milk, cheese, yogurt, and kefir
- Wild, line-caught, small omega-3 fish, including mackerel, sardines, anchovies, and salmon
- Organic unrefined or minimally refined herbs and spices

- Organic minimally refined condiments, like vinegar, mustard, and hot sauce
- Organic (ideally regenerative) minimally refined fermented foods like sauerkraut, kimchi, yogurt, natto, tempeh, tofu, and kefir
- Reverse osmosis or charcoal-filtered water

Water

Water makes up 90 percent of our blood, and clean water is of profound importance to our health. Unfortunately, it is becoming increasingly clear that this doesn't come from tap water. The Environmental Working Group (EWG) has a database where you can search the purity of your water based on zip code. The water in my community had 820 times the amount of arsenic recommended as safe. I recommend investing in a reverse osmosis filter of a high-efficacy charcoal filter (e.g., Berkey) to ensure you are getting a regular supply of clean water. Brita and similar inexpensive water filters typically use activated carbon filters, which are effective in reducing chlorine taste and odor, but they may not be as efficient in removing other contaminants like heavy metals, bacteria, and harmful chemicals.

Adequately hydrating with clean water is a significant part of the equation in becoming metabolically healthy and preventing obesity. According to Dr. Richard Johnson, professor of medicine at University of Colorado and author of the incredible book *Nature Wants Us to Be Fat,* even "mild dehydration stimulates the development of obesity." Interestingly, making fat tissue is a way for humans to store more water, called "metabolic water," which can be released in times of water scarcity. Think about camels: they can survive in the desert with low water supply in part because they store water in the fat cells of their fatty humps! How dehydration leads to obesity is one of the most fascinating stories in all of medicine. Dehydration activates a process in the brain called the polyol pathway, which stimulates the body to manufacture fructose. The fructose the body makes does two things: it stimulates a hormone called vasopressin, which tells our kidneys to retain water, and it causes us to print fat—meaning to literally manufacture more fat and fill our cells with it—through the disturbance of mitochondrial function. This then lets us store more "metabolic water" in that fat. According to Dr. Johnson, "people with obesity are ten times as likely to be dehydrated as their leaner counterparts." In a study in Germany, drinking just one additional glass of water per day reduced children's risk of becoming overweight by 30 percent.

Cut processed and ultra-processed foods from your diet—particularly those that contain the following:

- Refined sugars of any kind
- Refined grains of any kind
- Refined industrial vegetable or seed oils of any kind

A WORD ABOUT GRAINS

You might notice the absence of unprocessed grains from the "eat" list. I see no major benefit in adding grains in any form to the diet. Grains are a relatively modern food that provides some vitamins, minerals, and fiber, but much less than other foods on this list. For instance, 1 cup cooked quinoa has 5 grams of fiber per cup, 34 net carbohydrates, 8 grams of protein, and 160 milligrams of omega-3s—while just two tablespoons of basil seeds have 15 grams of fiber (three times as much as quinoa), 0 net carbs (meaning near zero glucose elevation), 5 grams of protein, and 2,860 milligrams of omega-3 fats (seventeen times as much as quinoa). In the context of the U.S. metabolic crisis—in which 93 percent of adults have problems with metabolism—avoiding carbohydrate-predominant foods with a lesser value of protective substances within them is a wise choice. Existing in the modern world—no matter how vigilant you are—means your gut lining will be compromised to some extent. Some of the concentrated proteins in modern grains can contribute to leaky gut, regardless of whether you have a strong sensitivity. Additionally, most grains in the U.S. are covered in toxic pesticides.

Conventional, Organic, Regenerative: What Does It Mean?

Conventionally Grown Food:

Conventionally grown foods make up 94 percent of food sales in the United States, and the term refers to foods not grown organically. Conventional farming uses one billion pounds of pesticides per year in the United States alone, many of which are known to cause damage to human and microbiome cells and are tied to obesity, cancer, and developmental illnesses, among many others. The World Health Organization has explicitly stated that glyphosate, the key ingredient in the most widely used pesticide, Roundup, damages our DNA and probably causes cancer. Conventional farming utilizes monocropping, the process of planting the same single crop repeatedly in one place, which strips the soil of key nutrients. Monocropping generally doesn't use cover crops, which are traditionally planted to protect the soil between plantings and replenish the soil with nutrients. Without cover crops, the soil overheats and loses water, becoming lifeless dirt instead of thriving living soil.

Additionally, we've replaced the natural replenishment of soil through cover crops and natural fertilizers, like manure and compost, with fossil-fuel-derived synthetic fertilizers. Huge amounts of natural gas and coal are used to directly make synthetic fertilizer. Research shows that long-term monocropping leads to "soil sickness" and a reduction in diverse bacteria. Conventional farming also utilizes mechanized tilling, an aggressive turning and agitating of the soil that kills the fragile ecosystem of microorganisms that allow our food to be as nutrient rich and resilient as possible. Conventional soil is depleted of microbial life, leading to topsoil depletion, water runoff, and toxic chemicals in the water and environment that are creating environmental catastrophes, like a dead zone the size of New Jersey in the Gulf of Mexico where the Mississippi drains.

Conventionally raised animals are subjected to confinement and pesticide-covered grain diets in CAFOs (concentrated animal feeding operations) that increase omega-6 fat content in their bodies. In the absence of diverse natural diets and movement, the squalid conditions lead to rampant infectious disease, so much so that 70 percent of antibiotics in the United States go toward conventionally raised animals. Astonishingly, 70 percent of conventional soy grown in the United States and nearly 50 percent of the corn go toward animal feed in a cycle that hurts our soil via conventional agriculture, then sickens animals by overloading their bodies with omega-6 fats, which then sicken humans who eat them.

Avoid conventionally grown foods at all costs: they hurt the soil, the environment, our water systems, farmer well-being, global biodiversity, your microbiome, and your cellular health. Eating nonorganic or nonregenerative food is promoting an environmentally devastating industry that uses extensive fossil fuels.

Organically Grown Food:

Organic farming refers to adherence to a strict set of standards overseen by the federal government that includes restrictions on the use of most synthetic fertilizers and pesticides. However, organic doesn't necessarily mean that the practices focus on regenerating thriving and biodiverse soil. Organically grown food is a significantly better option compared to conventionally raised foods because it minimizes the use of some of the most toxic chemicals in our soil and on our food.

Organic meat and dairy products come from animals who did not eat food grown with synthetic pesticides; however, this does not mean that the animal ate a natural diet. It very well may have eaten exclusively organic grain feed (like corn and soy), which is still omega-6 rich and promotes metabolic dysfunction in the animal. The best thing to look for on a label is "organic" *and* "grass-fed" or "pasture-raised" for meat and dairy, as this means the animal had access to pesticide-free natural diets like grasses and moved more freely.

Regeneratively Grown Food:

Regenerative food practices focus on soil health and biodiversity, utilizing diverse crop rotation, avoiding synthetic pesticides and fertilizers, minimizing tilling, and employing composting and other practices. Regeneratively grown food increases soil microbe count, enriches soils with nutrients, improves watersheds, decreases water runoff, and requires less water. Animals are incorporated into the regenerative farming ecosystem to roam freely in pastures and orchards and to naturally and gently agitate soil through grazing. In doing so, they replete and regenerate soil with nutrients and biodiversity from feces and urine. Regenerative farming leads to cleaner water and air, 30 percent less water use (since the healthy porous soil can store more water and it won't just run off), nutrient-dense foods, and enhanced carbon capture in the soil through significantly increased root-system growth. (Larger root systems are necessarily built by taking carbon from the environment to print carbon-based plant tissue.)

Animals raised regeneratively have higher levels of omega-3 fats by large margins, and their milk has six times more antioxidants and phytonutrients than conventional milk. (These nutrients are undetectable in milk from conventional cows.) Animals don't receive routine antibiotics (unless they are acutely ill) on regenerative farms, since the animals have resilient health from being able to move, eat, and socialize freely.

Some people argue that conventional farming is cheaper and more efficient than regenerative, and therefore necessary to feed our large population at scale. This argument is a narrow view focusing on extremely short-term gains that are only possible through Farm Bill subsidies. Conventional farming is fragile because it renders ecosystems fragile. Dr. Mark Hyman points out that we pay at least four times more for conventionally grown food that is artificially cheap: we pay for the taxpayer subsidies to prop up the unsustainable practices, for the food itself, for the detrimental health effects, and for the disastrous environmental outcomes. The winners are the ultra-processed food companies. Moving to regenerative farming practices at scale would slash our health care costs, rate of environmental damage, energy use globally, and reliance on fossil fuels. Additionally, by converting to regenerative practice, farmers are saving on input costs (like pesticides, insecticides, and pesticide-resistant seeds). In the film *Common Ground,* one farmer notes that he can save around $400 an acre on input costs with regenerative practices, translating to $2 million in savings yearly.

Choosing regeneratively grown foods is one of the most powerful choices you can make as a health seeker or environmentalist. Regenerative plants, cover crops, and healthy soil sequester carbon from the atmosphere and 3D print it into extensive root systems that grow immensely larger than conventional root systems that must battle through hard, lifeless dirt. The aggressive composting in regenerative farming practices produces little to no waste. It also drastically decreases the use of fossil fuels (which get converted to synthetic fertilizer), protects water systems from pesticide and fertilizer runoff (which kills marine life), and mitigates drought by capturing rainwater in porous, absorbent regenerative soil that would otherwise be lost to runoff. The Natural Resources Defense Council estimates that a 1 percent increase in healthy soil increases water storage capacity by over twenty thousand gallons per single acre.

DEFINING PROCESSED FOOD

Ultra-processed foods make up 60 percent of calories consumed by adults and 67 percent of calories consumed by children, and they drive Bad Energy diseases like obesity, high blood pressure, dementia, type 2 diabetes, and insulin resistance. And the impact is major. In a recent study of twenty thousand participants followed over fifteen years, more than four servings of ultra-processed foods per day conferred a 62 percent increased hazard for death during follow-up. Each additional serving of ultra-processed food increased all-cause mortality by 18 percent. We must understand what ultra-processed foods are and how to avoid them at all costs. (Spoiler alert: four servings of ultra-processed foods in a day is *not* as much as you might think; the total could look like a handful of pretzels, a serving of tortilla chips, a slice of store-bought bread, and a cookie.)

So what counts as ultra-processed food? The NOVA classification system splits foods into four categories based on how processed they are, according to the physical, biological, and chemical manufacturing processes used after "foods are separated from nature."

The categories include:

- Unprocessed and minimally processed foods
- Processed culinary ingredients
- Processed foods
- Ultra-processed foods

Unprocessed and Minimally Processed Foods

Unprocessed foods undergo zero alteration following their removal from nature—like eating an apple just off the tree. Whole foods that lack added ingredients, such as fruits, vegetables, eggs, nuts, seeds, dried herbs, spices, and raw cuts of meat, poultry, and fish, are generally regarded as minimally processed or unprocessed. Within the minimally processed food category, some processing may occur, such as washing, crushing, grinding, filtering, roasting, canning, boiling, vacuum sealing, freezing, nonalcoholic fermentation, pasteurization, or placing in containers. However, no part of the food has been stripped away or concentrated. Additionally, no extra salt, sugar, or other ingredients can be added.

In order to be metabolically healthy, unprocessed and minimally processed foods must comprise the vast majority of what you eat.

Processed Culinary Ingredients

Processed culinary ingredients include oils, butter, sugar, maple syrup, lard, and noncaloric ingredients, like salt. They are extracted from natural foods or nature by milling, drying, pressing, grinding, crushing, and refining. They are inherently "unbalanced," concentrated, and generally energy dense foods (salt being an exception) that are rarely consumed by themselves.

While certain processed culinary ingredients can be part of a health-optimizing diet, many can have negative effects on metabolic health.

Industrially extracted vegetable and seed oils like soybean oil and corn oils (the most common fats in the American diet), for instance, are harmful due to their concentrated omega-6 content, which can promote inflammation. In contrast, oils like olive oil and avocado oil, which are obtained by essentially squishing fatty whole fruits (rather than mechanically and chemically extracting oils from seeds or vegetables), are typically associated with positive health outcomes.

Processed Foods

Processed food manufacturing increases the "durability" and "sensory qualities" of foods by combining minimally processed foods with processed culinary ingredients to make "highly palatable" items. For example, this could include freshly made unpackaged whole grain breads, tomato sauce with added sugar, bacon cured with salt, fruit preserved in syrup, or vegetables or beans canned in a salty brine. The easiest way to identify processed foods is by looking for oils, salt, or sugar on the label.

Some processed foods can be part of a healthy diet, and again, it comes down to reading the label. For example, flaxseed crackers, like Flackers or Ella's Flats, may have just a few ingredients that are themselves healthy (like organic flaxseed, apple cider vinegar, and sea salt) and not heavily processed. You can visibly see the whole flaxseeds in the product. Additionally, grass-fed organic raw cheddar cheese, made just of unpasteurized milk and sea salt, is a well-sourced, natural processed food that can be part of a healthy diet.

With that said, most foods in the processed food category are problematic and include far too high levels of sugar, salt, and oil. This happens in foods you wouldn't expect, like ketchup, salad dressing, and peanut butter. Avoid any processed food with refined vegetable or seed oil, refined grains, added sugar, or an ingredient that is not an obviously recognizable food.

Ultra-Processed Foods

Ultra-processed foods are created in industrial factories by combining various extracted and adulterated parts from different foods with synthetic ingredients, like preservatives and food colorings. These are "Frankenfoods" you should never eat and never give to your children. These foods now comprise the vast majority of the calories we eat today in America. They should be zero percent of our diet. In a 2020 study of the impact of ultra-processed food consumption and chronic diseases, results show that the highest levels of ultra-processed food intake across studies increased the risk of overweight or obesity by 39 percent, waist circumferences by 39 percent, metabolic syndrome by 79 percent, and low HDL levels by 102 percent.

To make ultra-processed foods, manufacturers break down whole foods into parts and then often combine these parts with synthetic chemicals to create shelf-stable chemical imitations of less processed foods. Foods are first broken down into extracted parts like oil, sugar, starch, protein, and fiber. Foods may then undergo chemical modifications to further reengineer them, like using enzymes to extract natural flavors, colors, or proteins from ingredients. Manufacturers may add hydrogen to oil to make fat solid at room temperature and prevent the oil from going rancid, but these fats are known to cause inflammation and impair glucose regulation.

Ultra-processed foods include mass-produced versions of pastries, breads, cakes, cookies, nut milks, "nuggets" made of ground meat or soy, chips, crackers, granola bars, and other snack foods. Below is a short list of examples of ultra-processed foods. While these are considered normal foods in our culture, you should avoid them as strongly as if they were illicit drugs. Every item below has either refined sugar, ultra-processed grains, or industrially refined seed and vegetable oils—three classes of foods that need to be avoided for Good Energy. There are many brands that produce the food items on this list, but I am highlighting some of the most popular brands:

BEVERAGES:
1. Sweetened juice (e.g., SunnyD, Ocean Spray)
2. Energy drinks (e.g., Red Bull)
3. Flavored coffee creamers (e.g., Nestlé Coffee mate)
4. Nondairy milks (e.g., Oatly, Silk)
5. Flavored milks (e.g., Nesquik, Horizon Strawberry milk)

6. Fruit-flavored drinks (e.g., Capri-Sun)
7. Sports drinks (e.g., Gatorade)
8. Sweetened teas (e.g., AriZona and Nestea)
9. Soda (e.g., Coca-Cola, Diet Coke, and Coke Zero)
10. Artificially flavored water (e.g., Dasani Drops)
11. Fruit punch (e.g., Hawaiian Punch)
12. Flavored ice beverages (e.g., Slurpee, Icee)

BAKERY AND DESSERTS:

1. Cake mixes (e.g., Pillsbury)
2. Store-bought icing (e.g., Betty Crocker)
3. Chocolate bars (e.g., Snickers)
4. Cookies (e.g., Oreo, Chips Ahoy!)
5. Doughnuts (e.g., Krispy Kreme, Hostess Donettes)
6. Frozen waffles and pancakes (e.g., Eggo)
7. Packaged bread (e.g., Wonder Bread)
8. Sweet rolls and pastries (e.g., Cinnabon and Pillsbury)
9. Packaged cakes (e.g., Twinkies)
10. Muffins (e.g., Entenmann's)
11. Sweet crackers (e.g., Honey Maid)

CEREALS AND GRANOLAS:

1. Cereal bars (e.g., Nature Valley)
2. Instant oatmeal packets (e.g., Quaker)
3. Granolas with refined sugars (e.g., Kellogg's Special K Granola, Kashi GO)
4. Sweetened cereals (e.g., Froot Loops)
5. Toaster pastries (e.g., Pop-Tarts)

DAIRY:

1. Flavored yogurts (e.g., Yoplait and Go-Gurt)
2. Processed cheese slices (e.g., Kraft Singles)
3. Sweetened condensed milk (e.g., Eagle Brand)
4. Whipped toppings (e.g., Cool Whip, Reddi-wip)

MEAT AND POULTRY:

1. Chicken nuggets (e.g., McDonald's or Tyson)
2. Deli meats (e.g., Oscar Mayer and Boar's Head)
3. Hot dogs (e.g., Nathan's Famous)
4. Meatballs (e.g., Chef Boyardee)
5. Sausages (e.g., Jimmy Dean)
6. Bacon (e.g., Oscar Mayer)
7. Beef jerky (e.g., Jack Link's)

SNACKS:

1. Cheese puffs (e.g., Cheetos)
2. Chips (e.g., Doritos)
3. Crackers (e.g., Ritz)
4. Flavored popcorn (e.g., Smartfood)
5. Processed snacks (e.g., Combos or Dunkaroos)
6. Fruit snacks (e.g., Fruit Gushers, Welch's, Mott's)

FROZEN FOODS:

1. Frozen pizza (e.g., DiGiorno)
2. Frozen dinners (e.g., Hungry-Man)
3. Frozen burritos (e.g., El Monterey)
4. Frozen chicken wings (e.g., Tyson)
5. Frozen fish sticks (e.g., Gorton's)

SAUCES AND CONDIMENTS:

1. Barbecue sauce with added sugar (e.g., Sweet Baby Ray's)
2. Ketchup (e.g., Heinz)
3. Mayonnaise (e.g., Hellmann's)
4. Salad dressings (e.g., Hidden Valley)
5. Vegetable and seed oils (e.g., Crisco or Wesson)

PACKAGED MEALS:

1. Mac and cheese (e.g., Kraft or Annie's)
2. Hamburger helper (e.g., Betty Crocker)

3. Pizza rolls (e.g., Totino's)
4. Instant mashed potatoes (e.g., Idahoan)
5. Ramen noodle cups (e.g., Nissin Cup Noodles)
6. Lunch packs (e.g., Lunchables)

FROZEN DESSERTS:

1. Ice cream bars and sandwiches (e.g., Magnum and Nestlé Drumstick)
2. Popsicles (e.g., Fla-Vor-Ice)
3. Sorbet (e.g., Häagen-Dazs)
4. Sherbet (e.g., Baskin-Robbins)
5. Ice cream (e.g., Ben & Jerry's)

SOUPS AND BROTHS:

1. Canned soups (e.g., Campbell's Chicken Noodle)
2. Dry soup mixes (e.g., Lipton Noodle Soup)
3. Instant ramen noodles (e.g., Maruchan)
4. Bouillon cubes (e.g., Knorr)
5. Gravy mixes (e.g., McCormick)

SPREADS:

1. Chocolate hazelnut spreads (e.g., Nutella)
2. Peanut butter with added sugar (e.g., Jif)
3. Jelly and jam (e.g., Smucker's)
4. Marshmallow fluff (e.g., Fluff)
5. Sweet spreads (e.g., Smucker's Goober peanut butter and jelly spreads)

Many new packaged food brands are working to bring to the market healthier, sustainable versions of ultra-processed foods. Examples include organic frozen pizzas made with simple cauliflower and seed-flour crusts topped with mozzarella cheese and sugar-free tomato sauce, as well as packaged pastas made with organic legume or nut flours. Many packaged foods can be part of a healthy, Good Energy eating plan, but make sure to look closely at the labels to ensure you're buying organic ingredients without added sugars, refined grains, or seed and vegetable oils.

A Tale of Three Yogurts: Which is Ultra-Processed?

Ultra-Processed (Never Eat)

- **Dannon Light + Fit Yogurt.** Contains Cultured Nonfat Milk, Water, Fructose, Natural & Artificial Flavors, Modified Food Starch, Acesulfame Potassium, Sucralose, Citric Acid, Potassium Sorbate, Yogurt Cultures—eleven ingredients, chemicals known to disrupt the microbiome
- **Yoplait Kids Cup.** Contains Low Fat Milk, Sugar, Modified Corn Starch, Corn Starch, Natural Flavor, Potassium Sorbate, Red 40, Blue 1, Yellow 5, Vitamin A Acetate, Vitamin D3—eleven ingredients, zero active cultures, colorings known to be toxic and require warning labels in Europe. For example, in vitro experiments found potassium ascorbate to be genotoxic and have a negative effect on immunity, and some research links hyperactivity and inattention in children to coloring agents.

Minimally Processed (Good to Eat)

- **Straus Whole Milk Organic Greek Yogurt.** Organic Whole Milk, Yogurt Cultures—two ingredients, live active cultures, cows are pasture-raised on pesticide-free grass

Choose a yogurt that is organic, has minimal ingredients (ideally just milk and cultures), has no added sugar, and says "live active cultures" on the label.

Ultra-processed foods also have a massive environmental cost. For example, a one-liter bottle of grapeseed oil requires about 120 pounds of tiny grape seeds to produce, or about one ton of grapes. Frequently, ultra-processed foods are stored in plastic and other unsustainable materials that go into landfills. Most ultra-processed foods are made from crops that are grown conventionally, so on top of decimating our health, these foods are environmentally devastating and wasteful.

You might be thinking, *Isn't the cost of eating unrefined or minimally refined, sustainably sourced foods too high for most people?* Here's a possibly uncomfortable truth: you will either pay for healthy food up front or you will pay for preventable medical issues and lost productivity in the future. Medical issues are the cause of nearly 70 percent of U.S. bankruptcies. Adults with obesity experience 100 percent higher annual medical care costs. Those costs increase steeply as weight increases. People with type 2 diabetes incur average medical expenditures of almost $17,000 *annually*. People with chronic illnesses, like cardiometabolic disease, lose up to 80 annual work hours, with the annual cost of lost work productivity spanning up to $10,000. The odds of having been absent from work are 1.4 times higher in people with obesity compared to those without. Obviously, our health and food industries are letting us down: subsidizing ultra-processed food and initiating health care only when we are sick with metabolic diseases to "manage." It is a shortcoming of public policy that it is cheaper for a lower-income family to purchase a Coke than a bottle of water at many supermarkets (because the Coke has so many subsidized ingredients). We must change the incentive structures of our food and health system—but until then do whatever is in our power to reject ultra-processed food. Here are several tips to do this on a budget:

STOCKING THE GOOD ENERGY KITCHEN

Here are a few of my favorite ways to get organic food as cheaply as possible.

- Buy frozen organic fruits, vegetables, meats, and wild-caught fish in bulk, or buy fresh and freeze. I get four pounds of organic frozen cauliflower rice weekly at Costco for under $10, which makes close to eight meals.
- Cook large batches of organic beans or lentils in the slow cooker or stovetop. Bulk organic beans and lentils are often less than $4 per pound.
- Purchase the cheapest organic nuts and seeds in bulk. For instance, organic pine nuts can be upward of $44 per pound, while organic flax and chia seeds are often less than $6 per pound.
- Purchase whatever organic produce happens to be on sale. Doing so has had the added benefit of getting me to try new foods!

- Buy wild-caught canned fish, like salmon, instead of fresh fish.
- Join a community-sponsored agriculture (CSA) program or sign up for an organic produce delivery service that ships misshapen foods that otherwise would go to waste (like Imperfect Foods).
- Replace meat and fish with plant-based proteins, like beans and lentils, for some meals to cut costs.
- Talk to farmers at the farmers' market to get the best deals. Farmers will often reduce the price of certain items that they have in excess that week. Additionally, there are many farms that use no synthetic pesticides but have not gone through the costly and lengthy process to obtain official USDA organic certification. Their products will be chemical-free and likely cheaper than certified organic, and are a great option.

Good Energy Foods

Working off our list above of what categories of foods will—and will not—support Good Energy, we now need to zoom in on how to build a meal. Aiming for a Good Energy–supporting dietary plan is as simple as making sure you maximize five things and remove three things.

Every day (and ideally every meal) should include the following:

1. Micronutrients and Antioxidants

Micronutrients and antioxidants tell the mitochondria, "You are resilient."

Micronutrients are small molecules—like magnesium, zinc, selenium, and B vitamins—that serve four main functions in the cell supporting Good Energy.

- They are structurally incorporated into proteins to enable them to function properly.
  - *Example:* The micronutrient selenium gets incorporated into proteins called *seleno*proteins, which have key roles as protective antioxidants and in healthy immune cell function.
- They serve as cofactors that allow for chemical reactions in the cell, like those in the final stages of making ATP in the mitochondria.

- *Example*: B vitamins bind to protein enzymes in the mitochondria, creating slight shifts in the protein structure to allow for sequential steps in ATP production.
- They act as antioxidants to reduce damage from oxidative stress that can impair metabolic processes and mitochondrial function.
  - *Example*: Vitamin E can insert itself into cell membranes and donate electrons to neutralize reactive free radicals that can damage and destroy the fats in cell membranes, leading to chronic inflammation if left unchecked.
- They become precursors for key biologic processes.
  - *Example*: Vitamin B$_3$, also called niacin, is a precursor for NAD+ and NADP+, which are involved in more than five hundred chemical reactions in the cell, including serving as electron carriers in the mitochondria during the production of ATP.

Micronutrients facilitate the optimal action of many key biological processes, including how the body handles glucose. Unfortunately, our ultra-processed diets are more micronutrient depleted than ever, due to poor soil and excess processing.

Your roughly thirty-seven trillion cells can contain a thousand or more mitochondria, each with innumerable proteins embedded in their membranes that act as tiny molecular machines as part of the electron transport chain (ETC) assembly line of making ATP. Those ETC proteins require adequate levels of specific micronutrients to function correctly. These vitamins, minerals, trace metals, and antioxidants are crucial links in chain reactions that regulate every part of your body's metabolism. In many cases, these micronutrients are bound to these large protein complexes to create the "just right" molecular conditions that let the tiny biological machines work correctly.

Example: Micronutrient CoQ10 Supports Fertility

An example of how critical micronutrients are for Good Energy is CoQ10's role in fertility: CoQ10 is a micronutrient that is required for transferring electrons in the ETC, while also embedding in the cell membrane to offer antioxidant protection. After eggs are released from the ovary at ovulation, they undergo rapid "aging" and degradation as they make their way to the uterus, with many changes occurring to mitochondrial activity and mitochondria structure. CoQ10, which serves as a mitochondrial cofactor and improves mitochondrial function, significantly improves egg aging after ovulation. It reduces levels of oxidative stress and DNA damage and inhibits cell death pathways, thereby preserving egg (oocyte) quality. Give your mitochondria what it needs, and it will perform for you with flying colors, including supporting the health of a future baby.

Key Micronutrients for Good Energy:

MICRONUTRIENT	GOOD ENERGY BENEFITS	SOURCES
Vitamin D	• Enhances expression of insulin receptors and glucose transporter channels. • Increases the expression of mitochondrial genes involved in energy metabolism. • Reduces mitochondrial oxidative stress. • Regulates the expression of genes involved in inflammation and antioxidant defenses.	Fatty fish (salmon, tuna, mackerel), egg yolks, mushrooms
Magnesium	• Facilitates ATP synthesis by participating in the reactions that produce and utilize ATP in the ETC. • Reduces oxidative stress and enhances activity of mitochondrial enzymes. • Regulates glucose and fat metabolism by activating enzymes involved in glucose uptake, glycogen (stored glucose) synthesis, and fatty acid oxidation.	Nuts (almonds, cashews), seeds (pumpkin, sunflower), spinach, beans (black, kidney)
Selenium	• Serves as a cofactor for antioxidant enzymes, such as glutathione peroxidase. • Enhances expression and activity of insulin-signaling proteins. • Enhances thyroid function by promoting the synthesis and conversion of thyroid hormones, which regulate metabolic rate and energy production.	Brazil nuts, tuna, turkey, sardines, chicken, eggs

MICRONUTRIENT	GOOD ENERGY BENEFITS	SOURCES
Zinc	• Participates in the ETC as a cofactor. • Increases activity of antioxidant enzymes. • Regulates glucose and fat metabolism by activating enzymes involved in insulin signaling, glucose uptake, and fatty acid oxidation.	Oysters, beef, pumpkin seeds, beans (chickpeas, kidney), dark chocolate
Vitamins B_1, B_2, B_3, B_5, B_6, B_7, B_9, B_{12}	• Participate in various steps of energy metabolism, such as the breakdown of glucose before entering the mitochondria, the production of ATP in the mitochondria, and the synthesis of fatty acids and amino acids. • Act as cofactors for enzymes in the ETC and by regulating the expression of mitochondrial genes. • Regulate inflammation and oxidative stress by modulating the expression of genes involved in these processes.	• B_1: pork, brown rice, sunflower seeds, beans, nuts • B_2: milk, almonds, spinach, eggs, mushrooms • B_3: beef, chicken, peanuts, mushrooms, avocados • B_5: chicken, sweet potatoes, mushrooms, lentils, avocados • B_6: chickpeas, tuna, salmon, potatoes, bananas • B_7: eggs, almonds, sweet potatoes, spinach, broccoli • B_9: spinach, asparagus, avocados, beans (black, kidney) • B_{12}: beef, clams, salmon, milk, eggs
Alpha lipoic acid	• Acts as a cofactor for enzymes involved in the ETC. • Enhances glucose uptake and insulin sensitivity by activating proteins involved in glucose transport and insulin signaling. • Reduces inflammation and oxidative stress by modulating the activity of genes involved in these processes.	Spinach, broccoli, tomatoes, organ meats (liver, kidney)

MICRONUTRIENT	GOOD ENERGY BENEFITS	SOURCES
Manganese	• Participates in the synthesis of ATP in the ETC by stabilizing and activating protein enzymes. • Enhances antioxidant defenses by serving as a cofactor for antioxidant enzymes, such as superoxide dismutase. • Activates enzymes involved in glucose uptake and utilization.	Nuts (almonds, pecans), beans (lima, black), tea
Vitamin E	• Acts as an antioxidant. • Enhances insulin signaling. • Supports immune function, which indirectly supports metabolic health by reducing inflammation and infection.	Almonds, sunflower seeds, avocados, spinach, sweet potatoes
CoQ10	• Shuttles electrons between respiratory complexes during the synthesis of ATP in the electron transport chain. • Acts as an antioxidant by protecting against free radicals and reducing oxidative stress. • Improves glucose metabolism and insulin sensitivity by enhancing insulin signaling and reducing inflammation.	Organ meats (heart, liver), sardines, beef
Taurine	• Supports mitochondrial function by enhancing the expression of genes involved in energy metabolism and reducing oxidative stress. • Enhances insulin sensitivity by activating proteins involved in glucose transport and metabolism. • Regulates inflammation and oxidative stress by modulating the expression of genes involved in these.	Meat (beef, lamb), fish (mackerel, salmon), poultry (chicken, turkey), eggs
L-carnitine	• Facilitates the transport of fatty acids into mitochondria for processing, thereby promoting energy production and reducing lipid accumulation in tissues. • Reduces oxidative stress and improves the activity of mitochondrial enzymes. • Enhances insulin signaling and glucose uptake.	Red meat (beef, lamb), poultry (chicken, turkey), fish (cod, halibut)

MICRONUTRIENT	GOOD ENERGY BENEFITS	SOURCES
Creatine	• Converts to phosphocreatine, which can be rapidly converted to ATP during high-intensity exercise or energy-demanding tasks. • Enhances activity of mitochondrial enzymes and reduces oxidative stress. • Helps regulate inflammation and antioxidant genes.	Red meat (beef, lamb), fish (salmon, tuna), poultry (chicken, turkey), pork, eggs
Vitamin C	• Promotes expression of mitochondrial genes involved in energy metabolism and reducing oxidative stress. • Acts as an antioxidant by protecting against free radicals and reducing oxidative stress.	Citrus fruits (oranges, lemons), strawberries, broccoli, bell peppers, tomatoes, kiwi

Another key class of micronutrients is polyphenols, which are tiny plant chemicals that have incredible biologic effects, including acting as antioxidants and feeding the microbiome. While we typically think of fiber as being the food substance fermented by the microbiome, recent evidence suggests that the microbial transformation of polyphenols through fermentation can yield metabolites that can enter the body and promote a range of positive biological effects, including acting as protective neurotransmitters in the brain and directly reducing the growth of cancer cells, including stopping cancer cells from taking up glucose for energy. More than eight thousand known polyphenols exist in plants, and they offer a Swiss Army knife of benefits for cells. Of course, ultra-processing ruins this. When plants go through ultra-processing, like processing corn to make cornflakes, the polyphenols are largely lost.

Foods with the highest polyphenol count are dried spices and herbs, followed by cocoa, dark berries, seeds and nuts, many vegetables, coffee, and tea.

Eating a diverse array of foods from the list on pages 289–91 will ensure you get various micronutrients.

Best Antioxidant Sources

We've learned that antioxidant intake is a key aspect of promoting Good Energy by reducing oxidative stress. Foods with the very highest levels of antioxidants or polyphenols per 100 grams include the following:

- Almonds
- Allspice, dried
- Amla berries, dried
- Apples
- Artichokes
- Asparagus
- Bay leaves, dried
- Basil, dried
- Black beans
- Black chokeberries
- Black elderberries
- Black pepper, dried
- Blackberries
- Black tea
- Blueberries
- Broccoli
- Capers
- Caraway seeds, dried
- Cayenne pepper, dried
- Celery leaves, dried
- Cherries
- Chives, dried
- Chili, dried
- Cinnamon bark, dried
- Clove, dried
- Cocoa powder
- Coffee beans
- Cumin, dried
- Curry powder
- Dandelion leaves, dried
- Dark chocolate
- Dill, fresh or dried
- Fennel leaves, dried
- Fennel seeds, dried
- Ginger, fresh or dried
- Green mint, dried
- Green olives, with stone
- Green tea
- Hazelnut
- Kalamata olives, with stone
- Lavender, dried
- Mustard seed, dried
- Nutmeg, dried
- Oregano, fresh or dried
- Paprika, dried
- Peaches
- Pecans
- Peppermint, dried
- Pistachios
- Plums
- Pomegranate, whole
- Red lettuce
- Red onion
- Rose flower, dried
- Rosemary, fresh or dried
- Saffron, dried
- Shallots
- Spinach
- Strawberries

- Tempeh
- Thyme, dried
- Turmeric, dried
- Vanilla seeds

- Walnuts
- White beans
- Wild marjoram leaves, dried

2. Omega-3 Fatty Acids

Omega-3 fatty acids tell the cell, "You are safe."

We've learned previously that omega-3 fatty acids—including ALA, EPA, and DHA—are a type of polyunsaturated fatty acid, key for elements of cell structure, inflammatory pathways, and metabolic pathways. Omega-3s also contribute to artery elasticity.

Getting enough omega-3s also limits the impact of omega-6s, a fatty acid that, in excess, is associated with inflammation. The standard Western diet contains a ratio of as much as 20:1 omega-6s to omega-3s when it should be closer to 1:1. The higher ratio is largely due to high consumption of refined seed and vegetable oils (including canola, soybean, vegetable, safflower, sunflower, and corn oils—all high in omega-6s) and less consumption of omega-3-rich whole foods, like wild fatty fish, chia seeds, flaxseeds, and walnuts.

Chronic inflammation is a key aspect of Bad Energy. Many people talk about how omega-3 fats are "anti-inflammatory." What does this *really* mean? The first thing to understand is that the composition of omega-6 and omega-3 fats in the diet directly determines the ratio of these types of fats in your cell membranes, including all immune cells. In the cell membranes, these fats serve very different purposes. Immune cells can harvest omega-6 fats in the membrane to manufacture signaling molecules that tend to exacerbate and lengthen an inflammatory reaction. On the other hand, immune cells can use omega-3s to manufacture signaling molecules that decrease inflammatory genetic pathways and ultimately resolve the inflammatory processes. Omega-3s can directly decrease the activity of NF-κB—the master inflammatory pathway—to turn it down after an inflammatory episode.

Imagine a person with a high omega-6 concentration in the cell membrane of their immune cells. They get infected with a virus, perhaps the one that causes COVID-19. The body works to attack this virus. We expect collateral damage to the body—swelling, inflammation, oxidative stress, spewing toxic substances to kill virally infected cells. But once the person's immune cells kill the infected cells, all that warring needs to stop. And if the person has adequate omega-3s in their immune cell membrane, the cell will literally snip the omega-3s from the membrane and use them to manufacture resolvins and protectins, two types of specialized pro-resolving mediators (SPMs) to ease the war. But in the average American, where the omega-6 to omega-3 ratio is now extremely high, the fatty acid the cell grabs for and snips is much more likely to be an omega-6, which generates signals to *keep* the war going. This is chronic inflammation. Remember, the cells are blind and reach from whatever is around them. Your job with eating a better omega-3 to omega-6 ratio in food is to increase the probability that your cells manufacture the health-promoting, anti-inflammatory signaling molecules you need, like resolvins and protectins. How you feed yourself determines the likelihood of having chronic inflammation.

The best way to get omega-3s in your meals is to eat the following:

- Chia seeds
- Basil seeds
- Flaxseeds
- Walnuts
- Hemp seeds
- Sardines
- Mackerel
- Herring
- Anchovies
- Salmon
- Trout
- Fish roe or caviar
- Oysters

- Pasture-raised, 100 percent grass-fed game (venison, bison), beef, lamb, and eggs

3. Fiber

Fiber tells the microbiome, "I love you."

Fiber is a type of carbohydrate found in plants that is not fully broken down by the body and therefore does not get converted to glucose in the bloodstream. Instead, the gut microbiome ferments fiber into beneficial "postbiotic" by-products like short-chain fatty acids (SCFAs)—including butyrate, acetate, and propionate—that get absorbed into the body through the gut and regulate metabolism and improve insulin and glucose levels, regulate hunger and appetite, as well as promote anti-inflammatory effects in the gut and body. Fiber can help protect the gut's lining and mucus membrane, and slow digestion and absorption of nutrients. Colon cells are unique in that they use microbiome-derived SCFAs as a key fuel source, so the microbiome's adequate production of these molecules through fermentation of fiber is critical for a healthy gut lining. Without adequate energy, the gut lining can become a weak barrier between what is in the gut and what enters the bloodstream, a phenomenon called "intestinal permeability" or "leaky gut." When this happens, the gut becomes like a tattered piece of fabric (on the microscopic level), and harmful substances can enter the bloodstream and generate chronic inflammation, which we know is a root of many chronic diseases. As one research group noted, "The loss of (gut) barrier integrity is considered to contribute to inflammatory bowel disease, obesity, and metabolic disorders." In his book *Fat Chance*, Dr. Robert Lustig describes fiber as being "half of the solution" to the obesity epidemic. Despite this, the majority of people do not consume nearly enough fiber. The USDA's Dietary Guidelines for Americans state that over 90 percent of women and 97 percent of men do not meet the recommended daily intake of fiber, which is already set at an extremely low 25 to 31 grams per day (depending on age and gender). Ideally, we should aim to consume 50 grams or more of fiber daily.

The best ways to get fiber in your meals include eating the following:

- Chia seeds
- Basil seeds
- Flaxseeds
- Beans, especially lupini beans
- Tiger nuts
- Konjac root
- Artichokes
- Chicory
- Jicama
- Avocados
- Pistachios
- Raspberries
- Lentils
- Split peas
- Almonds
- Hazelnuts
- Pecans

The American Gut Project research showed that people with the healthiest microbiomes eat at least thirty different plant foods per week. Remember: conditions like depression and schizophrenia are so tied to poor gut bacteria that researchers can identify a person with depression or schizophrenia just by analyzing their gut bacteria composition. Get plant diversity and fiber.

In clinical practice, I have found that patients often have transformational improvement in their metabolic health and biomarkers when they aggressively increase fiber from natural foods. This is akin to magic for many. Beans and lentils have been shrouded in controversy because the Paleo diet, autoimmune protocol diet (AIP), and ketogenic diet eliminate these items out of concerns for inflammatory potential or carbohydrate content. For people with autoimmune issues and/or severe gut dysfunction, working with a functional medicine doctor can be beneficial to ensure that any foods you're introducing are supporting your healing journey, including beans and lentils. There may be compounds in beans and lentils that can promote inflammation *in the context of a damaged gut lining*, so some people may benefit from improving the integrity of the gut lining through a multi-modal diet *and* lifestyle strategy before introducing certain foods. However, for most people with good gut function, I recommend liberally including beans and lentils for their incredible polyphenol and fiber content. Personalized testing can help guide and empower you in all of this decision-making: for me, I eat beans and lentils daily, and I *know* they do not produce an appreciable glucose rise on my CGM data. Nor do they knock me out of a state of ketone production (based on finger prick ketone testing). My hsCRP (inflammation) levels are consistently less than 0.3 mg/dL (the lowest level possible), and my autoimmune markers are all negative on my lab testing. Given this, I can confidently say these foods are *not* leading to chronic inflammation or autoimmunity in my body. Rather than adhering to a dietary philosophy based simply on faith, test your biomarkers regularly and adjust your plan accordingly.

For someone who does see a large glucose rise with beans or lentils, it may be useful to either balance these foods with fat and protein, or aim to get additional fiber through lower carbohydrate fiber-packed foods like chia seeds, basil seeds, and flaxseeds. Over time with additional fiber and polyphenols, the microbiome and insulin sensitivity may change such that beans and lentils can be tolerated without a large spike.

4. Fermented Foods

Fermented foods tell the body, "You can do it."

Our gut microbiome plays a critical role in digestion, nutrient absorption, immune function, and mental health. Disruption to the balance of beneficial and harmful bacteria in our gut can lead to various health issues, including digestive problems, inflammation, and even mood disorders. Probiotic-rich foods contain live microorganisms, such as beneficial bacteria and yeast, that are like those found naturally in our gut microbiome. When we consume these foods, the live microorganisms can colonize and multiply in our gut, helping to maintain a healthy balance of beneficial bacteria and supporting overall gut health. Fermented foods are helpful because of their bacterial, *pro*biotic content. But they are also helpful because of the *post*biotics in the food. Postbiotics are the products of bacterial fermentation, like short-chain fatty acids (SCFAs). A major benefit of fiber-rich foods is that the bacteria in your gut will ferment the fiber to by-products, like SCFAs. But these SCFAs can also be present in fermented foods themselves as a by-product of the live cultures doing the fermenting.

Recent research shows that a diet high in fermented foods (around six servings per day) significantly increases microbiota diversity and decreases inflammatory markers. Six servings might sound like a lot. But adding a little bit here and there in every meal will be easier if you load your kitchen with various probiotic sources. I top almost every savory dish (like eggs, tofu scrambles, salad, stir-fries, or fish) with about half a cup of colorful sauerkraut or a dollop of spiced yogurt—logging an easy two to three servings of fermented foods. I also use tempeh as a protein source, season meals and sauces with miso, have yogurt in my midday snack and dessert rotation, and drink very low-sugar kombucha as a treat.

The best ways to get fermented foods in your diet include consuming the following:

- Sauerkraut (Note: pickles are different from sauerkraut and do not contain live cultures)
- Fermented vegetables (like fermented beets, carrots, and onions; again, these are not the same as pickles. Pickles get their sour flavor from being submerged in vinegar and sugar rather than through natural bacterial fermentation.)
- Minimally processed yogurt
- Kefir
- Natto
- Tempeh
- Kombucha (Note: I only recommend kombucha that has less than 2 grams of sugar per serving, ideally from honey or fruit. Read labels carefully.)
- Miso
- Kimchi

- Brine-cured olives
- Beet kvass
- Water kefir

5. Protein
Protein tells the cells, "Let's build!"

Dietary protein is an indispensable macronutrient that is essential for maintaining metabolic homeostasis. Protein is composed of amino acids, which serve as the structural and functional building blocks of numerous metabolic and physiological processes. Adequate protein intake is necessary for the synthesis and maintenance of skeletal muscle tissue, which plays a key role in regulating metabolic health by both being a glucose-absorbing sink as well as releasing hormones called myokines that can be anti-inflammatory and improve insulin sensitivity.

Various amino acids have been identified as critical for protein synthesis and the maintenance of skeletal muscle tissue. For example, leucine is an essential amino acid that stimulates muscle protein synthesis and has been shown to play a pivotal role in regulating muscle mass and function. Sources of leucine include animal-based proteins, such as beef, chicken, and fish, as well as plant-based sources, such as soybeans and lentils. Other amino acids, such as lysine and methionine, are also important for the regulation of muscle protein synthesis and the maintenance of muscle mass. These amino acids are found in a variety of protein sources, including dairy products, eggs, meat, and legumes.

Furthermore, protein intake has been shown to impact energy balance and body weight regulation through its effects on satiety, thermogenesis, and fat metabolism. High-protein diets have been shown to have positive effects on weight loss and prevent weight regain. Protein has a high thermic effect, meaning that it requires more energy to digest and metabolize compared to carbohydrates or fats. This increased energy expenditure can lead to greater energy balance and a potential reduction in body weight. Additionally, dietary protein has been shown to increase satiety and reduce food intake, which can lead to a reduction in overall calorie intake and improved body composition. Certain amino acids in proteins have a stimulatory effect on specific satiety hormones, like cholecystokinin and GLP-1.

The best ways to get more in your diet include eating the following:

* Meats: Beef, chicken, turkey, pork, and game meats like elk and bison
* Fish and seafood
* Dairy products: Milk, cheese, and yogurt are all good sources of protein and leucine. Greek yogurt is especially high in protein.
* Eggs: Eggs are a complete source of protein that contains all essential amino acids, including leucine.
* Legumes: Legumes, such as beans, lentils, and peas, are plant-based sources of protein that are also rich in fiber, vitamins, and minerals. They are a good option for vegetarians and vegans looking to increase their protein intake.
* Soy products: Soybeans and soy products such as tofu and tempeh
* Nuts and seeds: Hemp seeds, chia seeds, pumpkin seeds, almonds, sunflower seeds, flaxseeds, cashews, pistachios
* If using protein powders, choose organic and/or grass-fed or regenerative (if animal-based) with minimal ingredients, no added sugars, no colorings, no "natural flavors" or artificial flavors, no gums, and no ingredient names you aren't familiar with.

You'll find endless debates about protein—regarding bioavailability, completeness, the amount needed for optimal longevity versus optimal muscle growth, plant versus animal protein, and whether refined forms like protein powders are okay. I'm not going to resolve these debates here, but I recommend reading Dr. Gabrielle Lyon's book *Forever Strong* for a deep dive into protein. Protein cannot be an afterthought in our diet as it has been for decades, as so many of the critical metabolic processes in our bodies depend on it. As we get older and muscle mass naturally declines, we must actively fight this process with thoughtful protein intake and regular, consistent resistance training. The Recommended Daily Allowance (RDA) for protein is 0.8 grams per kilogram (0.36 grams per pound) of body weight, which doesn't account for activity level or dynamic metabolic needs (like recovering from illness). For a very active 79-kilogram (174-pound) person like myself, the RDA would suggest 64 grams of protein per day, or about 20 grams per meal. This is likely not enough. I favor a higher value of a minimum of 30 grams of protein at every meal to promote satiety, minimize blood sugar fluctuations, and provide my body with the necessary building blocks for protein and muscle synthesis. Aim for diverse, whole foods sources like those listed above.

Bad Energy Foods

If you remember one food principle in this book, remember that cutting the unholy trinity of these three ingredients from your diet will completely change your health and ensure you're making room for more Good Energy foods:

1. Refined added sugar
2. Refined industrial vegetable and seed oils
3. Refined grains

Let's examine why these three ingredients contribute so much to Bad Energy.

1. Refined Added Sugar

Refined added sugar causes astronomically more deaths and disability per year than COVID-19 and fentanyl overdoses combined. We need to see refined added sugar for what it is: an addictive, dangerous drug that has been included in 74 percent of foods in the U.S. food system and for which the body needs zero grams in a lifetime. Of all the levers most damaging our cells and preventing Good Energy, I believe the worst offender may be added sugar. This substance has become a mainstay of food that we and our children eat regularly. As Dr. Robert Lustig has noted, sugar shows up on labels in fifty-six different names and sneaks in everywhere.

While dozens of types of refined sugar are added to foods, chief among the offenders is high-fructose corn syrup, which is a brand-new substance (in the context of human history) wreaking havoc on the ability of our cells to make energy. Fructose employs a glucose-independent mechanism to compound the dysfunction of the cell's energy-producing capabilities. As we learned earlier, fructose (which is also found in fruit in its natural, unrefined form) shuts down our body's satiety signals to drive the consumer (historically, an animal preparing for hibernation in the winter) to eat more and store fat. But now we are in a constant fed state, and the industrial food manufactured with this additive shuts down our satiety cues and drives us to eat insatiably. Consider this: when a kid drinks one bottle of Coke, they ingest as much added sugar as they might have had in an entire year if they were living 150 years ago.

No Liquid Calories

Liquids make up 22 percent of the American diet, and almost all liquids, aside from water, black coffee, and unsweetened tea, contain empty calories that promote bad energy with no benefits. Not drinking your calories is one of the simplest and easiest cuts to reduce sugar and other chemicals that hurt energy regulation.

Eliminate all juice, soda, Frappuccinos, flavored milks, sweetened nondairy milks, Gatorade and other sports drinks, energy drinks, Slurpees, and sugary liquid toppings like syrup. Sugar that comes in liquid form is digested quickly and overwhelms the energy systems. (Homemade protein- and vegetable-packed blended smoothies like the ones on pages 309–10 are an exception.). Alcoholic drinks also destabilize blood sugar, in part by directly damaging mitochondrial function and generating oxidative stress, and should be minimized.

Instead, focus on drinking water; sparkling water; tea; coffee with no added sugar and either full-fat milk or unsweetened organic nondairy milk; or water with lemon and a pinch of sea salt.

Note on alcohol: While some studies show that people who drink small amounts of alcohol may have lower risk of type 2 diabetes, there is other research showing that there may be no safe level of alcohol for the brain and that even small amounts of alcohol (the amount in about one drink) can significantly reduce the recovery impact of sleep and nervous system regulation.

Heavy alcohol use increases oxidative stress, disturbs the microbiome, damages the liver, decreases fat oxidation in liver mitochondria (leading to stored fat in the liver), and generates inflammation. Limiting alcohol intake is necessary for optimal metabolic health. If you do consume alcohol, here are some strategies to follow for less negative impact:

- Always choose organic spirits and wine. For wine and champagne, try to additionally source biodynamically farmed wine. Conventional (non-biodynamic) wines can contain pesticides, additives, and sugars, many of which never need to be disclosed on the label.
- Avoid beer, which can increase uric acid levels.
- When making cocktails, avoid excess sugars like simple syrup, store-bought mixes, or excess fruit juice. If you are going to have a fruit-forward drink, opt for freshly squeezed lower glycemic organic fruit juices like lemon, lime, grapefruit, and muddled berries.
- Experiment with mocktails! There are many great brands of nonalcoholic cocktails cropping up, like Ghia and Seedlip.
- Dilute cocktails with sparkling water!
- Space out your last drink from bedtime by at least a few hours to minimize sleep disruption.

Understand that alcohol is a highly addictive and toxic substance that is normalized due to industry-influenced marketing and policy. If you choose to drink, choose your sources and timing wisely and limit it to a few drinks per month. Limiting exposure will diminish cravings for it.

2. Refined Industrial Vegetable and Seed Oils

When I was visiting my dad recently, I scanned the refrigerator. He had just made a trip to Whole Foods, and his fridge was stocked with organic items. At the front of the fridge was a bottle of Organic Almond Creamer. Looking at the nutrition label, I wasn't surprised: the second ingredient was refined sugar, and the third was canola oil, a refined seed oil. Next to this was organic hummus, and the third ingredient listed was canola oil.

My dad's house is full of health books. He makes a huge effort to eat healthily. He grows vegetables. But even with the best intentions—from the organic hummus to the artisanal almond milk—refined seed oils are a primary ingredient. Today, almost everyone is falling victim to hidden inflammatory oils and it is wrecking our health.

These industrially refined seed and vegetable oils include canola, corn, sunflower, soybean, grapeseed, safflower, peanut, and cottonseed. Look at almost any packaged food label from a large processed-food retailer, and you'll almost certainly see one of them.

The case against these refined vegetable and seed oils is very simple. These oils are extremely high in omega-6 fats, which skews our omega-6 to omega-3 ratio and increases inflammation in the body.

Since seed oils are cheaper to produce because of Farm Bill subsidies, they have taken market share in the American diet over fats that humans have relied on for thousands of years—such as olive oil, avocado oil, coconut oil, and animal-based fats (like butter, tallow, or ghee)—which are simply pressed from the flesh of a plant or rendered from the animal. Creating seed oils, on the other hand, requires intensive industrial processes and often involves extraction with chemical solvents like hexane, heating to over 150°F, bleaching, and dewaxing. (Watch a video of canola oil production to lose your appetite.)

Since 1909, our consumption of soybean oil (the most popular seed oil) has increased by a thousand times. Today, soybean oil is the largest source of calories for people in the United States—more so than beef, pork, and vegetables. Our soybean oil consumption, along with our following of the disastrous 1990s guidance to reduce fat in favor of refined carbohydrates, has robbed our diet of a key anti-inflammatory food (omega-3 fats) and substituted it with inflammatory oils and sugar.

3. Refined Grains

A "whole grain" is a type of grain that has all of its main parts: bran, germ, and endosperm. A corn kernel, an individual grain of brown rice, and a wheat berry are examples of whole grains, as no part of the whole grain has been removed. The bran is the outermost layer of the kernel and is generally rich in fiber, B vitamins, and minerals. The germ is the small, nutrient-dense part of the kernel that contains fat and micronutrients. Inside the bran is the endosperm, which is the majority of the kernel and contains the most starch. If you imagine a kernel as an egg, the bran is the shell, the germ is the yolk, and the endosperm is the egg white. Crush a whole grain and use it for making a product like bread and you get a "whole grain" processed item. But refining a whole grain to remove the bran and germ (leaving just the starchy endosperm), and you're in ultra-processed, dangerous territory. This is done because it can give the final product a chewier, fluffier texture (by removing the fibrous bran) and increases shelf life (by removing the germ, which contains fat that can go rancid). Since most of the vitamins are removed when the bran is removed, manufacturers will often "enrich" a refined grain product with synthetic versions of vitamins and minerals. As fiber is removed with the bran during refining, manufacturers may also add back in refined fiber products like inulin and pectin.

Ultra-processed grains are bad for health for many reasons. Without natural fiber, endosperm-predominant preprocessed carbohydrates are more rapidly absorbed into the bloodstream from the gut, which leads to increased blood glucose levels soon after eating. Fiber slows digestion and contributes to more stable blood sugar, while also supporting the health of the microbiome. Consuming refined grains can lead to a diet low in important nutrients and high in empty calories. They also are almost invariably conventionally grown with heavy pesticide use. In addition, many highly processed grain-based products are high in added sugars and unhealthy fats, as these often get combined in ultra-processed foods.

Research in over one hundred thousand adults followed for an average of 9.4 years showed that people who consumed the highest amount of refined grains (more than 350 grams per day) had a 27 percent higher risk of death and 33 percent higher risk of cardiovascular events (such as heart attack or stroke) when compared with those who ate the lowest intake of ultra-processed grains (less than 50 grams per day). To put it into perspective, 350 grams per day or more equates to about a serving of Cheerios (39 grams), two slices of bread (70 grams), a handful of pretzels (30 grams), cooked pasta (110 grams), and a Starbucks chocolate chip cookie (80 grams). You want to aim for *zero* grams of refined grains per day. The body does not need them, and they are damaging. I do not recommend whole grains either (brown rice, oatmeal, etc.), but they do have more nutritional value than refined grains.

Instead, choose alternatives made with nut flours or, better yet, swap for whole food substitutes. For example, make chia pudding instead of eating cereal, use butter lettuce leaves instead of tortillas for your tacos, and choose cauliflower rice instead of rice.

The following is a list of some easy and delicious grain alternatives:

REFINED GRAIN PRODUCT	GOOD ENERGY SWAP
White bread	• Bread made from nut flours (like almond) or coconut flour • Sweet potatoes cut lengthwise and baked can make a bread alternative • Coconut Flour Flatbread (recipe on page 325)
Flour tortillas or taco shells	• Seaweed sheets (nori) • Butter lettuce wraps • Collard green wraps • Jicama wraps (e.g., Trader Joe's) • Egg wraps (e.g., Crepini Organic Petit Egg Wraps with Cauliflower) • Lentil wraps (e.g., 2-Ingredient Lentil Wraps from ElaVegan.com) • Flax wraps (e.g., Flaxseed Wraps from SweetAsHoney.co) • Spinach-Chickpea Wraps (recipe on page 312)
White rice	• Cauliflower rice (buy frozen, or pulse cauliflower florets in food processor until rice-like; see recipe on page 354) • Broccoli rice (buy frozen, or pulse broccoli stems in food processor until rice-like) • Shirataki rice, made from high-fiber konjac root (e.g., Miracle Noodle brand) • Sweet potato rice (pulse sweet potato in food processor until rice-like)

REFINED GRAIN PRODUCT	GOOD ENERGY SWAP
Pasta	• Zucchini noodles • Sweet potato noodles • Beet noodles • Parsnip noodles • Note: the four noodles above are made with an inexpensive spiralizer device that I highly recommend purchasing to make a range of healthy noodles from vegetables. • Spaghetti squash (roast and scrape out squash flesh with a fork for noodle-like consistency) • Chickpea pasta • Lupini bean pasta (e.g., Kaizen Food brand) • Lentil pasta • Black bean pasta • Hearts of palm pasta (e.g., Trader Joe's, Palmini, and Thrive Market all make this type of pasta) • Konjac root pasta (also sometimes called miracle noodles or shirataki noodles; e.g., Thrive Market brand or nuPasta) • Kelp noodles (e.g., Sea Tangle Noodle Company)
Pizza crust	• Cauliflower crust (e.g., Cali'flour Foods) • Almond flour crust • Coconut flour crust • Pizza "bites" made with sliced eggplant • Sweet potato crust (e.g., Sweet Potato Pizza Crust from thebigmansworld.com)
Cakes, cookies, pastries	• Alternatives made with nut flours
Cereal or instant oatmeal	• Chia seed or basil seed pudding • Grain-free granola made with nuts and seeds • No-oat oatmeal made with nuts, seeds, and coconut flakes

By avoiding added sugar, industrial seed and vegetable oils, and processed grains, you avoid almost every ultra-processed food. And by doing this, you also avoid the innumerable additives in ultra-processed foods that directly damage us, like synthetic or ultra-processed preservatives, flavorings, emulsifiers, and colorings. Many of the additives in American ultra-processed foods are outlawed for use in other countries. For instance, potassium bromate, a dough conditioner in hundreds of types of baked goods, causes cancer ("*strongly* carcinogenic") in animals and is "possibly carcinogenic" to humans. In cells, it leads to free radical-based oxidative damage to DNA and fats and leads to mutations and breaks in the genome. Food coloring Red 40 is a synthetic food dye made from petroleum that is thought to induce neurotoxic effects through contributing to oxidative stress in the brain. It, along with the several other artificial food colorings on the market, are manufactured in processes that include many toxic chemicals like formaldehyde and have been shown to be contaminated with cancer-causing substances like benzidine. Red 40 alone has been linked to aggressive behavior in children, autism, and ADHD, and is thought to "aggravate mental health problems." Foods that incorporate Red 40 include Skittles, Fruit Punch Gatorade, Jell-O, Duncan Hines Butter Golden cake mix, Betty Crocker strawberry icing, Flamin' Hot Cheetos, Takis, and hundreds of other ultra-processed foods. Never eat food with "Red," "Blue," or "Yellow" in the ingredient list. There are so many natural alternatives for colors, like organic beet powder for red color, spirulina for blue color, or turmeric for yellow. Other common additives like titanium dioxide, brominated vegetable oil (BVO), propylparaben, acesulfame potassium, and many others are known to be directly damaging to cellular health, many through their impact on oxidative stress and mitochondrial dysfunction.

MANAGING GLUCOSE THROUGH DIET FOR GOOD ENERGY

We've covered five elements that are necessary to build a meal and dietary pattern that will help you build and maintain a body that is capable of making Good Energy. We've also covered three food categories to avoid. But there's an additional layer to explore, which is specifically focused on eating *strategies* to stabilize blood sugar day to day. These strategies serve to keep balance and optimal function throughout the body. As we learned in Part 1, erratic glucose levels are a big problem for our health and are one of the key negative outcomes of eating ultra-processed foods. Glucose levels that are increasingly variable over time are an indication that the body has lost "glucose tolerance," meaning that it is becoming insulin resistant and has Bad Energy. As we know, insulin resistance can result from all the factors that lead to Bad Energy outlined in Chapter 1, and of those factors, chronic overnutrition is largely reflected in the huge swings in glucose we can experience after eating foods with added sugars and processed grains.

Erratic, variable blood glucose is *both a cause and an effect* of Bad Energy. It is a *cause*, because overwhelming the body with huge influxes of glucose gums up the system and creates metabolic stress on the cell and mitochondria that leads to oxidative stress, mitochondrial damage, and resultant chronic inflammation. And as we learned, another extremely problematic feature of high glucose levels in the bloodstream is that high concentration of sugar sticks to things and causes dysfunction: glycation.

Erratic, variable glucose is also an *effect* of Bad Energy. *Any* process (like chronic stress, environmental toxin exposure, and sleep deprivation) that generates oxidative stress, chronic inflammation, and mitochondrial dysfunction contributes to insulin resistance and Bad Energy, which can then make the body less able to handle *any* level of incoming glucose from diet.

As a cause of Bad Energy, excess blood sugar exposure is one we need to dig into. The glucose levels in our diet are downright astronomical and one of the strongest levers in generating Bad Energy. Glucose is the only biomarker we can track in real time, letting us finely tune our exposures for the benefit of our health. Between refined sugars and refined grains and high starch foods (which turn directly into sugar), 42 percent of our calories are coming from foods that convert directly to sugar.

I cannot overstate how unprecedented this is—those calories are giving the body nothing of what it *actually* needs to function, so no wonder we have insatiable cravings and are so hungry. Imagine this: 42 percent of the seventy tons of food we are consuming in our lifetimes is *not* useful for building a healthy body or signaling for healthy cellular function. These useless foods are poisoning our microbiome and overwhelming our mitochondria, leading our cells to fill with fat and develop insulin resistance. The result is that glucose builds up in our bloodstream, wreaking havoc both inside and outside the cells. And, of course, the worst result of all: those overwhelmed mitochondria can't do their work, so we don't effectively make the energy to power our cells, so we get cellular dysfunction, leading to diseases of all kinds. Learning to eat for stable blood sugar is of paramount importance.

The following are nine strategies to keep post-meal blood sugar levels under better control:

1. **Don't Eat "Naked Carbohydrates":** Naked carbohydrates are carbohydrate-predominant foods that are eaten alone, like a banana (of which 92 percent of calories are from carbohydrates) or other fruits. Pair these carb-rich foods with healthy protein, fats, and/or fiber to slow digestion, increase satiety, and reduce the influx of glucose in the bloodstream. For instance, research shows that eating 3 ounces of almonds with a carb-heavy meal could significantly lower the post-meal glucose elevation.

2. **Sequence Meals for Optimal Metabolism by "Preloading" with Low-Glycemic Foods:** Eat non-starchy vegetables, fat, protein, and/or fiber before the higher carbohydrate part of a meal to lower post-meal glucose spikes. Unlike nearly every restaurant suggests, you should *avoid* bread and chips before your meal. This will spike your blood sugar, which can lead to *increased hunger*. In one study, consumption of about 20 grams of protein and 20 grams of fat about thirty minutes before eating carbohydrates significantly decreased post-meal glucose elevation in both nondiabetic and insulin-resistant individuals. Try these simple ways to preload meals:

   - Always order a salad filled with greens and some protein (egg, chicken, cheese) before eating a starchy entrée. Make sure the dressing has no sugar.
   - Ask the waiter *not* to bring bread or chips before a meal.
   - If your plate includes a starch (e.g., potato or pasta), protein (e.g., chicken or fish), and vegetable, start with the vegetable, then eat the protein, and then end with the starch.
   - Eat a handful of nuts, a hard-boiled egg, or some chopped veggies about a half hour before sitting down to a meal or going to an event.

3. **Eat Earlier:** Amazingly, the exact same meal will likely cause a lower glucose spike if it's eaten in the morning instead of late at night. Our

bodies are naturally more insulin resistant at night, so in a sense we get "more bang for the buck" by eating carbohydrates earlier in the day, when we can process them better. A study in the *British Journal of Nutrition* with healthy, normal-weight participants wearing CGMs showed that eating high-glycemic food later in the evening will cause a significant increase in both insulin and glucose levels compared with eating the exact same meal earlier in the day. In this study, evening meals were consumed at 8:30 p.m., and morning meals were consumed at 9:30 a.m. Avoid high-glycemic meals and desserts at night.

4. **Tighten the Eating Window:** Eating in a narrower window during the day leads to lower glucose and insulin spikes compared to eating the exact same amount of food spread out over a longer period of the day. Time-restricted feeding (TRF) involves eating all your food and calories for the day in a limited window. A 2019 study in *Nutrients* showed that when eleven overweight, nondiabetic individuals practiced TRF for just four days, where all calories were eaten in a six-hour window, they significantly lowered fasting glucose, fasting insulin, post-meal glucose peaks, and mean glucose levels compared to when they ate the *exact* same food over a longer, twelve-hour window. To put TRF into practice, start by trying to limit the time when you eat to twelve hours (e.g., 8:00 a.m. to 8:00 p.m.), and then tighten the window to ten hours (e.g., 8:00 a.m. to 6:00 p.m.) and eventually to eight hours (e.g., 10:00 a.m. to 6:00 p.m.). As your body becomes more metabolically efficient through Good Energy living, TRF becomes easier because your body becomes more adept at processing stored fat for energy.

5. **Avoid Consuming Liquid Sugar:** Any sugar that is delivered to the GI tract in liquid form will be absorbed fast, potentially causing glucose spikes. Liquid sugar sources include soda, juice, and drinks with added sugars like Frappuccinos, sweet tea, and the many alcoholic beverages that contain sugar. One exception is a well-balanced blended smoothie, filled with vegetables, fat, low-glycemic fruits, and protein. These types of smoothies can often be consumed without an appreciable glucose rise, based on Levels data. See pages 309–10 for recipes.

How About Artificial Sweeteners or Natural Nonnutritive Sweeteners?

- Research has found that consuming artificial sweeteners, such as aspartame (Equal), sucralose (Splenda), and saccharin (Sweet'N Low), can lead to higher weight, microbiome disturbance, and alteration of GI hormone levels, and they can cause insulin release. Avoid these completely.
- Natural nonnutritive sweeteners like allulose, monk fruit, and stevia, as well as sugar alcohols like erythritol, are all better options than sugar or artificial sweeteners. However, these natural sweeteners can still trigger the reward pathways in the brain that drive cravings for sugar. They can also cause bloating and other GI symptoms (especially sugar alcohols). Use them sparingly, and wean to none over time.

6. **Add Fiber to All Meals:** Fiber slows digestion, promotes microbiome health, and lowers post-meal glucose rises. A study in *Diabetes Care* of eighteen individuals with type 2 diabetes looked at the differences in metabolic markers between four weeks of a higher-fiber, lower-glycemic-load diet as compared with four weeks of a lower-carbohydrate, higher-fat diet. They found that on the higher-fiber diet, the participants experienced a significant drop in LDL cholesterol, post-meal glucose levels, and post-meal insulin levels, as well as blood triglycerides three hours after lunch. This study's fiber sources included legumes, vegetables, fruit, and whole grains. Other good sources of fiber include chia seeds, flaxseeds, other nuts or seeds, avocados, beans, high-fiber fruits or vegetables, lentils, and tahini. Aim for at least 50 grams of fiber per day.

7. **Use Food Adjuncts, Like Vinegar and Cinnamon, to Lower Glucose Responses:** Apple cider vinegar is known to have a glucose-lowering effect when taken before or with a meal, and the effect can be pronounced, with some studies showing a 50 percent reduction in post-meal glucose in healthy individuals. There are several ideas of why this happens,

including the possible impact of vinegar on slowing how fast the stomach empties food, thereby making you feel fuller longer. Additionally, vinegar may modulate the activity of insulin, allowing for improved insulin sensitivity and glucose uptake. In cell culture studies, the acetic acid in vinegar may also suppress the activity of a class of gut enzymes called disaccharidases, which break down sugars for digestion, thereby lowering the total sugar absorbed from food. Just two teaspoons of vinegar have been shown to reduce post-meal glucose levels by 23 percent when eaten with a meal of complex carbohydrates; but of note, this effect was negated for consumption of simple sugars (which include dextrose, glucose, and fructose), presumably since these are not processed by disaccharidases that can be potentially inhibited by vinegar.

Similar to vinegar, cinnamon may improve glucose levels and insulin sensitivity in people with and without type 2 diabetes. Natural compounds in cinnamon, including methylhydroxychalcone polymer (MHCP) and hydrocinnamic acid, may mimic insulin's activity or enhance insulin receptor activity and contribute to glucose being taken into cells and packaged into a healthy storage form called glycogen. Cinnamon is rich in plant chemicals that reduce oxidative stress, which may also contribute to its metabolic benefits. A study of forty-one healthy adults randomized participants to consume 1 gram, 3 grams, or 6 grams of cinnamon mixed with food for forty days. All doses of cinnamon led to a drop in the post-meal glucose levels, but this was largest for those taking 6 grams, for whom post-meal glucose levels dropped around 13 percent, from a post-meal mean of 106 mg/dL on day one to 92 mg/dL on day forty.

8. **Walk for at Least Fifteen Minutes After Meals:** This simple step can reduce the glucose impact of your meal by up to 30 percent and is an unbelievably high-yield habit to incorporate after as many meals as you can.

9. **Eat Mindfully and with Gratitude:** Research has shown that by addressing mealtime behaviors and thought patterns while eating, it can change

the metabolic response to food. Mealtime behaviors like paying attention to the sensory and spiritual dimension of food, paying attention to the dining atmosphere, and awareness of emotional eating have been shown to be part of plans that lower hemoglobin A1c levels over twelve weeks in patients with type 2 diabetes. Additionally, research has shown that eating your meals faster is associated with a significantly increased risk of type 2 diabetes, with one study showing a twofold increase in risk for type 2 diabetes among those who eat faster and another showing that incidence rates of metabolic syndrome among fast eaters were over four times higher than for slow eaters! The proposed reason for this is because speedy eating may cause you to consume more calories before feeling full. It's astonishing to think that just slowing down and appreciating the spiritual dimension of food could impact blood sugar, but research suggests that it can.

———————

The pathway to Good Energy starts with your fork. The journey begins by simply putting more of the helpful molecular information on this utensil. The transition to an ultra-processed diet over the last hundred years has been disastrous for our physical and mental health, and our journey to Good Energy moves us away from an ultra-processed diet toward whole, unprocessed, nutrient-rich foods grown in thriving, healthy soil. But food is not the only unprecedented threat our cells are facing, and the following chapters will explore other factors to be aware of.

Recap: Creating a Good Energy Meal

Good Energy Foods:

1. Micronutrients and antioxidants (see pages 157–62 for comprehensive lists)
2. Omega-3 fatty acids (see pages 163–64 for top foods)
3. Fiber (see page 165 for top foods)

4. Fermented foods (see pages 167–68 for top foods)

5. Protein (see page 169 for top foods)

Bad Energy Foods:

1. Refined added sugar

2. Refined industrial vegetable and seed oils

3. Refined grains

To view the scientific references cited in this chapter, please visit us online at caseymeans.com/goodenergy.

CHAPTER 7

Respecting Your Biological Clock

Light, Sleep, and Meal Timing

Empty bags of blood were already covering the operating room floor as I walked in.

I was in my second year of residency, and I was "on call," meaning that I was the only ENT surgeon awake covering three major hospitals for all issues related to my specialty. I had already been up for twenty-four hours and was trying to sneak a couple of minutes of rest in the break room when my pager went off.

At least fourteen doctors and nurses were running around the operating room in a frenzy as I came in. A woman's neck was splayed open on the table, and multiple trauma surgery residents were trying to stymie bleeding with their hands and clamps. She had been stabbed numerous times in the neck while at home, and her arteries were gushing blood. The attending trauma surgeon asked me to scrub in and help her explore the neck. I put on surgical gear and prepared to assist.

Within minutes, I was fishing through the gashes in the woman's neck, looking for any significant tears of vessels that could be repaired. I was immersed in this task for minutes until I looked up to realize that others in the room had stopped and were stepping away from the body. The patient was dead. Looking at the raw, tattered, exposed skin on the neck from the stab wounds, I envisioned what had happened to this woman less than an hour before: the violence, the anger, the fear, the screaming, the blood, the sharpness of the knife.

I considered myself an extremely empathetic person. I had been honored with the Gold Humanism Award at Stanford, my house was littered with personal development books, and I was nicknamed the "peacemaker" in my family. But during that moment, my most pressing thought was the need to go to sleep.

I called my supervising physician to alert him to the situation. He quickly cut me off and barked, "Are you seriously waking me up to tell me about a dead person?" and hung up. I was stunned at the time, but in retrospect, his response was understandable: this man was getting woken every night by residents, still had a full operating room schedule every day, and was similarly desperate for sleep, even thirty years into the job.

By my fifth year, when I was a chief resident, I looked back on my time in residency as if it were a blur. For most days, I stood in a windowless operating room, stealing sporadic sleep when I could find small breaks and shoving packaged food into my mouth at all hours of the day and night. I later learned that sustained disruptions to the ingrained sleep needs of our bodies result in measurable brain damage, emotional dysregulation, metabolic issues, and even memory deficits.

My residency years are an extreme case. But, in similar ways, our modern, Western, technology-driven culture distorts our natural schedules—our circadian rhythms. We no longer sleep or eat at times and with patterns in line with how our cells are biologically programmed to thrive. These changes to a natural schedule of eating and sleeping represent a profound contributor to Bad Energy.

In the past hundred years, average sleep duration has decreased 25 percent. Until several thousand years ago, humans spent most of their lives outside or in exposed shelters—there was no true "indoors." We've only had artificial light for about 0.04 percent of human history. Today, modern education and work environments expect kids and adults to sit at desks in sealed rooms with limited sunlight for most of the day. Then we go back to our homes, where we largely remain indoors. Sadly, in the modern world, a successful life looks like living inside a box, working inside a box, staring at lighted boxes, and being buried in a box. We are largely separated from our life-giving forces: the sun and the earth.

I'm not suggesting we go back to prehistoric times and ban artificial light, homes, or digital technology. But I think society should step back and appreciate how new and biologically disruptive these inventions are and how closely they are linked to our profound rates of mental and physical dysfunction rooted in Bad Energy.

Over millions of years, we have developed very complex chronobiology—a pattern of biological activity based on time—that has been coded into our cells through features like "clock genes" and specialized brain regions responsive to light. While our cells have their own internal clocks, they must synchronize with external light cues to make sure things stay on track. The two main external synchronizing cues are the timing of exposure to light and the timing of exposure to food. Our chronobiology sets off the dominoes each day of when we should wake up, when we should eat, when we will best metabolize food, when we release hormones, how our genes are expressed, and when we should sleep.

Humans are *diurnal* animals, meaning that our biology is set for activity and feeding when it is light out, and for sleeping and fasting during the dark. Plenty of *noct*urnal animals have flipped biology (in which they are active at night and sleep during sunlight). But that's not us. In our modern world, however, we have completely desynchronized our behavior from our chronobiology. We now eat late and flood our eyes with artificial light late into the night. To the trillions of cells expecting one set of activities at a certain time but experiencing another, this is mass cellular confusion. And it manifests as the symptoms and diseases many of us suffer from today.

Research shows clearly that our modern erratic sleep schedules, light exposure, and eating schedules directly lead to mitochondrial dysfunction, oxidative stress, and chronic inflammation—the three hallmarks of Bad Energy.

Today, most people—and even most doctors—go through life without deeply considering their circadian rhythm. But step back and think about how little sense this makes. If the battery of an electric car can run for four hundred miles and requires eight hours to fully charge, you operate the machine within those parameters. If you instead charge the car for six hours and expect it to travel seven hundred miles, you'll be sorely disappointed at its output. What's happening to our cells is that simple. We have decimated the schedule that the stunning machines of our bodies are encoded to run on. Then we throw up our hands in confusion as to why so many people experience fatigue, insomnia, brain fog, sluggishness, or anxiety. So we reach for the prescription pad to "treat" these conditions, further disrupting our circadian rhythm.

Of course, we've all heard the perfunctory calls for getting enough sleep, but understanding the *why* is necessary for long-term behavior change. And shockingly, we rarely ever hear about how getting direct sunlight into our eyes at the right times is profoundly important for metabolic and overall health, despite masses of research that shows this. Most of what we hear about the sun is that we should *avoid* it, to our huge detriment. Nobody should go through life without understanding the schedule our cells are wired for and how profoundly important this is for our energy regulation.

And this understanding comes down to three interconnected factors: sunlight, sleep, and when we eat.

WE ARE MADE OF SUNLIGHT

This isn't a metaphor. Almost all energy we consume from food comes directly from the sun. For most of us, *photosynthesis* is a term we learned in middle school and promptly forgot. But remember this miraculous fact: the energy transferred from the sun—traveling ninety-two million miles through space—is stored in the chemical bonds of glucose molecules generated in plants. Even if you stick to a more carnivorous diet, many animals we eat are herbivores, so most of the energy we receive from food can be traced to the sun. It's our life source.

Let's also not forget that photosynthesis creates oxygen, which every cell in our body needs to create energy.

The reason we have life on Earth is because of the sun. That we aren't taught about the three key ways it is crucial to our body's functioning is a shameful medical blind spot.

Turning the Machine On

Since the dawn of the simplest life-forms, a regular pattern of sunlight and darkness has been a consistent environmental stimulus driving our biology. Human cells are encoded to be on a twenty-four-hour sleep-wake cycle, entrained to function in two separate modes: activity-feeding mode during sunlight, followed by resting-starvation mode during darkness. The biology of these two phases is very different, with different genetic expression, metabolism, and hormonal activity. Light exposure dictates which phase we're in. Giving the body mixed signals with erratic or irregular light and dark exposure leads to dysfunction and disease.

Sun entering our eyes is the body's "on" switch. The amount of light a human is exposed to outside on a clear day is a hundred times more than the amount inside with artificial light. Even sitting under a shaded tree, a human is exposed to over ten times or more light than when sitting inside with artificial light. One study showed that lux—a measure of light intensity—is generally lower than 100 indoors and can be higher than 100,000 outdoors. Despite the transparency of windows, glass is still a physical barrier to photons reaching your eyeballs and key information getting to your cells. Just as food is molecular information that dictates how cells function, light can be thought of as energetic information that dictates to the body what time it is and therefore how the cells should function. Modern children now spend only about one to two hours experiencing light intensities greater than 1,000 lux, an unnatural travesty contributing to metabolic disease, obesity, vision problems (which have risen dramatically in recent decades), and more. Unsurprisingly, the amount of time spent outdoors confers significant protection against being overweight and developing chronic diseases.

When light hits the photoreceptors in our eyes, it triggers an electrical impulse sent along from one cell to the next. These reactions lead to the brain's suprachiasmatic nucleus (SCN), which is a master conductor of our body's many functions. The little three-millimeter holes in the skull that the optic nerves travel through are the primary way our body knows what time it is. These optic nerves are just waiting to transmit that light signal to turn "on" the body's proper biology in the morning. But modern living largely prevents us from spending much time outdoors in the morning.

While the SCN—and nearly every cell in the body—has its own internal twenty-four-hour pattern of activity, light "synchronizes" our internal cellular clocks, confirming the time and orchestrating the release of the hormonal and genetic processes that are responsible for all aspects of our biological activity. These activities include energy production, melatonin release, digestion and hunger, and stress hormones.

"Irregular photic signals"—meaning experiencing light during naturally dark times or being indoors when it is light outside—can profoundly disturb our metabolism and increase the risk for all sorts of Bad Energy diseases.

More light in the morning and less at night signals to the SCN what time of day it is and sets our bodies up to time genetic and hormonal signals appropriately. Simply put: a key way that you regulate your hormones, metabolism, weight, and risk for disease is by *showing* your cells what time it is by exposing your eyeballs to direct sunlight throughout the light part of the day and by hiding your eyeballs from as much light as possible when the sun is down.

Directing Energy

Experts studying sleep and diabetes have been aware since the 1960s that insulin sensitivity and glucose tolerance undergo a rhythmic cycle throughout the day. This phenomenon is believed to be caused by the influence of melatonin, a hormone that is secreted by the brain during darkness and induces drowsiness, on insulin sensitivity.

Studies suggest exposure to bright light during the day is also crucial for maintaining insulin sensitivity. In a study conducted in Brazil, obese women who received bright light therapy three times a week for five months after daytime exercise experienced a notable reduction in insulin resistance and fat mass compared to women who did the same workouts but did not receive light exposure.

Moreover, scientists from the University of Geneva discovered that even minor changes in light exposure (such as an hour of light exposure in the middle of the dark cycle or light deprivation for two days) can have a significant impact on insulin resistance. This finding may help explain why people who are exposed to light at inappropriate times are more likely to develop metabolic disorders like diabetes.

Sunny Mood

Sunlight has been found to have an impact on mood, which is interconnected with our metabolic health. Decreased sun exposure has been known to trigger depression in some individuals, while in others, the mood changes may be more subtle. Research has established a connection between reduced sunlight exposure and lower levels of serotonin, which regulates our mood. There is also a correlation between more exposure to natural light and higher levels of serotonin. This could be attributed to the fact that natural light enhances serotonin-1A receptor binding in the brain and can potentially stimulate serotonin production in the skin. Studies also suggest that increased serotonin signaling can reduce appetite and improve glucose control.

SLEEP

Want to kill a puppy? Subject it to sleep deprivation for just nine days.

Want to give yourself prediabetes? Reduce sleep to four hours a night for just six days.

Every time you skimp on the quantity, quality, or consistency of sleep, you inch toward the grave—and toward metabolic symptoms and diseases— by generating oxidative stress, mitochondrial dysfunction, chronic inflammation, plus a big helping of microbiome dysfunction. You could eat a perfect "Good Energy" diet, but if you don't sleep, your cells will spew out excess free radicals, send out danger signals, recruit the immune system, struggle to make energy, and become insulin resistant. Lack of quality sleep is a profound "danger" signal to the body, throwing off proper metabolism and promoting fat storage.

Lack of sleep also creates a vicious cycle. Once you develop Bad Energy—from any constellation of the many contributors (food, sleep, stress, being sedentary, toxins, etc.)—it has a negative impact on your ability to *get* good sleep. People with metabolic diseases have more trouble with sleep, worsening their conditions. You must break this cycle for a symptom-free life, and society—to have a healthy and well-functioning culture—needs to overcome the modern pervasive phenomena of poor sleep. Sleep-deprived cells are engines of Bad Energy.

Looking specifically at Bad Energy processes, we see that sleep affects all of them.

- **Mitochondrial Dysfunction:** A study of chronic sleep deprivation in mice, where mice could rest for four hours per twenty-four-hour period over four months, deliberated that "the structure of mitochondria was *destroyed* by long-term sleep deprivation." Electron microscopy images of the healthy versus sleep-deprived mitochondria in the paper show that the latter look like comical misshapen blobs compared to the healthy version. "Destroyed mitochondria," unsurprisingly, rapidly led to heart failure in mice because an underpowered heart muscle will fail. What's more, additional research in mice shows a significant decrease in the activity of the mitochondrial electron transport chain—the key final steps in making ATP—after seventy-two hours of sleep deprivation.

- **Oxidative Stress:** Sleep deprivation has been shown to increase free radicals and subsequent oxidative stress all over the body, including in the liver, gut, lungs, muscles, brain, and heart. In a recent paper from the premier medical journal *Cell*, sleep deprivation in animal models led to a significant accumulation of damaging free radicals in the GI tract, associated with early death. Free radical accumulation gradually increases with each day of sleep deprivation and gradually decreases after stopping deprivation. Since reactive oxygen species are a natural by-product of metabolic processes, researchers have hypothesized that one of the key functions of sleep is to help neutralize free radicals accumulated during the day.

- **Chronic Inflammation:** Even modest sleep restriction—from eight hours to six hours per night for a week in a laboratory setting—can significantly increase pro-inflammatory chemicals in the blood, including IL-6 and TNF-α, both of which are the body's danger signals that are known to induce insulin resistance.

What's more, gene expression studies in mice show that chronic sleep deprivation increases the expression of 240 genes and decreases the expression of 259 genes, and many of these are related to metabolism.

Amazingly, sleep deprivation can profoundly alter microbiome composition, and researchers think that the impact of this dysbiosis is part of what mediates the Bad Energy hallmarks, like chronic inflammation. In a lab, you can deprive a mouse of sleep and then transfer that mouse's microbiome to a mouse that isn't sleep deprived and doesn't have a microbiome, and the latter mouse will develop chronic inflammation throughout the body and in the brain, as well as cognitive impairment.

In humans, a tight link between sleep deprivation, gut dysfunction, and oxidative stress exists. In a survey of hundreds of college students, almost 90 percent slept fewer than seven hours per night, and 42 percent suffered from bowel disorders. In these students, sleep restriction decreased the gut bacteria that produce the SCFA butyrate that we learned about in Chapter 5, which serves as fuel for gut cells, impacts the expression of genes involved in energy metabolism, and positively regulates mitochondrial function. Remember, a healthy and strong gut barrier is protective against chronic inflammation by preventing foreign substances from leaking through the gut lining. The intestinal microbiome is acutely sensitive to a lack of sleep and may be responsible for fueling the Bad Energy fire that leads to many of the consequences of sleep deprivation. We need to sleep not only for ourselves but also for our microbiome!

Additionally, we've learned that chronic overnutrition is a key driver of Bad Energy, and sleeping too little will vastly increase your likelihood of overeating by altering hunger and satiety hormones. In one study, twelve healthy young men who had their sleep restricted for two days had an elevation in the hunger hormone ghrelin and a decrease in the satiety hormone leptin. They also reported increased hunger and appetite, especially for calorie-dense, high-carbohydrate foods. Other research has shown that experimental limitation of sleep will induce a significant increase in the consumption of protein, fat, and overall calories, plus weight gain, and abdominal fat increases. To protect against the urge for overfeeding and hunger: sleep.

Today, you often hear medical leaders say the causes for the increase in obesity are "complicated." This infuriates me. The main causes are straightforward: the explosion of highly processed food coupled with the systematic erosion of healthy sleep, which causes the dysregulation of hormones, making us want to eat more.

We wonder why we feel terrible after not sleeping well for just one night, and hopefully, this section helps flesh it out: it's like putting a bomb inside your cells.

Obstructive Sleep Apnea

Close to a billion people globally are estimated to be suffering from obstructive sleep apnea (OSA), a sleep-breathing disorder characterized by symptoms such as daytime sleepiness, nighttime snoring, and periods of obstructed breathing at night. Due to its impact on sleep quality and quantity, a diagnosis of OSA greatly increases risk of metabolic sequelae like heart disease, heart failure, arrythmias, type 2 diabetes, obesity, dementia, and stroke. In the other direction, obesity puts people at much higher risk of OSA, as excess tissue and weight in the neck, throat, lungs, and abdomen can all contribute to airway and breathing obstruction at night, and rates of OSA are increasing as overweight and obesity rates increase. Some research suggests OSA prevalence has increased by up to 55 percent from 1993 to 2013, in lockstep with rising rates of obesity. According to *JAMA*, "patients with mild OSA who gain 10% of their baseline weight are at a sixfold increased risk of progression of OSA, and an equivalent weight loss can result in more than 20% improvement in OSA severity." If you snore or have been told you stop breathing or choke at night, experience daytime sleepiness and fatigue, have disrupted sleep, or are having stagnating health progress, make sure to get tested for OSA. Weight loss can significantly reduce or eliminate OSA for many patients.

Light hitting the eyes is an "on" signal for many bodily processes. And exposure to dark prompts the release of melatonin in preparation for sleep, a time of fasting when metabolic activity shifts dramatically, with a 15 percent drop in metabolic rate and when we burn through stored fat and glucose for energy. During sleep, the brain undergoes changes in electrical activity and cerebral blood flow that support memory consolidation, cognitive function, and metabolism. Professor Matthew Walker has noted in his book *Why We Sleep* that the *Guinness Book of World Records* still recognizes "Most Motorcycles Driven over the Body While Lying on a Bed of Nails" but has stopped recognizing attempts to break the sleep deprivation record because these attempts are just too dangerous.

We are not made to go without regular, consistent sleep in a single time zone. And until the last split second of human evolution, we likely never did. Railroads were popularized just 120 years ago, air travel just 65 years ago. Our great-grandparents and everyone before them rarely traveled out of a time zone in their lives. And when the sun went down, they didn't have much else to do other than sleep.

We accept irregular and inconsistent sleep as a hallmark of modern life. But I don't think we appreciate that it is a completely new phenomenon. Almost half of all people in the United States say they feel sleepy during the day between three and seven days per week. And 35.2 percent of adults report sleeping on average for fewer than seven hours per night. As many as 30 percent of adults meet the definition of obstructive sleep apnea (OSA), a condition inextricably linked to insulin resistance as both cause and effect.

At sixteen hours of no sleep, the body begins experiencing mental and physiological deterioration. At nineteen hours of no sleep, a person is as cognitively impaired as someone with a blood alcohol level at the legal limit of .08 percent. It gets much worse from there, as I saw in hospitals.

Lack of sleep dramatically impairs cognitive ability. A University of Pennsylvania study showed that if participants experience four hours of sleep for six nights, they experience a 400 percent increase in the number of microsleeps they experience during the day. The study defines "microsleep" as a period of no conscious response or motor response during a task.

Most worrying is that the participants did not realize they were experiencing microsleeps when they were occurring.

Even more concerning is if that sleep-deprived person is controlling a knife deep inside your unconscious body. Research shows residents working thirty-six-hour shifts will commit 36 percent more serious medical errors and make 460 percent more diagnostic mistakes in the intensive care unit than a well-rested doctor. They will also be significantly less empathetic to patients' pain at the end of a twenty-six-hour shift. After a thirty-six-hour shift, a resident is 73 percent more likely to stab themselves with a needle or cut themselves with a scalpel. When a sleep-deprived resident finishes a long shift and gets in their car to go home, they are 168 percent more likely to be involved in a motor vehicle incident resulting from fatigue.

The fact that doctors are some of the most sleep-deprived and least knowledgeable people about sleep is a huge problem. Doctors receive, on average, seventeen minutes of education on childhood sleep and three hours total of sleep education across four years of medical school. You can assume your doctor knows virtually nothing about sleep, despite good sleep being one of the most effective tools in preventing and reversing diseases of all kinds. When a doctor pays lip service to "getting sleep" and sends you on your way, they aren't being direct enough. Every medical leader should be speaking urgently and plainly: every person should prioritize the quantity, quality, and consistency of sleep like their life depends on it.

Quantity

We need to get seven to eight hours a night of good-quality sleep for our bodies to be protected from Bad Energy physiology. Sleep deprivation almost immediately impacts our ability to make energy, with studies showing that sleep deprivation decreases ATP production in several brain regions in mice. No one wants a brain with less energy to run itself.

One study found healthy, normal-weight individuals who slept fewer than 6.5 hours per night had to produce 50 percent more insulin than normal sleepers to achieve similar glucose results—placing the short sleepers at significant risk of developing insulin resistance in the long term. Remember, prediabetes and type 2 diabetes *are* insulin resistance—a root of nearly every other chronic symptom and disease.

Just a couple of nights of low sleep can severely impact insulin sensitivity. In one study, eleven healthy young men were examined after being subjected to six nights of sleep deprivation, where they were limited to only four hours of sleep per night. Following the deprivation period, the participants were given a full week of twelve hours of sleep per night. This study showed that the participants experienced impaired metabolism and insulin resistance during the low-sleep period. In particular, their capacity to remove sugar from their bloodstream was 40 percent slower than when they were adequately rested. Interestingly, this relatively short six-night sleep deprivation period led to metabolic changes in the young men that made them exhibit glucose responses characteristic of prediabetes.

Cortisol (a key stress hormone) tells our body that something "stressful" is happening. It also partially controls the regulation of glucose and insulin. Unfortunately, in cases like chronic sleep deprivation or chronic psychological stress, chronic cortisol stimulation causes damage. Cortisol decreases insulin sensitivity, meaning cells are less likely to use glucose. When cells don't use glucose, it remains in circulation, elevating blood glucose levels and further fueling inflammation and glycation. Getting only four hours of sleep for six days can increase evening cortisol levels, which in turn can elevate blood sugar.

The research consistently points to the "magic number" of getting seven to eight hours of sleep. Warning signs blare if you average below seven hours per night. Interestingly, the risk for metabolic dysfunction increases if you average *more* than eight hours by disrupting your sleep-wake cycle.

Children are often subjected to truncated sleep resulting from early school start times. For them, the relationship between Bad Energy and sleep deprivation is especially distressing. This culturally sanctioned sleep deprivation sets kids up for a lifetime of metabolic illness. Several studies have shown that children who do not get sufficient sleep for their needs at a given age experience higher insulin levels, insulin resistance, higher fasting glucose, and higher BMI. What's more, the magnitude of short sleep for a young child has a linear relationship with the risk of obesity a few years later in childhood.

Quality

Minimally interrupted sleep is also a critical component of metabolic health. Reduced sleep quality is linked to Bad Energy conditions such as type 2 diabetes, obesity, heart disease, Alzheimer's disease, and stroke.

One study followed over two thousand adult men for eight years and found that subjects who reported difficulty maintaining sleep had a twofold to threefold higher risk of developing type 2 diabetes.

And in the short term, studies showed a link between sleep quality and the immediate ability to manage blood sugar efficiently the next day. In these studies, the better sleep quality a person had, the more likely they were (on average) to have a lower blood glucose response to breakfast the next morning, compared to those who had poorer sleep. Poor sleep quality, measured by sleep fragmentation, may affect glucose responses by changing cortisol and growth hormone levels, both of which have a strong impact on insulin sensitivity, metabolism, and glucose levels.

Sleep quality can also be assessed by the amount of time spent in deep and REM sleep, which are metabolically restorative for the body and are impacted by lifestyle factors like late meals, alcohol, late caffeine intake, and light at night. Recent research looking at cancer mortality, cardiovascular mortality, and all-cause mortality over twelve to twenty years showed that mortality was 13 percent higher for every 5 percent reduction in REM sleep. Based on this study, the threshold we really want to meet for lower risk is 15 percent or more REM sleep per night. But more is better. The lowest-risk individuals had more than 20 percent REM sleep.

Consistency

In recent years, I have been surprised to learn how keeping a consistent bedtime matters profoundly to our metabolic health. Our biology is set up for regular, consistent rhythm, so it's not too surprising, but the magnitude of the impact is.

Research has found that social jet lag of greater than two hours in people sixty years or younger yields an approximately twofold increased risk of metabolic syndrome and diabetes or prediabetes. Social jet lag is a measure of sleep consistency looking at the difference in bedtime and wake time between workdays and days off as measured by the "midpoint" of sleep. For example, if a person sleeps from 10:00 p.m. to 6:00 a.m. on weekdays, the midpoint of their sleep is 2:00 a.m. If they sleep from midnight to 10:00 a.m. on weekends, their midpoint is 5:00 a.m. This represents three hours of social jet lag, doubling the risk of metabolic disease. Almost half of U.S. adults report at least one hour of social jet lag. Similar associations are seen in night shift workers, who experience significantly higher rates of type 2 diabetes.

The impact of poor sleep consistency has also become clear through research on the health effects of daylight savings time (DST), where an entire population is forced to shift their sleep and wake time by one hour twice a year. Research has shown that these biyearly shifts are associated with increased heart attack, stroke, hospital admissions due to arrhythmias, missed medical appointments, emergency room visits, inflammatory markers, high blood pressure, car crashes, and mood disorders, as well as changes in gene expression, including in clock genes. The American Academy of Sleep Medicine has released a position statement advocating for getting rid of seasonal time changes, as this one-hour shift appears to "incur significant public health and safety risks" and "misalignment between the biological clock and the environmental clock."

We ignore the science of circadian clocks at a societal level, most disastrously when it comes to kids. During puberty, teens experience a shift in their circadian rhythms that causes them to naturally want to stay up later and sleep in longer. However, most schools still have start times that are very early in the morning, some before 8:00 a.m. This can be incredibly damaging to the metabolic health of teens, as research has shown that insufficient sleep can lead to insulin resistance, weight gain, and an increased risk of type 2 diabetes, and up to 45 percent of teens are getting inadequate sleep.

Studies have also shown that delaying school start times to match the natural circadian rhythms of teenagers can have significant benefits. A study published in the *Journal of Clinical Sleep Medicine* in 2017 proposed that when middle schools and high schools shifted their start times to 8:30 a.m. or later, students experienced improvements in sleep duration, daytime sleepiness, and academic performance.

Artificial Light

We've all heard that artificial light at night can disrupt our sleep, and the reason is that this light at unnatural times signals to your SCN and cells that it is daytime when it's not, confusing our deeply ingrained biological clock. Light at night is so strongly detrimental to our health that it is now considered an "environmental endocrine disruptor," meaning that it can *directly* alter hormone signaling, just as a medication or toxin could do. As a hormone disruptor, light can starkly alter melatonin production, increase inflammatory responses, and elevate circulating stress hormones. A study in the *International Journal of Obesity* showed that even when controlling for food intake, artificial light at night helps to explain about 70 percent of the excessive body mass prevalence among people worldwide. This sounds shocking until we think about how profoundly new and disruptive artificial light is to our biology, with this recent invention completely changing the secretion of several hormones in our bodies in the blink of an eye in 1806. That's when the first incandescent bulb was turned on. The advent of the first home TVs in 1938 and then computers in 1971 vastly exacerbated the issue.

Research has found that increased exposure to light late in the evening is associated with increases in insulin resistance and glucose levels, with one study linking higher light intensities at night to a 51 percent increase in type 2 diabetes in elderly subjects. What's more, research shows that being exposed to indoor room light of just 200 lux as opposed to dim light of less than 3 lux before bedtime causes later melatonin release onset by ninety minutes, and presleep levels of melatonin were reduced by 71.4 percent. Some of the known functions of melatonin include inducing sleep, suppressing cancer, supporting bone health, acting as an antioxidant, providing neuroprotection, protecting against mood disorders, and serving as an anti-inflammatory molecule. Melatonin is also involved in pathways related to healthy reproduction and egg quality. Given this, disrupting melatonin with excessive artificial light at night is a lifestyle factor to take seriously.

Even ambient light in our bedrooms has an effect. In one study of more than one hundred thousand women, exposure to light while sleeping was strongly associated with a higher BMI, higher waist circumference, and higher waist-to-hip ratio.

Meal Timing

Earlier in the chapter, we discussed how properly timed light exposure plays a key role in telling your brain's SCN what time it is, so it can set up the proper genetic, hormonal, and metabolic activity for the day. Another key signal for telling your cells what time it is involves *when* you eat. If we eat during the dark period of the twenty-four-hour cycle—when our physiology is biochemically ready to support rest and fasting—we experience a desynchronization of our metabolic processes, which increases the risk for metabolic problems. In animal studies, when mice are fed their normal diets but during the time when they're meant to be asleep, they rapidly gain weight. The misalignment between feeding time and the body's natural circadian cycles induces glucose intolerance, altered gene expression, and weight gain.

Human circadian biology primes us to be more insulin sensitive and generate more heat from metabolizing food in the morning instead of the evening. Overall, research suggests that we do much better by front-loading the day with food—especially higher carbohydrate foods—and stopping eating as early as possible in the evening. One study showed that eating food later in the evening (at 8:30 p.m.) caused a significant increase in both insulin and glucose levels compared with eating the exact same meal consumed in the morning (at 9:30 a.m.).

Unfortunately, U.S. adults display erratic eating patterns that are completely out of line with our natural circadian biology. As modern Americans:

- We have up to eleven eating events per day.
- Only 25 percent of food intake occurs before noon.
- 35 percent of intake occurs after 6:00 p.m.
- More than half of us eat over a period of fifteen hours or more a day.
- On weekends, eating windows are shifted to later.

Erratic daily food patterns and ultra-frequent food intake predispose us to metabolic dysfunction. In contrast, choosing to eat at consistent times, and cutting off the last food intake earlier in the evening, is an example of time-restricted feeding (TRF), which represents a promising approach for the prevention and therapy of metabolic disturbances. Research conducted on overweight individuals without diabetes revealed that practicing TRF for just four days can considerably reduce fasting glucose, fasting insulin, and mean glucose levels.

TRF is under the umbrella of fasting, which is an intentional restriction of food. Far from a health fad or hip wellness trend, fasting is a practice that has been part of our history and biology, given that we didn't always have constant access to food. Our bodies are primed to function optimally when they must flip-flop between discrete periods of eating and discrete periods of not eating. Remember, the two primary fuel sources for your cells to make ATP are glucose and fat.

- Glucose circulating in the bloodstream and stored in chains in the muscle and liver is more readily accessible for quick energy (like a debit account).
- Fat is a long-term energy storage source to tap into when glucose is low (like a savings account).

The problem today is that almost everyone is in a constant fed state—fueling their bodies off glucose instead of fat, from first thing in the morning (with a carb-heavy breakfast) till late at night (with dessert). This constant feast—with no famine—keeps our body in glucose-burning mode and deprives us of the benefits of utilizing fat for fuel, making those fat-burning pathways less efficient.

When people say they are hungry (or even "hangry"!) after not having a meal for a few hours, likely this reflects metabolic inflexibility: a problem switching from glucose burning to fat burning. Metabolic inflexibility results from the body's reliance on carbohydrates and glucose for energy because it's rarely given an opportunity to flip into fat burning. When we prepare our bodies to transition more effectively, we can alleviate some of the unpleasant symptoms, such as nausea, irritability, and fatigue, that we experience when our glucose levels are low. Additionally, this adaptability can enhance our ability to burn fat, particularly following a high-fat meal. Conversely, when our bodies become accustomed to constant glucose intake, they become less proficient at burning fat and lose metabolic flexibility. Metabolic inflexibility is linked to metabolic syndrome, type 2 diabetes, and chronic inflammation.

Most normal-weight humans can go well over a month without eating a single morsel of food with minimal negative health consequences just by tapping into their natural, healthy fat stores. One extremely obese man— Agostino Barbieri—fasted for 382 days without eating a piece of food. He came out the other side healthier. Obviously, this was an extreme case given Barbieri's severe obesity, but it makes the point that our perceptions around the time we can go between eating are incorrect.

Fasting lets your body practice—and over time, improve—its process of switching between burning available carbohydrates and glucose (when you eat) and burning fat for energy (when you're not eating). Insulin normally promotes fat storage and restricts fat breakdown, so when we fast, we allow insulin levels to fall and let fat get mobilized for energy. Fasting is also a stressor on the body, so it should be used with intention and thoughtfulness, particularly in menstruating women. *The Complete Guide to Fasting* by Dr. Jason Fung, *Fast Like a Girl* by Dr. Mindy Pelz, and *Women, Food, and Hormones* by Dr. Sara Gottfried are great books to learn more about fasting protocols.

No matter which fasting style you follow, you should try to reduce your daily eating window to avoid food in the late evening, and try to eat your last food before dark as often as possible. This tweak alone will be life-changing.

RESETTING YOUR RHYTHM

Unfortunately, our Western cultural norms are in direct opposition to optimizing chronobiology. Schools, the medical system, and workplaces are ignorant of the profound and inescapable impact of our sleep and meal timing on our cellular function. So you must take things into your own hands and be a counterculture circadian warrior in your journey to generate Good Energy. Doing so will involve hard choices that may seem like a sacrifice. But waiting on the other side for you is better mental and physical health.

If factors in your household or living situation are preventing you from getting enough sleep, you need to take steps to rectify them if you want to minimize any symptoms you have. If a pet is jumping on your bed, preventing you from sleeping through the night, you should consider intensive pet training or finding a new home for your pet. If your partner snores so loudly that you can't sleep, they should address the problem, and you might consider earplugs or sleep in a different room until it's resolved.

Many of you may be thinking, *I would sleep more, but I have trouble sleeping!* You wouldn't be alone: around a third of all adults experience insomnia. Many factors that lead to Bad Energy are the same factors that lead to insomnia, and when you work toward Good Energy habits, you are improving your chances at good sleep. For instance, a high intake of ultra-processed foods, which we know contributes to metabolic issues, also confers fourfold higher odds of having insomnia. Artificial light contributes to Bad Energy and insomnia. Chronic stress contributes to Bad Energy and insomnia. Eating late at night contributes to Bad Energy and insomnia. It's all connected.

Good Energy results from good sleep, but as we know, many other factors contribute to Good (or Bad) Energy. So if sleep is a struggle for you, start with some of the *other* pillars of Good Energy (food, movement, stress management, toxin avoidance, etc.), and you may find that sleep gets a lot easier, creating a positive and compounding virtuous cycle.

Tips for Protecting Your Circadian Rhythm

1. Understand Your Sleep Patterns

- Get a baseline assessment of your sleep quantity, quality, and consistency by wearing a sleep tracker. My preferred sleep tracker is Fitbit (more examples in Part 3).
- Quantity: Assess your average sleep duration per week and whether it is less than seven hours per night. Do you have days that tend to be outliers for getting more or less sleep?
- Quality: Most sleep trackers will tell you how long you take to fall asleep and how much time you spend awake each night. Additionally, trackers will help you understand whether you are getting adequate REM and deep sleep, and what factors (like alcohol, eating late, nighttime light exposure, etc.) may be negatively impacting your sleep.
- Consistency: Assess whether you are experiencing social jet lag of more than one hour by figuring out the midpoint of your sleep window and comparing it day to day throughout the week.
- Once you understand your baseline, create a strategy to work toward a more consistent bedtime and wake time, as well as a goal for increasing the quantity of sleep to at least seven hours per night without any outliers.

2. Find Accountability for Your Sleep Goals

- Once you set goals for bedtime, wake time, and quantity of sleep per night, share them with a friend, partner, or coach and commit to sending them your sleep data daily to ensure you stay accountable. I like to put my money where my mouth is with my accountability partner. If I don't adhere to my sleep goals, I must go clean my best friend's house! New digital services, such as Crescent Health, pair you with a sleep coach to stay accountable.

3. Log Your Food Temporarily to Understand When and What You Are Eating

- Food logging is an excellent way to understand exactly what and when you are eating. When I reviewed my own food logs with a nutritionist, I realized for the first time that I had a small snack almost every night at 11:00 p.m. Logging my food helped me set realistic goals for my eating cutoff time.
- I track my food in the Levels app while wearing a continuous glucose monitor and in MacroFactor when I'm not. Both are seamless ways to know exactly what and when I'm eating.

4. Pick a Cutoff Time for "Last Call" on Daily Eating

- Set a reasonable goal for when your last bite of food will be. Start with something achievable (for instance, if you eat something at 9:30 p.m. most nights, set your first goal for 9:00 p.m.). As you reach the goal for two weeks straight, bump it up a half hour or so every two weeks until you reach your final goal.

5. Work to Minimize Bright, Artificial Light After Dark

- Purchase red light bulbs for the main rooms you spend time in after dark, such as your bedroom, bathroom, kitchen, and family room. Using red light instead of standard bulbs will minimize the blue light your brain receives. If these bulbs are impossible to obtain, install dimmers on your lights and dim them to minimal brightness after dark.
- Use blue light–blocking glasses after dark. I use Ra Optics.
- Turn your screens to "night mode" after dark. This mode reduces the intensity of blue light your screen emits.
- Aim to stop looking at screens—even backlit e-readers—during the hour before bed. If you want to read for work or fun, print out the material, use a non-lit screen (like a reMarkable tablet), or read a paper book.

6. Create a Light-Free and Sound-Free Bedroom

- Remove all light and sources of noise from the bedroom. Even small amounts of light from windows, alarm clocks, or TVs can significantly disturb sleep. Invest in blackout curtains.
- Invest in well-fitting earplugs and a comfortable eye mask.

7. Get Outside in the First Hour of the Day

- Your body needs to know when it is day and night to function properly. Your brain will set you up for a Good Energy day if it knows when it is daytime. But you have to "show" your brain sunlight.
- Within one hour of waking, get outside, no matter what. Don't stare directly at the sun, but make sure the photons have a direct path from the sky to your eyeballs—with no windows or sunglasses in the way. It doesn't matter if it's raining or snowing or if it's cloudy or sunny—being outdoors gives you vastly more solar energy than if a window is blocking the sunlight. You may need to invest in the right outdoor gear so that you have no excuse to avoid this. For instance, when I moved to a snowy town, getting comfortable snow pants, tall waterproof boots, and a long parka allowed me to quickly suit up for a comfortable walk despite months of freezing (and sometimes blizzarding) conditions.
- Ideas for implementation: I like to use the two to three minutes while I'm brushing my teeth to walk around my front yard. Doing so ensures I get sunlight in the first ten minutes of the waking day. Make a habit of walking around the block while you drink your coffee or take your first morning call. Even spending ten minutes outside in the first hour of the day can have a significant positive impact on synchronizing your body's internal clock with the sunlight.

8. Spend *Significantly* More Time Outdoors During Daylight Hours

- Aim to get outdoors more frequently throughout the day by scheduling moments to pop outside.

- Learn to take pride in how many cumulative hours you can spend outside in twenty-four hours. Bonus points if you're exposed to natural areas like parks or forests, which independently boost health.
- Try to move activities you regularly do indoors to the outdoors, like eating meals, reading, taking phone calls, catching up with your partner at the end of the day, or playing with your kids. Get creative.

To view the scientific references cited in this chapter, please visit us online at caseymeans.com/goodenergy.

CHAPTER 8

Replenishing What Modernity Took Away

Movement, Temperature, and Nontoxic Living

———

The first two years of med school consist of wall-to-wall lectures. At Stanford Medical School, we sat for eight hours per day in a dark subterranean classroom, with ten minutes of breaks between classes. During these breaks, we could sneak a meal at the adjacent café, which served pizza, cheesy pasta, sandwiches, fries, and chips.

Even at this time, before my full awakening regarding metabolic health, I found something discordant about budding doctors *sitting* all day while learning about cardiovascular disease, diabetes, and hypertension. I read a *New York Times* article that described sitting for long periods of time as a "lethal" activity for our health because of increasing metabolic and cardiovascular dysfunction. I installed a makeshift standing desk in the back of the lecture hall made from an IKEA storage tub turned upside down on top of a desk. This sparked curiosity among my classmates. So I sent a survey to students about their interest in standing desks in classrooms, and to my surprise, most students responded. One hundred percent of respondents said medical school causes them to sit too much. Nearly 90 percent said standing options in classrooms would increase their quality of life.

Emboldened, I reviewed dozens of academic studies showing the deadly impact of excess sitting and presented the findings to the medical school administration, along with survey results from students. I explained how installing standing desks would be great marketing to promote Stanford's innovative image, as well as support medical student health and well-being. My proposal was rejected. I was told I needed formal evidence to support that this would be a valuable intervention. I agreed. Thus began my two-year journey of a grant-funded, ethics board–approved interventional study of the impact of standing desks in classrooms. I implemented a trial with Stanford medical students and conducted structured interviews and surveys. I pursued training in qualitative research coding and interpretation and analyzed the data. The results were clear: students reported increased alertness, attention, and engagement during the intervention and wanted standing desk options in classrooms.

Two years after my first meeting, I stood before the Stanford Medical School administration and presented the data they had requested. Again, the proposal for standing desks was rejected. I was told that the new Li Ka Shing building—a $90 million architectural marvel donated by the richest person in Hong Kong—had design guidelines and safety codes. There would be no standing desks.

At nearly every medical school in the country today, young doctors, in their first two years, still spend most of their time sitting for long periods. We now know sitting is one of the fastest ways to ensure increased risk for the exact diseases med students are learning how to treat. Up to 73 percent of physicians are overweight or obese, and the leading causes of death for doctors are all the largely preventable Bad Energy killers, with heart disease, cancer, and stroke at the top.

Our obsession with sitting represents a greater theme contributing to Bad Energy: our desire to be comfortable. We like to sit and we like comfortable temperatures—which is understandable. Unfortunately, these two comforts of modern life aren't conducive to optimal cellular physiology or longevity. We celebrate our comfortable, seated, climate-controlled world as a win—and to some extent, it is! But the reality is these factors of modern life conspire to lull our cells into a state of cellular complacency.

Don't push the body much, and it will break down. Push a body too hard for too long and it will also break down. But push a body *just* past the point of comfort—specifically with movement and temperature—and magic happens: the cells rise to the occasion, adapting and turning on dormant pathways to make us more resilient, happier, and healthier, especially if we follow that stress with time to adapt, recover, and amplify resilience pathways.

Many complex biological systems improve their function when their environments push them a bit. For example, the most phytonutrient- and antioxidant-rich plants are grown in the harshest, rockiest climates, like those of the steep mountainsides of Sardinia. These plants activate their own antioxidant stress resilience pathways to survive, which translates into potent health benefits for us when we eat them. Outdoor cats exposed to harsher environments have significantly less obesity than indoor cats. And 50 percent of domesticated dogs over age ten develop cancer, yet this rarely happens to dogs or wolves in the wild. Depression afflicts 75 percent of domesticated dogs but is rare in wild animals. While 40 percent of modern humans will get cancer, our closest relatives—chimpanzees—rarely get it, despite sharing nearly 99 percent of our genes.

Something about a more natural, wilder life is good for our biology. Is it possible that the comforts of domestication are hurting us?

As modern life has stripped away basic realities of historical life—like regular movement and large swings in external temperature—massive industries have cropped up, getting us to pay to add them back in. Among the offerings are fitness classes, gyms, cold plunges, saunas, and light therapy. The constant stress we feel to exercise and purchase these "healthy" products is a perverse trick. It is ironic that we pay for the luxury of comfort and then are sold solutions to remedy the resulting deficiencies. The Good Energy solution is not just incorporating more biohacking "protocols" and tools into your day, which often add stress as more boxes to check. The solution is about changing your mindset to see controlled discomfort and adaptive stressors as critical biologic information and about building your days to incorporate such stressors as the default. It's also about being skeptical, and frankly critical, of our "normal" built environments and cultural norms around movement. These norms include sitting at desks all day; having sitting areas serve as the centerpieces of our homes; being shuttled constantly in cars, on scooters, and on escalators and elevators; and getting upset if our thermostat is more than a few degrees from 70°F.

In addition to harming us by shielding us from these stressors, industrial modernity has also taken away our opportunity to live in a nontoxic world that protects our cells from being overburdened and damaged. Approximately eighty thousand synthetic chemicals are now used by industry, filling our air, water, food, and homes with substances that interact with our cells, many in ways that are either known to be harmful to our cells or have unknown effects. Many of these substances are part of a class of chemicals called *obesogens*, meaning they are known to directly impair Good Energy processes and contribute to accumulation of fat and obesity. We throw our hands up in confusion at the plummeting mental and physical health of our population, while simultaneously bathing our cells (and those of our fetuses and children) in a constant invisible "chemical soup" of lab-created toxins that directly impair neurotransmitters, the microbiome, mitochondria, our genetics, and our hormones.

This chapter examines the Bad Energy effects of our move to an indoor lifestyle and away from the natural world, and what we can do to start feeling better today.

MOVEMENT

Despite the miraculous capabilities of the human body as the only bipedal primate, we *choose* to spend nearly 80 percent of our time sitting. The 2008 Pixar movie *Wall-E* portrays a dystopian future with obese humans zooming about in robotic hover-chairs, seeking entertainment via holographic screens, consuming packaged food delivered by robots, and never needing to lift a finger. This, sadly, is close to our current reality.

People in the United States have a desire to be fit, with sixty-four million belonging to fitness centers and spending nearly $2,000 on average on health and fitness per person annually. But we are getting sicker every year. Despite a doubling of fitness center memberships since the year 2000, obesity has gone up 10 percent in that time. Our nation has the most gyms of any country in the world, yet we are among the fattest. The CDC reports that over 75 percent of U.S. adults do not engage in the recommended amount of activity, and 25 percent are not active *at all*.

What explains this disconnect between our clear desire to be healthy and our disastrous failure to develop movement habits? I believe the answer lies in the fundamental concept of "exercise." We have characterized exercise as an isolated bout of activity—separate from the rest of our daily life—and an item on the to-do list. Our metabolic processes function best when movement is a regular, consistent part of our lives, not a task to be performed in an hour or two. Until very recently, continual movement was essential for daily survival: hunting, gathering, and traveling long distances on foot. As recently as 1820, 79 percent of Americans worked in the physically demanding job of agriculture. There was no SoulCycle, Barry's Bootcamp, or gyms on every city street corner in 1900, yet the obesity rate was close to 0 percent.

Today, just 1.3 percent of people in the United States are employed in agriculture. We now sit or lie down virtually *all* the time. Unlike many cities in Europe and Asia, most American urban areas are designed for cars, not people. Astonishingly, parking takes up about one-third of the land area in U.S. cities. If you live in a low walkability area, prediabetes incidence is 32 percent higher, and the likelihood of developing type 2 diabetes is 30 to 50 percent higher. If you're lucky enough to live in a highly walkable city, the rates of obesity and overweight magically drop from 53 percent to 43 percent. The CDC reports that the average U.S. adult today takes between 3,000 to 4,000 steps per day, which is less than two miles. Compare this with modern hunter-gatherer populations, who take closer to 20,000 steps a day and spend less than 10 percent of daily hours sitting (and notably, have the lowest level of heart disease of almost any population ever studied). Dan Buettner's book *The Blue Zones* demonstrates that the populations that live the longest don't "exercise" in the modern sense of a targeted, focused spurt of activity. Movement is just naturally built into their daily life. Again, our challenge is not how to fit more fitness classes in. It's how to design our daily lives to make movement the norm, which is simple but requires creativity and boldness.

Spurts of focused physical activity *are* certainly great for health. But optimal metabolism results from regular low-level physical activity, which continuously stimulates cellular pathways that promote Good Energy physiology. Excess sitting is associated with all three hallmarks of Bad

Energy: more inflammation, more oxidative stress, and more mitochondrial dysfunction. And just squeezing in a workout once a day doesn't counteract the problems with sitting too much. Research suggests that prolonged sedentary time is associated with bad health outcomes, regardless of physical activity. Sitting itself is the monster, no matter whether you exercise. Dr. Andrew Huberman recently noted that "even if we get our 180 minutes of zone 2 (moderate) cardio per week, the benefits are largely (or entirely) erased by sitting more than five hours per day." If exercise is going to improve metabolism in a major way, it's going to look very different from today's fitness industry. Instead, it's going to look like regular movement reentering the fabric of our everyday lives.

We're made for movement: our muscles, bones, and joints work together in a finely tuned orchestra, allowing us to run, jump, climb, and lift with remarkable precision and efficiency. Unfortunately, we're squandering these miraculous gifts.

Muscle Contraction Is Medicine

The reason that moving regularly is important is because a body in which muscles are contracting frequently (even at low intensities for short periods) is experiencing totally different physiology than a body where the muscles are worked in only a one- to two-hour exercise block per day (no matter how intense that block). Muscle contraction is miraculous medicine. At a basic level, muscle cell activity kicks off two processes: it prompts the entry of calcium into cells, and it depletes ATP. The increase in calcium and dip in ATP set off a slew of signaling pathways that ultimately push the cell to process glucose or fat to make *more* ATP to keep fueling the muscle. At the center of this is a key protein called AMPK, which is like an "energy sensor" in cells. Sensing a decline in ATP as muscle contractions use it up, AMPK activates and stimulates the incredible PGC-1α, which increases fat burning, glucose uptake, and the creation of more mitochondria (to make more ATP).

In addition, AMPK also stimulates mitophagy, whereby cells clear out old, dysfunctional mitochondria to make room for healthy, new mitochondria. Without effective mitophagy, we accumulate poor-quality mitochondria that produce excessive free radicals, generating one of the key hallmarks of Bad Energy: oxidative stress. And while exercise induces some free radicals, the stimulation of PCG-1α promotes the expression of several antioxidant genes, thereby increasing the oxidative defense systems in the body. Exercise can also acutely increase inflammation, but research has shown that muscle activity decreases chronic inflammation over the long run. In fact, research increasingly shows that muscle is an anti-inflammatory hormone-secreting organ. It releases myokines, immune-modulating proteins, into the blood that limit the inflammatory response. In the case of both oxidative stress and inflammation, the controlled stressor of increased movement and exercise leads the body to lower levels of both over time.

Muscle contraction is vital to metabolic health because it disposes of excess glucose, and incredibly, muscle can do this *without* needing insulin to stimulate the entry of glucose into the cells. In fact, when exercising, people with type 2 diabetes—despite being extremely insulin resistant—can clear glucose from the blood at levels near or identical to people without diabetes, all because they can clear glucose *without* needing to use insulin. Why? Exercise stimulates AMPK, which directly signals for glucose channels (GLUT4 channels) to travel from the inside of the cell out to the cell membrane to let glucose in.

By clearing glucose from the blood without requiring as much insulin secretion, exercise increases our body's sensitivity to the hormone. In fact, studies show that a single exercise session can increase insulin sensitivity for at least sixteen hours.

The ability of GLUT4 transporters to clear glucose from the blood isn't marginal. According to Levels data, adults often see a 30 percent lower glucose spike when they take a gentle walk after eating a high-carbohydrate meal. Muscle contraction is a silver bullet for processing excess food energy that otherwise can clog up our cells and lead to dysfunction. Exercise stimulates the production of more and healthier mitochondria to generate Good Energy, upregulating antioxidant defenses and quelling inflammation over the long term.

Just Move More

Moving more frequently means more glucose clearance from the blood continuously throughout the day. Every time you stand up from your desk and take a five-minute walk or do thirty air squats (bending your knees so that you mimic a sitting position while keeping your feet flat on the ground), remember that you are giving your body a signal that brings glucose channels to the membrane to keep clearing glucose to make ATP. You can see how different this situation is from someone who sits all day and exercises for an hour in the evening. All day, the muscles lack a signal to soak up and use excess glucose, leaving it circulating in the bloodstream and requiring insulin to get it into cells.

Your daily movement doesn't need to be hard to be effective, but it needs to be frequent. A study of eleven participants completed four movement regimens:

- No exercise
- Twenty minutes of jogging before breakfast, lunch, and dinner
- Twenty minutes of jogging after breakfast, lunch, and dinner
- Short spurts of jogging for just three minutes every half hour throughout the day.

All three movement patterns added up to sixty total minutes of jogging per day. But the results showed something fascinating: the short three-minute bursts of jogging every half hour significantly reduced post-meal glucose spikes, compared to the longer pre- and post-meal jogs.

You don't need to jog to see this effect; walking works, too: a study of seventy healthy, normal-weight adults looked at three similar scenarios:

- Sitting for nine hours
- Walking for a thirty-minute period once per day and then sitting
- Regular activity breaks of walking for one minute and forty seconds every thirty minutes.

While both activity groups walked a grand total of thirty minutes per day, the study showed that people who took the short walks every thirty minutes had the lowest post-meal glucose peaks and insulin levels. Here's an analogy to drive the point home: If your body needs about 90 ounces of water per day for optimal function, it wouldn't make sense to chug it all in thirty minutes, and not drink the rest of the day. Sipping the 90 ounces throughout the day would obviously be much better. Same with movement. You might find those constant "stand up" reminders on the Apple Watch and other wearables annoying, but those recommendations are backed by solid science and might be the most important prompt these wearables can offer.

Be Hot

A catchy term has arisen to refer to more movement through the day outside of exercise: non-exercise activity thermogenesis (NEAT). NEAT refers to any spontaneous physical activity that is not the result of voluntary exercise. I find it odd that we've had to give this concept a fancy name and acronym. Before the urbanization of work and the transition to a desk-based existence, NEAT was just life. NEAT includes activities of daily living that require movement, like cleaning, grocery shopping, gardening, puttering around the house, walking from the car to a store, going upstairs, using a standing desk, and playing with kids—even fidgeting counts. Unsurprisingly, available data support that more NEAT could be an essential tool for body-weight control.

Treadmill desks are an example of attempting to fit more NEAT into the day. Researchers hypothesize that if you have obesity, using a treadmill desk at slow speeds for just 2.5 hours per day could lead to a weight loss of 44 to 66 pounds in a year. This hasn't yet been proven with data over a full year. But research has shown that using a treadmill desk at work for just 2.5 hours per day for ten days led to an average drop of 2.6 pounds of fat mass and an increase of 2.2 pounds in lean mass (muscle).

It's worth thinking more about the *thermogenesis* part of non-exercise activity thermogenesis, which refers to how exercise is "heat generating."

Why is this relevant? When we contract our muscles, we need more ATP for energy, which means we split it from adenosine *tri*phosphate into ADP, or adenosine *di*phosphate, releasing a phosphate. When that phosphate splits off, the energy from the chemical bond is either used to fuel cellular activities (like muscle contractions) or dissipated as heat. The more we make and use ATP, the more heat we generate, which is why people who have higher muscle mass tend to generate more heat at baseline. Some studies have shown that exercise training can raise baseline body temperature. Concerningly, Stanford research shows that our body temperatures on average have gone down by close to 2 percent since preindustrial times, corresponding to lower metabolic rates. I find it disturbing that our temperature, as a species, is consistently declining. Heat is a marker of our life force, our mitochondrial function, our engine, our Good Energy, our yang, our light, and it's dimming because we're sitting. You can stoke your internal fire by simply moving more (and building more muscle).

Marketing over Science

Like the mass confusion about what to eat, the mass confusion about the "right" form of movement and exercise can be paralyzing for consumers, while fueling an $800 billion global fitness economy that has us continuously doubting our strategy. I think this creates a defeating lack of confidence in the average person that hurts the larger mission to get us to be more active. The United States as a whole is the largest fitness consumer, yet our population's health worsens yearly. Nearly three hundred thousand scientific studies on physical exercise have been published in the last ten years, yet we've never been fatter or more sedentary. We have blindly relinquished common sense in pursuit of "evidence." The top podcasts in the country debate the nuances of exact minutes per week and time of day to do zone 2 training versus high-intensity interval training (HIIT), lactate thresholds, eccentric versus concentric training. But only 28 percent of Americans meet the *basic* guidelines for physical activity. All this information is interesting, but let's not miss the forest for the trees: it's not like there's an epidemic of exercising *too* much in America.

Here's the reality: Research has shown that *all kinds* of physical activity benefit metabolic health and slash the risk of metabolic diseases. In large populations, when total energy expenditure is the same, people who do the most walking (relatively low intensity) *and* those who do the most vigorous activities (relatively high intensity) profoundly reduce their type 2 diabetes risk to a comparable degree.

Simply walking about 10,000 steps per day (as compared with lower amounts) is associated with the following:

- 50 percent lower dementia risk
- 50 to 70 percent lower risk of premature death
- 44 percent lower risk of getting type 2 diabetes
- 31 percent (or more) lower risk of obesity
- Significant reductions in cancer occurrence, major depression, gastric reflux, and sleep apnea

Zero medications or surgeries can do for chronic disease prevention what walking about 10,000 steps a day can do. Despite this, physicians rarely prescribe exercise to patients. If a medication could slash Alzheimer's risk by 50 percent, it would be front-page news and prescribed to every patient. But this "drug" does exist—it's walking! Yet less than 16 percent of doctors prescribe movement to their patients, and 85 percent of practitioners report zero training in prescribing exercise.

Even when the science on movement is clear, the medical system does not adjust. Take, for example, the impact of physical activity on COVID-19 outcomes. A study of 194,191 people with COVID-19 showed that people who were consistently inactive prior to contracting the coronavirus were 191 percent more likely to be hospitalized and 391 percent more likely to die than those who were the most active ("most active" meant logging an average of just 42.8 minutes of moderate to strenuous physical activity per day). The benefits of exercise held even for those with preexisting conditions. Given that mitochondria are the coordinators of cell immunity and cell survival, mitochondrial function was implicated as early as 2020 as a key factor in the likelihood of getting COVID, dying from COVID, and experiencing long COVID. Researchers made recommendations to "urgently" pursue preventive avenues to "strengthen the mitochondria" for best COVID outcomes, with the leading recommendation being exercise (in addition to fresh foods, breathing practices, and general preventive medicine practices). None of this science made it into public health recommendations or any formal guidelines.

As a thought experiment, imagine if we took just a fraction of the $4 trillion of annual health care spent and put it toward incentivizing more movement: making cities more walkable; putting treadmills throughout office buildings; subsidizing short hourly movement breaks in every school, hospital, and workplace; or even outright paying at-risk populations to move more!

Keep It Simple

With food, we covered three simple rules that get you quite far: don't eat added sugar, don't eat industrially processed vegetable and seed oils, and don't eat highly processed grains.

With fitness, I also suggest three simple rules.

1. Walk at least 7,000 steps per day and space these steps out throughout the day. Work up to 10,000 per day.
2. Get your heart rate above 60 percent of your maximum for at least 150 minutes a week. (That's 30 minutes, five days a week.)
3. Lift heavy things multiple times per week in a way that hits every major muscle group.

Are there important personalized and nuanced diet and movement strategies beyond these simple rules? Of course. But here's the key: following these simple guidelines will make you feel so much better and facilitate the awe, curiosity, and energy to go deeper. When you experience the benefits of cutting refined sugars, grains, and industrial oils from your diet, I can almost guarantee that you'll start researching more whole-food recipes and exploring other books and podcasts for more personalized nutrition strategies. And if you commit to walking at least 7,000 steps a day and doing 150 minutes per week of aerobic exercise as nonnegotiable, you'll inevitably explore different varieties of fitness and find the routine that's right for you. Start with the basics, and in the form of *any* activity you enjoy, and make sure you're hitting your goals. When you do this, the next levels tend to bloom like a stunning flower.

I want to drill deeper on the recommendation for logging that 150 minutes of activity with elevated heart rate per week. Zone 2 aerobic training is defined as an activity that generates a heart rate at 60 to 70 percent of your maximum heart rate (often defined as your age subtracted from 220). Think of a brisk walk or light jog that you can continue for an hour without much difficulty. Consistent zone 2 exercise confers powerful metabolic benefits by stimulating mitochondrial health without excessive strain on the body. The benefits of zone 2 are proof that you don't have to run your body into the ground for effective metabolic workouts. Zone 2 typically feels oddly easy. But the proof is in the research: sustained moderate exercise increases the number of mitochondria, improves glucose uptake, increases the efficiency of your heart, and reduces the risk for nearly every chronic disease.

How do you know you're in zone 2? Many fitness trackers, including Apple Watch, now show zone scores based on your age and weight. Or you can use the talk test: when you're on the upper edge of zone 2, you shouldn't be able to say a sentence out loud without slowing down to catch your breath.

While you can stay in zone 2 for the entire 150 minutes each week (again, the key part of this habit is doing *anything* consistently), there is evidence that getting your heart rate higher for short bursts by incorporating HIIT can have powerful metabolic benefits. The American College of Sports Medicine defines HIIT as any kind of workout that alternates short bursts—anywhere from five seconds to eight minutes of intense activity—where your heart rate reaches 80 to 95 percent of its maximal capacity, with equal or longer periods of rest or physical activity, where your heart rate is at 40 to 50 percent of your max.

Lastly, I implore anyone working to optimize their metabolic health or weight to incorporate resistance training (otherwise known as strength training or weight training). Resistance training simply means intentionally making your muscles work against a weighted force, which could be functional movements such as lifting or pushing heavy things in your home or at work, lifting or pushing weights, or using your body weight as a force to work against (think pull-ups or push-ups). Since we know that muscles play an important role in clearing glucose from the blood, muscle mass correlates with insulin sensitivity. A study from the NIH reported that "resistance training has a favorable effect on metabolic syndrome since it decreases fat mass, including abdominal fat. It also enhances insulin sensitivity, improves glucose tolerance, and reduces blood pressure values." Think of a thick layer of muscle covering your skeleton as a metabolic shield and a gateway to a longer and happier life. In my experience, incorporating resistance training can be transformational for people who are feeling "stuck" in their progress toward metabolic optimization or weight loss. Focused weight training is especially important for women entering middle age, who can greatly benefit from a metabolic boost as metabolism takes a big hit with the natural decline of estrogen at menopause. Muscle expert and geriatrician Dr. Gabrielle Lyon goes as far to say, "We aren't over fat; we are undermuscled." The idea is that if you focus attention on *building* more muscle rather than just *losing weight*, you'll be much better off in succeeding in improving body composition and metabolic health. And since muscle mass naturally (and rapidly) declines each decade beginning at age thirty, and low muscle mass is a risk factor for premature mortality, we need to start weight training early in life and continue for life. It's never too late to start.

GOOD ENERGY BIOMARKERS AND MOVEMENT

When you're striving to be part of the 6.8 percent of metabolically healthy Americans, regular movement will help you get there. Research shows that exercise improves all five of the following basic biomarkers of metabolism:

- **Glucose Levels Above 100 mg/dL:** Twelve-week exercise programs of either high-intensity running (40 minutes per week) or low-intensity running (150 minutes per week) both brought participants' blood sugar from the prediabetic range (100 mg/dL or greater) to the nondiabetic range (<100 mg/dL).

- **HDL Cholesterol Less Than 40 mg/dL:** A 2019 review of the literature showed that exercise increased HDL cholesterol, "with exercise volume, rather than intensity, having a greater influence." Meanwhile, "raising HDL levels pharmacologically has not shown convincing clinical benefits."

- **Triglycerides Above 150 mg/dL:** Numerous studies have demonstrated that physical activity effectively lowers triglyceride levels. In a 2019 study, an eight-week moderate aerobic exercise program significantly reduced triglyceride levels in participants. Furthermore, even a single session of intense aerobic exercise has been found to decrease triglyceride levels the following day. This positive effect could be due to the increased activity of hepatic lipase in the liver, an enzyme that facilitates the absorption of triglyceride from the bloodstream.

- **Blood Pressure of 130/85 mmHg or Higher:** Research has shown the effects of exercise among populations with high blood pressure were similar to the effects of commonly used medications.

- **A Waistline of More Than 35 Inches for Women and 40 Inches for Men:** Not surprisingly, regular exercise can help decrease obesity by increasing energy expenditure and promoting weight loss. Research shows a clear inverse relationship between the amount of movement people do each week and the size of their waistline: more movement, smaller waist circumference. What's more, lower activity (fewer than 5,100 steps per day) yields a 2.5 times higher risk of central obesity than higher activity (more than 8,985 steps per day).

TEMPERATURE

We know that too much stress on the body all the time is bad, but controlled *increases* in specific stressors can cause adaptations that lower our chronic levels of oxidative stress and inflammation.

A valuable mechanism to stress cells into positive adaptation is exposing them to extreme temperatures. You've probably heard about cold plunging. It's been gaining a cult following among the biohackers, despite the upward of $5,000 price tag for many of these specialized tubs. Getting cold or hot isn't something we could control for much of human history. "Indoors" is a very new concept, and air-conditioning and central heat are even newer. Our ancestors from the nineteenth century had inconsistent heating—and no cooling systems—in their homes. Extreme heat and cold between seasons and even in a single day was the norm for most humans for much of history. In the Sahara Desert, for example, temperatures can reach up to 122°F during the day and drop to 50°F or below at night. In the Rocky Mountains, temperatures drop from 80°F during the day to 40°F or lower at night.

Our modern lives of "thermoneutrality" makes for bored mitochondria. Mitochondria are heat-generating structures, like furnaces, but if we don't stimulate them to do the work to generate heat and ATP, they won't do as much. Our mitochondria are so bored and abused that our species appears to be cooling. Body temperature seems to have dropped by as much as 1.06°F over the past two hundred years, possibly because of a generally lower metabolic rate. In recent years, we've seen compelling research showing how adding large temperature fluctuations back into our lives brings metabolic benefits by stimulating vascular activity, increasing the cells' ability to generate their own heat, and increasing our cells' antioxidant capacity.

Heat and Cold

Our bodies have several mechanisms for regulating our internal temperature when we're exposed to cold. One way is through shivering, where the muscles contract rapidly, splitting ATP molecules and, in doing so, producing heat. Another way is through non-shivering thermogenesis, where our body produces and utilizes more of a special type of metabolically healthy fat (called brown fat) to help keep us warm.

Brown fat is different from the white fat that most people are familiar with. While white fat stores energy, brown fat burns energy to produce heat. It is sometimes referred to as "thermogenic fat." Brown fat is brown because it is filled with mitochondria and expresses high levels of a protein called uncoupling protein 1 (UCP1). UCP1 is unique to brown fat and allows it to produce heat instead of ATP. The UCP1 protein is a channel that lets protons that were destined for driving ATP production instead leak out from the inner membrane of the mitochondria, dissipating as heat instead of generating ATP. Brown fat levels increase in winter as the body adapts to stay warmer. Interestingly, HbA1c levels (a marker of average glucose levels) tend to be *lower* in the winter, when temperature is colder and brown fat levels are higher, although a causal relationship between HbA1c and brown fat has not been established.

Studies have shown that brown fat readily takes up and utilizes glucose and that people with more brown fat tend to have lower body mass and lower glucose levels. In fact, a 2021 study found that the prevalence of type 2 diabetes in people with obesity and with brown fat was nearly half that of people with obesity without brown fat, about 8 percent versus 20 percent, respectively.

Exposing yourself to cold can activate your brown fat, which can help you manage your blood sugar levels. Research shows that sleeping in a room at 66°F for a month can increase insulin sensitivity and double the activity and volume of brown fat in healthy men. Even short periods of cold exposure can improve insulin sensitivity and glucose disposal, especially in people with brown fat. In one study, wearing cooling vests for five to eight hours increased resting energy expenditure by 15 percent in subjects with brown fat. Whole-body glucose disposal also increased by about 13 percent for subjects with brown fat, but there was no significant change for those without brown fat. Cold acclimation can also improve metabolic health, even in people with little brown fat. A ten-day cold acclimation program led to a 43 percent increase in insulin sensitivity in men with type 2 diabetes compared to their levels under normal temperatures. The program also increased the activity of the GLUT4 glucose channel.

Researchers have also found that higher brown fat levels are related to lower glycemic variability, helping maintain stable whole-body glucose levels even when a person is not exposed to cold. In a 2016 study in *Cell Metabolism*, participants were given a 75-gram glucose drink in a comfortable 75°F room. The researchers found that brown fat activation and resting energy expenditure both rose in response, even though the participants weren't exposed to cold, as the brown fat's glucose uptake and processing generated heat. The paper suggested that a brown fat deficiency could be a clinical indicator of the development of blood sugar dysregulation. Simply put, we want much more brown fat, and the best way to get it is to expose the body to cold and inspire it to adapt.

Studies on deliberate heat exposure show that it has positive impacts on metabolic health. Researchers surmise that regular sauna use produces "a general stress-adaptation response" that is "possibly analogous to the . . . responses of exercise." Heat exposure can also increase the production of a protein called heat shock protein 70 (HSP70). HSP70 is involved in a variety of cellular processes, including stress response and inflammation. Research has suggested that HSP70 may play a role in improving insulin sensitivity and reducing inflammation.

Additionally, heat exposure has been shown to increase the production of nitric oxide, the molecule that helps to relax blood vessels and improve blood flow. Improved blood flow can enhance glucose uptake in skeletal muscle, which can improve insulin sensitivity. These mechanisms have led research findings to show that heat exposure is linked to reduced blood pressure, improved cardiac function markers, decreased total and LDL cholesterol levels, and decreased fasting blood glucose levels.

An observational study of Finnish men found striking reductions of metabolic conditions in people who regularly used saunas: "reductions [in] sudden cardiac death (63%) and all-cause mortality (40%) as well as for dementia (66%) and Alzheimer's disease (65%), in men who used a sauna 4–7 times per week compared to only once per week."

Cold and heat exposure can lead to a significant improvement in mood. Research has shown that cold-water submersion can increase dopamine levels by 250 percent. Cold exposure has been shown to activate the sympathetic nervous system and release neurotransmitters like norepinephrine, which can increase alertness and mood. Repeated sauna use has been shown to lower cortisol, the main stress hormone.

Heat seems to also upregulate our antioxidant defenses, positively impacting the oxidative stress that contributes to Bad Energy.

Before you go running to purchase an expensive sauna and ice bath, I would recommend trying one of these free or inexpensive ways.

1. At the end of your showers, turn the water to cold for two minutes. This is how my coauthor, Calley, started doing regular cold exposure, and he came out of the shower feeling great and ended up looking forward to it.
2. Jump into cold bodies of water. From October to about April in Oregon, the river and lakes near my house are all extremely cold, so I frequently jump in with friends. Now, nearly everywhere I go that has cold water, I'll take a dip, from glacier lakes in Montana or Wyoming during hiking trips, to the ocean in Northern California, to unheated pools in winter.
3. Find a cold-plunging or sauna group in your town on Meetup, social media, or Google.
4. Take a hot yoga class, like Bikram or Modo Yoga, which keeps the temperature above 100°F during the class.
5. Get outdoors and move when it's hot outside (but make sure to stay hydrated, consume enough food and electrolytes, and don't get sunburned.)
6. Find a local gym or community center with a sauna or hot tub.

How much to do? Exact numbers are unclear and will differ between people, but in a review of the research, Dr. Andrew Huberman recommended fifty-seven minutes of hot sauna per week and eleven minutes of cold exposure per week "as reliable thresholds to derive major benefits on metabolism, insulin and growth hormone pathways."

SYNTHETIC CHEMICALS AND ENVIRONMENTAL TOXINS

Synthetic chemicals and environmental toxins envelop us and are a key, grossly underrecognized driver of Bad Energy. Since World War II, over eighty thousand synthetic chemicals have entered our environment and approximately fifteen hundred new chemicals are released each year, many of which have never been tested for safety in adults, children, or fetuses.

Artificial chemicals and toxins are now found in dangerous levels in our air, food, water, homes, and soil and present a constant assault on our cells that directly impair the microbiome, gene expression, hormone receptors, the folding of our genome (*epigenetics*), intracellular signaling pathways, neurotransmitter signaling, fetal development, enzyme activity, hormonal control of eating behavior, thyroid function, resting metabolic rate, liver function, and more. These chemicals are drivers of all three hallmarks of Bad Energy: oxidative stress, inflammation, and mitochondrial dysfunction—and the link is now so well defined that many of these chemicals are being classified as *obesogens*, meaning that they are known to impair metabolism in such a way that they causatively contribute to obesity and insulin resistance. Dr. Robert Lustig, professor emeritus of neuroendocrinology at UCSF, believes that at least 15 percent of the obesity epidemic is directly tied to environmental chemicals.

Examples of obesogens include household disinfectants and cleaners, fragrances and perfumes, air "fresheners," makeup, lotions, shampoos, deodorants, body wash, household paint, the ink on receipts, plastics, vinyl flooring, food preservatives and colorings, many pharmaceutical drugs, clothing, furniture, children's toys, electronics, flame retardants, industrial solvents, car exhaust, and the pesticides that cover our food. The emerging understanding of the obesity-promoting qualities of industrial chemicals tells us that eating an ultra-processed food like Cheerios means that you may be getting a *quadruple* dose of Bad Energy potential: one in the ultra-refined food itself, one in the additives and preservatives, one in the pesticides, and one in the plastic packaging. Wash it down with conventional milk and a glass of unfiltered water and you compound the issue.

Many of these synthetic chemicals support industry interests but not cellular health. Adding chemicals to products increases shelf life, allows for the cheapest packaging, or gives a product a scent without using natural essential oils—but they also pose significant harm to humans. While the GRAS (generally recognized as safe) designation given by the U.S. Food and Drug Administration (FDA) is intended to allow for the commercial use of substances deemed safe for use in food and other consumer products, this oversight is grossly inadequate. Companies are able to *self-determine*

GRAS status via their own review of scientific literature, and the program is entirely voluntary, meaning that a company does not need to get the FDA's approval if *the company* determines that the chemical in question is GRAS—talk about conflict of interest! Many chemicals that have been given GRAS status at one time are now clearly linked to serious health issues such as cancer, neurologic problems, metabolic disruption, or infertility, including artificial sweeteners, propylparaben (an antimicrobial preservative found in lotions, shampoos, and food), butylated hydroxyanisole (BHA, a food preservative), and brominated vegetable oil (a food additive). Moreover, GRAS is predicated on the idea that chemicals exist in isolation and ignores the *synergistic* adverse effect of layering hundreds of these chemicals on a human body simultaneously, every day, which is the overt reality of our world. GRAS is not protecting you, and you should focus on consuming and using products that are as natural as possible in all domains of life.

The Endocrine Society has come out strongly for increased precautions around synthetic chemicals, stating "strong mechanistic, experimental, animal, and epidemiological evidence" for the impact of hormone-disrupting environmental chemicals on "obesity, diabetes mellitus, reproduction, thyroid, cancers, and neuroendocrine and neurodevelopmental functions." They add that while "ten years ago, there simply was not the body of evidence that there is today about the . . . disease consequences of endocrine disrupting chemicals," the state of evidence now "removes any doubt."

The following list describes nine classes of chemicals in the environment that are known to hurt human health directly through metabolic mechanisms:

1. **Bisphenol A (BPA)**—commonly found in plastic products such as plastic water bottles, food containers like cans, and thermal receipts, BPA is a known hormone disruptor that accumulates and sticks around in fatty tissue. (Of note, studies have found that a thermal receipt—like the type you might get at a grocery store—can contain 250 to 1,000 times more than a can of food.) It increases the risk of obesity, insulin resistance, type 2 diabetes, male and female infertility, and chronic

inflammation. Studies have suggested that BPA reduces antioxidant capacity, increases oxidative stress, and impairs mitochondrial dynamics.

2. **Phthalates**—commonly found in cosmetics, fragrances, nail polish, lotion, deodorant, hair spray, gel, shampoos, toys, plastics, and artificial leather, phthalates are hormone disruptors that are "significantly related" to insulin resistance, high blood pressure, earlier menopause, pregnancy loss, birth complications, genital development and semen quality, early puberty, asthma, developmental delay, and social impairment. Phthalates induce mitochondrial toxicity and increase oxidative stress in a dose-dependent manner, meaning that the more exposure, the worse the effects.

3. **Parabens**—commonly used as preservatives in moisturizers, shampoos, makeup, deodorant, shaving cream, foods, beverages, and pharmaceuticals, parabens are absorbed through the skin and oral ingestion and have been shown to be present in several body fluids and human tissues like blood, breast milk, semen, placental tissue, and breast cells. Parabens are problematic in how they bind to hormone receptors like those of our sex hormones (estrogen, progesterone, and testosterone) and stress hormones—thereby altering hormonal activity—and impact the metabolism of hormones. Hormones dictate all aspects of our biology, like neuronal development, immune function, thyroid function, metabolism, fetal development, and reproduction. Parabens directly bind hormone receptors and impart functional changes to the delicate balance of hormones regulating our lives and feelings. Parabens have been associated with DNA damage in sperm, sperm death, and infertility. Unfortunately, current wastewater treatment technology does not effectively remove parabens.

4. **Triclosan**—commonly used as an antimicrobial agent in personal care products, such as toothpaste and hand sanitizer, triclosan is absorbed into the body through skin and mouth tissues. It has been linked to hormone disruption, immune system impairment, thyroid problems, and antibiotic resistance, mostly in animal studies. Triclosan has been found in human body fluids, with peer-reviewed research suggesting

that "humans are unequivocally exposed to significant and potentially unsafe levels." Triclosan causes "universal disruption of mitochondria" as a mitochondrial uncoupler, leading to changes in mitochondrial shape to a dysfunctional "doughnut" shape, inhibition of the electron transport chain, mitochondrial splitting or "fission," prevention of mitochondria from moving around the cell effectively, and reduction of proper calcium levels in mitochondria (which are required for function). Overall, triclosan's multifarious impacts on the mitochondria negatively impact ATP production and increase oxidative stress.

5. **Dioxins**—a group of "highly toxic" compounds that are by-products of industrial processes (like bleaching paper pulp and making pesticides) and burning trash, coal, oil, and wood. These "persistent organic pollutants" (POPs) don't readily degrade and persist in our environment while accumulating in animal fat. According to the World Health Organization, more than 90 percent of human exposure is through fatty animal foods like fish, dairy, and meat. Through animal and human research, dioxins are known to cause developmental and reproductive problems, skeletal deformity, kidney defects, reduced sperm count, increased rate of miscarriages, immune system disorders, lung cancer, lymphoma, stomach cancer, and sarcomas. Dioxins may impact human health by generating "mitochondrial stress signaling," which activates the NF-κB pathway, and can induce chronic inflammation and disturb microbiome activity.

6. **Polychlorinated Biphenyls (PCBs)**—Fortunately, PCBs have been banned. However, these slowly degrading chemicals are still "ubiquitous environmental contaminants" found in air, water, soil, and fish worldwide and through interactions with PCB-containing products or equipment made before 1977. Considered dioxin-like, PCBs were widely used in making hydraulic and lubricating fluids, flame retardants, plasticizers, paint, adhesives, lubricating fluids, and other industrial products. Like many synthetic chemicals, they "bioaccumulate and biomagnify as they move up the food chain,"

meaning that if you eat a food like a bottom-feeding fish that may regularly dine on PCB-laden sediment or other PCB-containing fish, the level of PCBs in the fish could be as much as one million times higher than the water it lives in. In cell culture studies, PCBs are toxic to neurons due to impairment of the mitochondrial electron transport chain, impairment of the initial breakdown of glucose in the cell (a process called glycolysis), and, ultimately, reduction in ATP production.

7. **Perfluoroalkyl and Polyfluoroalkyl Substances (PFAS)**—commonly found in nonstick cookware, grease-proof coatings for paper and cardboard food packaging (like microwave popcorn bags, fast-food wrappers, and take-out containers), firefighting foams, and coatings for carpets and fabrics, these are often referred to as "forever chemicals" because they do not readily decompose or get excreted from the human body. A key source of PFAS in the environment is drinking water. Research has shown that PFAS possibly increase the risk of cancers of the liver, breast, pancreas, and testicles in animals, and cancers of the testicles, kidneys, thyroid, prostate, bladder, breast, and ovaries in humans (although some data conflicts). When PFAS accumulate in tissues of the body, they damage mitochondria, which contribute to the recruitment of immune cells and the development of chronic inflammation. They also generate oxidative stress by both creating more free radicals and impairing the activity of antioxidants.

8. **Organophosphate Pesticides**—5.6 billion pounds of pesticides are used each year globally, despite being strongly linked to oxidative stress, cancer, respiratory problems, neurotoxic effects, metabolic problems, and adverse child development. These pesticides cover our food and enter the water system, with the USDA estimating that the drinking water of fifty million people is contaminated with pesticides and agricultural chemicals. This not only hurts consumers but especially discriminates against farmers and children. Acute pesticide poisoning (APP) is estimated to affect 44 percent of farmers every year, for a total of 385 million cases per year worldwide and approximately twenty thousand deaths. Children are uniquely at risk from pesticides because

of pesticides' impact on their tiny bodies during critical developmental windows, and they can be exposed through the air, food, water, pets, and touch by playing on carpet, upholstered objects, lawns, grass in parks, and eating conventional and processed food. Forty-five percent of all reports of pesticide poisoning to poison control centers involve children. Studies have suggested that organophosphate exposure may affect mitochondrial function by inducing oxidative stress and impairing mitochondrial respiration. Do not use pesticides, like Roundup, on your lawn, and avoid conventionally grown foods. As with many chemicals, the liver primarily metabolizes pesticides before they are excreted in feces or urine. Protecting liver, gut, and kidney function is paramount to the effective elimination of many toxic synthetic chemicals, which Good Energy habits can help.

9. **Heavy Metals**—commonly found in contaminated soil, water, and food, heavy metals like mercury, cadmium, arsenic, and lead are naturally occurring substances that can be toxic when concentrated at high levels through manufacturing and industrial processes. Excess heavy metals can cause various health problems, including neurological damage, developmental delays, cancer, and other health issues. Research has shown that metals can both increase oxidative stress and lead to mitochondrial dysfunction.

A common theme among many of the most dangerous chemicals in our modern world concerns plastic production and food preservation. We must limit our societal use of plastics: We have now produced nine *billion tons* of plastic since it was patented less than two hundred years ago, the vast majority of which is now trash, littering our oceans, rivers, and streams, leaching toxic Bad Energy chemicals into our water, soil, food, and even our air. The rise of ultra-processed and packaged food—and the hoards of toxic "preservatives" we now use to make them shelf-stable—is a phenomenon less than one hundred years old. These recent problems could quickly scale back with collective effort and will, and they must.

Contaminated water is another key theme, and I don't believe it's an overstatement to say that drinking water is unsafe to drink without filtering for most Americans. The Environmental Working Group (EWG)'s database that analyzes water contaminants based on zip codes shows that it's not uncommon for substances like arsenic to be over *one thousand times* the EWG health guideline in many cities. Research estimates that tap water is contaminated with PFAS for over two hundred million Americans. The fact that our water is poisoned with chemicals that diminish our body's capability to power itself can sound dispiriting. But to me, it is empowering to understand in plain language that many institutions impacting our health are broken, so we can be motivated to protect ourselves and work toward better solutions.

Regarding water, health leader Dhru Purohit has aptly popularized the truism: "Either you have a filter, or *you* become the filter." This applies to all aspects of our environment: we either thoughtfully source pesticide-free food, filter our air, filter our water, buy less-toxic toys and furniture, stop touching receipts and thermal papers, minimize plastic use, and eliminate conventional household products and personal care products with synthetic scents and obesogens, *or* our bodies and poor organs become the filters for the thousands of synthetic chemicals that these products contain. Without this vigilance, we damage our bodies and force our cells to manage the overwhelming task of responding to these threatening toxic substances rather than letting the cells do their work of producing Good Energy to let us thrive. Minimizing the toxic burden in your environment through simple swaps and filters is easy, inexpensive, and high yield for metabolic health.

Principles for Replenishing What Modernity Took Away
Exercise Principles:
- Moderate intensity movement for at least 150 minutes per week
  - Calculate your max heart rate by subtracting your age from 220, and then determining what 64 percent of this is, which is the floor for moderate-intensity movement.
- Log 10,000 steps per day.
  - Measurable on any fitness tracker.

- Move a little bit during at least eight hours every day.
  - Measurable on any fitness tracker.
- Aim for resistance training three times per week.
  - Incorporate exercises that fatigue the arms, legs, and core every week. You can resistance train with body-weight exercises or with weights.

Temperature Principles:

- Get at least one cumulative hour per week of heat exposure.
  - This can be through a dry sauna, infrared sauna, or a heated exercise class like hot yoga.
- Get at least twelve cumulative minutes per week of cold exposure.
  - This can be through cryotherapy, cold showers, or cold immersion in a cold plunge tub or cold body of water (like a lake, river, or pool in winter).

Toxins Principles:

- Filter air and water in your home.
  - Using an activated charcoal filter and reverse osmosis are the best options for water, and a HEPA filter for air.
- Eat unprocessed organic or regeneratively grown food.
- Avoid plastics wherever possible; opt for glass or other materials instead.
  - Take stock of the plastic products in your home, closet, and kitchen and work to minimize.
- Swap out home care and personal care products for clean alternatives with transparent ingredients that you know.
  - A great first step is to remove any products in your home that have scents and replace with unscented products or eliminate entirely: air "fresheners" in the car and home, detergents, fabric softener, dish soap, dishwashing liquid, laundry sheets, shampoo, conditioner, body wash, body soap, deodorant, shaving cream, perfume, lotion. The scents in all of these products are overtly toxic. Unscented organic castile soap (like Dr. Bronner's) can replace hand soap, body

soap, body wash, and dish soap; vinegar and water can replace all-purpose cleaning sprays; and organic jojoba oil or coconut oil can replace lotions.

• Check the EWG databases for toxicity ratings on various consumer products.

• Support the body's natural detoxification pathways that involve the liver, gut, kidney, skin, and circulatory system by practicing Good Energy habits.

To view the scientific references cited in this chapter, please visit us online at caseymeans.com/goodenergy.

CHAPTER 9

Fearlessness

The Highest Level of Good Energy

Humans have evolved to experience potent feelings of fear, anxiety, sadness, and judgment, and for good reason: these feelings help keep us safe by generating unpleasant sensations to get us to respond in the face of a real threat to our survival. Without the ability to respond to threats in our surroundings, we'd quickly perish. Throughout human history, most of the threats we've been exposed to would be in our immediate surroundings, like a natural disaster, a snake slithering into your dwelling, or an invading army. But in the span of just a century, we now have the technological capability to be exposed to the threats facing *any* person, *anywhere* in the world, twenty-four hours a day, all live-streamed to a screen in our hands. Overnight, the traumas and fears of eight billion others have all become *ours* to process.

This is potentially the most abnormal thing we face as modern humans, more than the ultra-processed food, the excess sitting, the constant artificial light, or the thermoneutral existence. The human mind and body were never meant to experience constant terrorizing messaging, and we now cannot avoid it (billboards, newspapers, social media, TV!). And we also can't seem to look away, because we are biologically hardwired to pay attention to threats. Technological connectivity has ushered in an era of full-blown digital terrorism that we are, oddly, glued to. As CNN's technical director was caught saying about the news, "If it bleeds, it leads." When the stories are morbid, they get attention. On top of this, all humans will experience personal challenges and traumas throughout our lives, and in the face of our cultural stigmatization about mental health care, we have limited resources to process them. With all this, we are getting crushed:

- Close to 40 percent of U.S. women report a diagnosis of depression in their lifetime, and a full third of Americans report an anxiety disorder in their lifetime.
- Three-quarters of young Americans feel unsafe daily.
- A survey published in February 2023 by the CDC revealed that in 2021, 57 percent of high school girls reported experiencing "persistent feelings of sadness or hopelessness in the past year," a significant increase from the 36 percent reported in 2011.
- Seventy-six percent of Americans reported health impacts from stress in the past month, with the main drivers of that stress being health concerns.
- Many other leading surveys show a pronounced increase in depression, particularly among adolescents around the 2011 period (which happens to be the year Instagram burst onto the scene).

It's easy to gloss over these statistics, but take a moment to take them in: in a time when life expectancy and standard of living seem to be higher than ever, *hundreds of millions* of people in the wealthiest country in human history—including children—are suffering from sadness, fear, and profound stress. There has always been suffering in the world, but now we can *see* exponentially more of it than ever, all at once, on screens we hold in our beds and at the dinner table.

In response, modern humans have looked for salvation and coping anywhere we can get a hit of dopamine-fueled "pleasure" and distraction: things like processed sugar, alcohol, soda, refined carbs, vapes, cigarettes, weed, porn, dating apps, email, texts, casual sex, online gambling, video games, Instagram, TikTok, Snapchat, and the relentless novelty of experiences. As Johann Hari, author of *Stolen Focus,* has said, "We've created a culture where really large numbers of people can't bear to be present in their daily lives and need to medicate themselves throughout the day." The impact of our modern psychological reality—and the unhealthy coping mechanisms—is that our cells' ability to produce Good Energy is dimmed, creating a vicious cycle that robs us of the full potential of our human experience.

A cell living in a body experiencing chronic fear is a cell that cannot fully thrive. When our cells sense sustained danger, they divert resources to defense and alarm pathways instead of normal functions that generate sustainable health. Given this, no matter how pristine your dietary intake is, how much you're moving, how much sunlight you're getting, or how many hours of quality sleep you're getting, if the cells are bathed in a stew of stress created by the way psychology translates to biochemistry (via hormones, neurotransmitters, inflammatory cytokines, and neurologic signals), all the other healthy choices will fall flat.

It is our most fundamental job to take stock of the persistent fear triggers in our life and work to heal them or limit their exposure. We do this through psychological modalities like boundary setting, introspection, meditation, breathwork, therapy, plant medicine, spending time in nature, and many others outlined at the end of this chapter.

Don't confuse setting boundaries to what information you allow in your ears and eyes with putting your head in the sand; it's understanding and protecting your biology so you don't implode. This allows you to show up with maximal energy to positively impact the world.

Everyone's threat signals are going to be different. It could be chronic work stress from a challenging relationship with your boss. It could be residual childhood trauma from a strained relationship with a parent. It could be a feeling of lack of safety in your home or neighborhood. It could be a news article about a murder that happened twenty-five hundred miles away. It could be from a sense of danger from a virus sweeping across the globe. It could be from news of war five thousand miles away. It could be about rights or liberties being threatened by a political agenda. It could be from a worry about not being good enough, pretty enough, or smart enough. Take stock of your own so you can protect your cells from constant psychological harm and create an environment of peace for them.

THE FEAR MACHINE THAT KEEPS US SICK AND DEPENDENT

In medical school, I was taught that *anything*—no matter the cost, side effects, or societal toll—is justifiable to prevent death, even if it only squeaks out a few more painful, vegetative days. The message patients receive from hospitals and pharma companies isn't that "we are going to keep you healthy and help you have the best possible life"—it is that "we are going to keep you alive."

Attend your annual physical. Get your screenings. Take your pills. Get this surgery. And if you don't, *you just might die.* The fear of death is weaponized to get patients to do *anything*: more meds, procedures, operations, and specialists. The subtext is that if you say no, delay treatment, or take a more natural route, you just might die sooner. These dynamics are especially powerful in the modern West, where—unlike many indigenous and Eastern cultures—we tend to be culturally avoidant of talking about death or having curiosity about it, leading it to be an existential fear for many. So many of the texts that have stood the test of time—spanning Rumi, Khalil Gibran, Hafiz, Marcus Aurelius, Yogananda, Seneca, Lao-tzu, Thích Nhất Hạnh, and more—implore us to examine death and trust that it is both natural and not to be feared. Somehow these messages haven't remotely made it to the mainstream health care ecosystem, where death is unacceptable.

For me, death was my greatest fear from childhood and into adulthood and the one I have had to address head-on to unpeel the layers shielding me from Good Energy. I have spent more of my life worrying about the ways I or my family could die than about any other issue. Death was the reason for my mind racing countless nights. Death is why I got into medicine.

A set of experiences with my mother beginning in early 2020 changed my perspective on worry—particularly about death—forever. Concerned about her rising glucose and cholesterol levels, I took her to Sedona for "Dr. Casey's Bootcamp" of proven actions to improve metabolic health: extended fasting, cold plunging, exercise, morning sunrise hikes. It was a year before we'd discover her pancreatic cancer.

Having not eaten for three days and on a ketone high, I felt euphoric as my mom and I looked at the towering Red Rock Mountains together. My mom and I had hiked to the top of a ridge in the dark for a full-moon drum circle that we'd heard about from a local art gallery, and she and I danced together in the moonlight with abandon.

Looking at the towering rocks, I couldn't get the idea out of my head that the mountains and I were made of much the same thing. The atoms that make up my body have been on the earth since its creation some 4.6 billion years ago. And for a brief sliver of time, my mitochondria produce ATP to power the organization of these atoms into my tissues, organs, and ultimately *me*.

In Sedona, my mom and I talked about how the ideas of "self" and the finality of death were illusions. In reality, large portions of our bodies are dying on a regular basis—we each shed more than a *pound* of cells each day. Our cells make up to 88 percent of dust in our homes. In medical school, I looked at slivers of body parts on slides under the microscope and was surprised to see the full spectrum of life and death happening inside what *seemed* like an "adult" living body. But at the microscopic level, cells were dying, dividing, being born, aging at vastly different rates. At the cellular level, we die and are reborn trillions upon trillions of times in one "lifetime." The discarded matter from our bodies returns to the earth and eventually creates new things. Fossil fuels, which supply 80 percent of the earth's energy today, are nothing more than the remains of animals and plants that existed millions of years ago. We are literally powering our cars and homes with the atoms that made up our ancestors.

It is merely a limitation of our visual systems that we don't see these innumerable reactions happening every second in our body and the constant creation and re-creation that makes up our world.

I speculated with my mom about whether the discarded pieces of myself would be taken up into a delicious piece of broccoli that feeds a child. Or maybe I would supply some carbons that will be pounded into a perfect diamond. Or maybe I will donate some atomic dust to a gust of wind that helps form mountain ranges that are yet to exist. Probably all the above, plus other forms I can't even conceive of.

The impact we have on others—the people we love, the people we mistreat, the people we teach, the people who read our writing—literally changes their biology and lives forever. As my mom and I danced and hugged under the moonlight, I thought about how this loving experience with her was literally changing the physical neural pathways and biology in my body through neurotransmitter and hormone release, reinforcing synapses, and transferring microbiomes to each other. My experience of her—and all people with whom I choose to interact—will physically encode itself in me.

On January 7, 2021, I received a Facetime call from my mother while I was preparing dinner, tears streaming down her face as she told me that she was dying, that she had to leave me, and that she would not meet my future children. She relayed that she had learned earlier that day that her vague stomach pain had actually been widely metastatic stage 4 pancreatic cancer and she had softball-sized tumors all throughout her belly.

Over the next thirteen days, the final days of my mom's consciousness, she received hundreds of letters about the impact she'd had on people's lives. I will never forget the gratitude and poignant emotion on her face as she sat reading them, while outside on the porch overlooking the Pacific. Every note was from a human who'd been biochemically changed because of my mother's impact on them. Just as we had talked about in Sedona, I could feel that she was fundamentally immortal due to her impact on everyone in her life and her energetic ripple effect in the universe, which every one of us is connected to and contributes to by our sheer existence. She was without fear as she held my hand and told me that she could feel her life force rapidly retreating.

Days after she died, we buried her in a natural cemetery along the coastline. How profound to lower her beautiful body into a small patch of dirt among the endless expanse of the ocean. This woman—whom my brother and I had lived inside of, our source, who built my body and consciousness, who traveled the world, and who impacted thousands of people—disintegrated into the earth to feed the trees and flowers and mushrooms above her in an eternal cycle. Worrying about the years her physical body existed on Earth seemed so irrelevant. All my years of anxiety about my mortality and the mortality of my family had been wasted energy. Death is uncontrollable and it is OK. I feel that because when I held my mother as she took her last breath, *she* was OK. In her final waking moments, she whispered to me that we are here to protect the energy of the universe. That it all—the life, the death—was perfect.

Lowering my mother into the soil, I felt the deepest sense that my mother and I—and everything and everyone else—are inextricably intertwined, and nothing about death can change that. Despite the human-made forces creating the overwhelming perception of separation, scarcity, and fear in order to exert power, create dependency, and extract money from humans and nature—just as the forty-two specialties of medicine obfuscate the reality of one body—we can push back and we can embody a different truth of total connectedness and limitlessness. I felt Rumi's words wash over me: "*Don't grieve. Anything you lose comes round in another form*" and "*Why think separately of this life and the next when one is born of the last?*" And in the solidification of that belief, I felt the next layer of Good Energy open for me: fearlessness.

The grip of existential worry and chronic low-grade fear that had lived in me from early childhood started to be processed and released, and in that, I felt my health baseline shift and I felt compelled to continue the journey of becoming empowered by my true nature as a dynamic, eternal process, a concept I'd never been taught in my medical training. My mind was relaxing and my cells were becoming free to do their best possible work.

HOW THE MIND CONTROLS METABOLISM

Why is overcoming chronic fear so critical to Good Energy? Because in many ways, our mind controls our metabolism. When it comes to Good Energy and the brain, it's a vicious cycle: a lack of healthy habits weakens the brain's defenses to chronic stress, and chronic stress and fear can directly cause more metabolic dysfunction that worsens mood and resilience. Consider that 75 to 90 percent of human diseases are related to activation of stress-related biology, and much evidence points to a common pathway between psychological stressors and metabolic dysfunction. Your cells "listen" to all your thoughts through biochemical signals, and the message they are getting from chronic stress is to halt the production of Good Energy. In fact, intense acute stress and chronic stress trigger all the hallmarks of Bad Energy:

1. **Chronic Inflammation:** In mice, just six hours of acute stress leads to a "rapid mobilization" of the immune system, with the increase in concentration of inflammatory cytokines. Cytokines are specific immune chemicals involved in early attacks of infections and wounds, as well as gene expression of pathways related to immune cell migration (the way immune cells get to the place they need to go to fight). Stressful thoughts trigger neuroinflammation (inflammation in the brain). Neuroinflammation leads to metabolic dysfunction in the brain and predisposes us to metabolic diseases, like depression and neurodegeneration. It also impacts the whole body by kicking off the "stress arm" of the nervous system—the sympathetic nervous system (SNS) or fight-or-flight system. Overactivation of the SNS drives insulin resistance, hyperglycemia, and mobilization of inflammatory cells and cytokines throughout the body, further compounding Bad Energy everywhere. Longer periods of psychological stress, like childhood abuse, are associated with elevated levels of the inflammatory cytokines CRP, TNF-α, and IL-6. One researcher notes that chronic stress–induced inflammation represents the "common soil" of a wide variety of metabolic diseases like cancer, fatty liver disease, heart disease, and type 2 diabetes. Remember, inflammation directly leads to Bad Energy by blocking the expression of glucose channels, blocking the insulin signal from transmitting inside the cell, and promoting the release of free fatty acids from fat cells, which can then be taken up by the liver and muscle and generate insulin resistance.

2. **Oxidative Stress:** In 2004, a study examined the blood of fifteen medical students both before and after their significant exams to measure oxidative stress biomarkers. The findings showed that the students had lower levels of antioxidants leading up to the exams and experienced

higher levels of DNA and lipid damage from oxidation. These results suggest that their cells were subjected to oxidative stress during the stressful period. There is evidence to suggest that work-related stress also contributes to oxidative stress. For example, a study in Japan demonstrated a correlation between 8-hydroxydeoxyguanosine (8-OH-dG), an oxidative stress marker, and female workers' perceived workload, psychological stress, and sense of impossibility in reducing stress. Similarly, a study in Spain found a relationship between high levels of work-related stress and malondialdehyde, another oxidative stress biomarker. In rats, chronic stress induces oxidation of fats and decreases antioxidant activity. This correlated with higher LDL cholesterol and triglycerides, lower HDL, and, ultimately, plaque development in the rodents' arteries. Interestingly, animal studies have shown that ingested antioxidants may protect against stress-induced mitochondrial dysfunction, "indicating the existence of stress-sensitizing and stress-buffering factors for the effects of induced stress on mitochondria." Similarly, when mice are engineered to overexpress mitochondrial antioxidant enzymes, they seem to have increased capacity to handle stressors.

3. **Mitochondrial Dysfunction:** While almost all research on psychosocial stress and mitochondrial function has been done in animals, the results indicate a clear theme that "chronic stress induced through a form of psychosocial stressor decreases mitochondrial energy production capacity and alters mitochondrial morphology." This showed up as reduction in the function of mitochondrial proteins, lower rate of oxygen consumption (which is needed to make ATP in the mitochondria), and lower mitochondrial content.

4. **High Glucose Levels:** Elevations of stress hormones resulting from acute psychological stressors can lead to *diabetogenic effects*, meaning that they immediately raise blood sugar rapidly while also causing fat cells to break down fat and release it into the bloodstream, which promotes insulin resistance. During stress, the body mobilizes a "quick" and robust source of energy, so stress hormones prompt the rapid

breakdown of stored glucose from the liver (glycogenolysis) and increase production of glucose from the liver (gluconeogenesis). As stress hormones trigger the rapid breakdown of triglycerides (stored fat) in fat cells, one of the breakdown products is glycerol, which can be transported to the liver to manufacture glucose via gluconeogenesis. Researchers believe that repeated acute stress responses could "induce repeated exposure to transient hyperglycemia and hyperlipidemia, and insulin resistance, which could evolve toward type 2 diabetes onset in the long term." Levels members often report being surprised by the impact a stressful day at work can have on their blood sugar, and how increases in blood sugar can indicate stress.

5. **Worse Metabolic Biomarkers:** Chronic stress is associated with obesity, lower HDL, increased visceral fat, larger waist circumference, and higher blood pressure, LDL, heart rate, insulin levels, and triglycerides. What's more, cortisol levels have been shown to be a predictor of elevated levels of HOMA-IR, a key marker of insulin resistance.

Traumas Crush Good Energy

It's not just the day-to-day low-grade stressors that add up to problems for health. Traumatic events also have a long-term impact on our metabolic health. A significant body of research shows that stressful events during childhood, called adverse childhood experiences (ACEs), can have long-term effects on the regulation of stress hormones in our bodies. These can include emotional or physical neglect or abuse, household dysfunction, insults or put-downs, bullying, crime, death of a loved one, severe illness, life-threatening accidents, and natural disasters. Research suggests that up to 80 percent of people experience one or more of these events, and they contribute to increased risk of developing conditions such as obesity, diabetes, heart disease, and metabolic syndrome. In one study, children who were maltreated (as defined by maternal rejection, harsh discipline, physical or sexual abuse, or multiple changes in caregivers) were 80 percent more likely to have high inflammatory marker levels (CRP), while social isolation conferred a 134 percent higher risk of having elevated metabolic biomarkers. Early life adversity has been consistently associated with dys-regulation of the stress regulation pathways in the body that persists into adulthood, which can predict stress-related chronic illness like metabolic diseases. What's more, childhood abuse may be related to altered reward processing in the brain and may predispose to excess food intake and food addiction into adulthood.

So often in my practice, I would ask patients if they were "stressed" or had past traumas, and they would flatly say no. But in digging into the details over a two-hour visit, they often had significant childhood adverse experiences that had not been fully processed. Many times, they also reported feeling trapped in their job, being overburdened by caregiving responsibilities without adequate support, experiencing strained family relationships with parents, spouses, extended family, or children, social and financial anxiety, loneliness, a history of intimate partner violence, and many other traumas or negative situations in their lives that they didn't necessarily label as "stress" or "trauma" but that were still very real and present.

Training Our Brain to Heal

No matter what has transpired in our lives or what is going on in the world around us, we have to find a way to *feel safe* in order to be as healthy as possible. "Being safe" is somewhat of an illusion: I, you, and everyone we love are going to die. But *feeling safe* is something we can cultivate inside our minds and bodies through intentional practice. This is lifelong work, and there will not be a single path for everyone. A first step is awareness of the impact of chronic threat triggers and life traumas on our health. We then have to improve the "hardware" (the physical structure and function of the body) and the software (the psychology and frameworks). To improve the hardware, it involves all the Good Energy habits: food and lifestyle strategies that create a biological reality in the body most conducive to mental health. To improve the software, it involves pursuing modalities that help manage and heal the stressors, traumas, and thought patterns that limit us and contribute to our poor metabolic health and thriving.

Eating healthily, sleeping well, and working out might seem like trivial matters if you are facing existential dread or depression, but I promise you this: if you get your heart rate up for at least 150 minutes a week and follow the food principles in Chapter 5, you will notice an improvement and your brain will be more equipped to navigate the stresses of life. If you sleep an adequate amount, your world will automatically look far more awe-inspiring. Focus on the *inputs*—the habits—and the results will begin to happen. Especially in a place of stress or fear, it can be very hard to get motivated to do any of this work. A good first step is to find *anything* healthy from this book that feels inspiring and give it a shot, because small wins beget more wins.

We are animals in cages right now, surrounded by encroaching threats that are entering our homes and daily lives through technology, chemicals, and more. Since our brains use a disproportionate 20 percent of the energy in the body despite being just 2 percent of total weight of the body, dysfunction at the cellular level hits the brain extra hard. Focus on Good Energy habits, and slowly but surely, Good Energy will take over your life.

The Work

Healing trauma, developing unconditional self-love, feeling limitless, and making peace with death are tall orders. The following fifteen strategies are research-supported modalities that can help:

1. Form a Relationship with a Mental Health Therapist, Coach, or Counselor

We have doctors for our physical health, mechanics for our cars, trainers for our workouts, accountants for our taxes, lawyers for our contracts, and financial advisers for our investments, and yet we still find it niche or stigmatizing to get professional help for the most important aspects of our lives: our minds. I implore you to ignore any cultural messaging and stigma around "mental health" and instead view therapy, counseling, or coaching as one of the highest leverage investments you can make to maximize your life. If you shy away from the concept of "mental health," think of it as a "brain coach" or "brain optimizer." One hour per week of introspection and unpacking feelings with a professional could make the difference between being imprisoned by repetitive maladaptive thought patterns and being psychologically free. Finding a great therapist can take time; don't get discouraged if you don't click with the first one.

Online services like BetterHelp.com simplify getting paired with a therapist. Or ask people in your community, whom you find resilient and happy, if they have a therapist they've worked with and liked.

2. Track Your Heart Rate Variability (HRV) and Work to Improve It

Use wearables like Whoop, Apple Watch, Fitbit, Oura, HeartMath, or Lief to monitor HRV and identify triggers that lower HRV. With Lief, you can see your HRV in real time and can note which experiences cause HRV to drop (indicating more stress) and which interventions—like taking a deep breath—help when HRV is low.

3. Practice Breathwork

Breathwork is a powerful way to stimulate the vagus nerve and activate the parasympathetic nervous system (PSNS), which is the "rest and digest" arm of the nervous system. Activating the PSNS can help calm you down rapidly. You can also try simple breathwork techniques—like *box breathing*, which is a relaxation technique involving taking slow, deep breaths in a pattern of inhaling, holding, exhaling, and holding again for a count of four seconds for each phase. You can find many guided videos on You-Tube, as well as on apps like Open and Othership.

4. Practice Mindfulness Meditation

Consistent mindfulness meditation for eight weeks, with daily sessions as short as twenty minutes, has been shown to significantly decrease several metabolic biomarkers, including uric acid, triglycerides, ApoB, and blood sugar, while also improving mood, anxiety, and depression. These changes are likely a result of meditation's impact on lowering stress hormones and the positive metabolic effects that result. Both NF-$\varkappa$B gene expression and hsCRP are reduced in people who practice mindfulness meditation compared to the general public. Expert meditators can lower the expression of pro-inflammatory genes and change epigenetic pathways in a single extended meditation session. Through the activity of our minds, we can literally change our genetic expression, blood glucose levels, and immune system activation.

Mindfulness meditation can seem extremely intimidating and hard, but it needn't be. Meditation can be as simple as sitting quietly and just mentally noting whenever a thought pops into your head. As each thought emerges, notice it, note *thought* in your head, let it go, and reset. In doing that, you flex the muscle of returning to the "present moment." In a ten-minute session, you might have one hundred thoughts pop into your head. Having so many thoughts pop up might seem like a failure, but noticing them is actually the work. The alternative is that you *don't* notice as they pop into your head, and you let them take you on a ride on the "train of thought" without your ever noticing. By simply noting the thought, you get *off* the "train of thought" and back to the present moment. In doing this, you solidify the understanding that your identity is separate from the rush of stressful thoughts running through your brain. Most of us spend the entirety of our life jumping from thought to thought, never getting off the "train," thinking that this is "reality" or "you." It's not: you can simply step off and reset into the present moment, and this is like waking up from a dream and stepping into a blissful spiritual space.

The voices in our head—the fear, anxiety, anger, sadness—are *not* us. Many get frustrated with meditation because they "aren't good at it" and "get distracted." The point of meditation *is distraction*. Meditation shows us that no matter how hard we try, our head will produce thoughts and that we can choose to let those thoughts pass or change them. We then can take this insight to our daily life, letting us disassociate from the weight of the out-of-control inner voice, so we can more clearly tune into our limitless spiritual nature, while also being more present to fully experience playing with our kids, taking a walk, or having a conversation with a loved one.

Another way to practice mindfulness at any moment is to close your eyes and scan every sensation in your body: your heartbeat, your butt on the chair, any areas of warmth or cold, your toes on the ground, the air moving into your nose and lungs. Because this body scan forces you into the present moment, it takes you away from mental states of anxiety or stress.

My favorite meditation apps are Calm and Waking Up, and there are many guided meditations on YouTube. Even a ten-minute meditation can transform a day.

Devices like Muse can help you train your meditation practice and help you know when you are reaching a more relaxed brain state with biofeedback.

5. Try Movement-Based Mindfulness Practices, Like Yoga, Tai Chi, or Qigong

Research has shown that mind-body interventions that deal with both physical and mental well-being, like yoga and qigong, can improve depression, anxiety, and stress. They also increase activity of the PSNS, lower cortisol, reduce inflammation, and change genetic folding and expression (epigenetics), all of which can positively impact metabolic issues.

6. Spend Time in Nature

Some doctors are now prescribing "nature pills"—prescriptions to spend time in nature—because evidence shows that it lowers stress hormones significantly, and it increases the PSNS and mood. Even going to a city park has measurable impacts on health and stress markers.

In closely observing nature, we get the opportunity to meditate on the profound harmony, interconnectedness, and cycles that thread through the natural world. We see many polarities and cycles that surround us to create life, health, and beauty: polarities like sleeping and waking, night and day, cold and hot, parasympathetic and sympathetic nervous system, high and low tide, alkaline and acidic. Cycles like spring to summer to fall to winter, new moon to first quarter moon to full moon to last quarter moon, and menstruation to follicular phase to ovulation to luteal phase. These rhythms surround us in nature, and they are our best teachers in achieving fearlessness, because they show us that the world is *fundamentally harmonious* even when things swing between different states. But in the modern world, living inside and so separate from nature, we have begun to ignore, fight, or suppress polarities and cycles, under the illusion that they are suboptimal and we can outsmart them. Through industrial agriculture, we've asked the soil to give us endless summer. Through widespread use of oral hormones for everything from acne to PCOS to contraception, we've trivialized the stunning—and life-creating—rhythmicity of women's bodies, as well as the cycle's potent utility as a biofeedback tool of a woman's overall health. Through around-the-clock artificial light, we've created the illusion that we don't need night. Through thermostats, we've pushed a thermoneutral existence where we're never too hot or cold. The results haven't been good. We have forgotten that we get the best out of natural systems not through dominance, oppression, and overworking, but through respect, care, and gentle support.

In our busy, distracted, industrial lives, we've become separate from nature, and therefore we've become fearful and controlling of its natural rhythms and realities, getting stressed by a sense of scarcity when we aren't in the phase or pole of our liking. The "yin" periods of cycles and polarities appear unproductive and wasteful, so we squash and rush them, thinking we're brilliant for creating a world of constant "yang." How foolish we are. Attention toward and awe for nature is the best teacher in gaining comfort with death and anxiety based on a sense of scarcity. When you look up and really spend time with nature and learn from it with humility and awe, you realize that you have nothing to fear. Don't allow yourself to be separated from your source: soil, sun, water, trees, the stars, and the moon. Get outside often to feel more peace.

7. Read Inspirational and Thought-Provoking Books and Texts About Mindset, Trauma, and the Human Condition

I keep these authors' works all throughout my house as a constant reminder of the "bigger picture." Audiobooks and podcasts work great for this as well.

I highly recommend the following books about mindset, mental health, and reshaping our relationship with stress and trauma: *Mindset, A Return to Love, Untethered Soul, How to Do the Work, Brain Energy, Hacking of the American Mind, Brain Wash, How to Change Your Mind, Waking Up, The*

Four Agreements, You Are More Than You Think You Are, The Book of Boundaries, Getting the Love You Want, 4,000 Weeks, and *Attached.* Many of these books are great on audio, and I find that listening to ten minutes of books, podcasts, or texts that address mindset and mental fortitude while I'm getting ready for the day puts me in a positive headspace.

Authors and poets who address the human condition, mortality, eternity, and continuity with nature that I recommend are Mary Oliver, Pema Chödrön, Paramahansa Yogananda, Michael Pollan, Clarissa Pinkola Estés, Seneca, Marcus Aurelius, Robin Wall Kimmerer, Rumi, Lao-tzu, Khalil Gibran, Hafiz, Walt Whitman, W. S. Merwin, Thích Nhất Hạnh, Diane Ackerman, Alan Watts, Lewis Thomas, Ram Das, Rainer Maria Rilke, Deepak Chopra, and Wang Wei.

8. Try Aromatherapy

Clinical research supports that natural scents can be powerful triggers of relaxation. Lavender oil is well studied and especially potent in minimizing stress and helping with sleep, as outlined in the peer-reviewed paper "Lavender and the Nervous System." Rub a few drops of lavender essential oil between your hands, cup your face, and inhale deeply a few times.

9. Write

If you're feeling down or stressed and can't get "unstuck," set a timer and write about any problems for five minutes. Writing is also an incredible way to channel creativity and to connect with "the bigger picture." Many studies have shown that writing is a way to lower distress and improve clinical benefit in patients with anxiety or inflammatory diseases. "Positive affect" journaling for twelve weeks, which may include focusing on writing about positive emotions like gratitude or reflection on how someone else has helped you, has been shown to reduce mental distress in patients with medical issues and anxiety, while improving resilience and social integration.

Books I recommend for starting a regular writing practice include *The Artist's Way* by Julia Cameron, *The War of Art* by Steven Pressfield, *Big Magic* by Elizabeth Gilbert, and *The Creative Act* by Rick Rubin.

10. Intentionally Focus on Awe and Gratitude

Focus on awe, abundance, and gratitude every day. My best days start with a blank sheet of paper where I list all the things I'm grateful for, helping engender a profound sense of abundance that calms me and helps me act from a place of security rather than fear.

Take walks where you intentionally focus on finding the awe in things around you: a cloud rapidly moving across the sky, a fruit tree in a neighbor's yard, a weed sprouting out from a crack in the concrete, the moon beaming down at you, snow falling from above, a bird sitting on your fence. Let yourself be humbled by taking in things that are much bigger than you and totally out of our control, like mountains, sunsets, rivers, oceans, and forests.

Until recent history, humans were less distracted by constant assaults on our attention that trigger our dopamine and keep us coming back for more. We had space to be humbled by the grandeur of nature and life cycles, with animals, harvests, the sun, the moon, birth, and death being experienced as cosmic powerful forces. We've been robbed of this connection to our bodies and nature and need to make conscious efforts to train our brains back to being able to see and appreciate the majesty of all of it. Miracles are hiding in plain sight everywhere, obscured by the "distraction industrial complex" in the zero-sum game of attention. It is an act of rebellion and independence to refocus your attention on awe.

Rick Rubin shares in *The Creative Act*, "Zoom in and obsess. Zoom out and observe. We get to choose." I spent a lot of mental energy concerned about gun violence because I see it plastered on every screen around me, and sometimes I let it control a lot of my mind space and behavior, obscuring my ability to "see" the awe-inspiring beauty around me. We should never ignore societal problems or avoid working to improve them. But by allowing ourselves to create space for our attention to dwell on awe, we can generate physical and mental health that lets us show up most potently and limitlessly to help bring *more* energy and commitment to positively impacting the world and overcoming devastating societal trends.

11. Practice Active Self-Love

Be mindful of negative self-talk and find ways to become your biggest supporter and the greatest love of your life. Sometimes the biggest form of threat in our lives—and that our cells "hear"—is our own voice berating ourselves for our perceived shortcomings. Often we might just be mimicking damaging voices that berated us in our past or from culture that we internalized. Actively change the narrative. You have the power to talk to yourself with kindness and support, telling yourself messages like: "I love you so much. You are resilient and have gotten through so much in life. I'm proud of you for taking the time to read a book about health." Speak to yourself (and your cells) as you would speak to a newborn in your arms, a life that need not do anything to deserve unconditional love and care. If this is a struggle, loving-kindness meditations and professional therapy can help.

12. Be Less Busy

Embrace "JOMO," the Joy of Missing Out. Get comfortable with periods of unstructured time, alone, without constant distractions. Find pleasure in saying no when you aren't completely excited about a particular activity or event. A good metric of when to skip something is when it's not a "whole body YES," a term coined by leadership coach Diana Chapman, author of *15 Commitments of Conscious Leadership*. When missing out feels uncomfortable, remind yourself of the abundance of opportunities in life, such that "missing out" is really a scarcity-based illusion. Every *no* to something you feel lukewarm about is a *yes* to time that can be spent doing something more meaningful.

13. Cultivate Community

Loneliness, which one-third of U.S. adults feel frequently, can directly contribute to poor metabolic health, according to a 2023 article published in *Frontiers in Psychology*. Given that social connections are evolutionarily valuable for survival, loneliness is thought to have "evolved as an alarm signal, akin to hunger or thirst, to seek out social contact to promote survival." The link between loneliness and poor metabolic health is not fully understood, but may be due to dysregulation of the balance of SNS and PSNS and increased stress signaling, which can dampen the function of the mitochondria. Positive social connection can counteract this possibly through the release of oxytocin, a hormone and neurotransmitter that may protect against stress and suppress the release of stress hormones.

14. Commit to a Digital Detox

Research suggests that excess smartphone use is associated with negative "psychiatric, cognitive, emotional, medical, and brain changes." Reducing smartphone use by just one hour a day has been shown to decrease depressive and anxiety symptoms and improve life satisfaction. Choose activities that *force* you to be away from your phone, devices, social media, and the news. Such activities might include paddleboarding, surfing, swimming, rafting, wilderness backpacking, or rock climbing. Leave your phone behind when you leave the house, like going to the grocery store, to a concert, or on a long hike. Have a friend change your social media passwords and not give you the passwords back until a specified time. Or take the suggestion from Johann Hari's book *Stolen Focus* and buy an impenetrable kSafe that will keep your tech locked for whatever time you specify.

15. Consider Psilocybin-Assisted Therapy

If you feel called, I also encourage you to explore intentional, guided psilocybin therapy. Strong scientific evidence suggests that this psychedelic therapy can be one of the most meaningful experiences of life for some people, as they have been for me.

If the word *psychedelics* makes you cringe, I used to be in your position. I spent my childhood and young adult life being extremely judgmental about the use of any type of drug. But I became interested in plant medicine and psychedelics after learning more about their extensive traditional use, analyzing the groundbreaking research from University of California–San Francisco and Johns Hopkins, and reading *Waking Up* by Sam Harris and *How to Change Your Mind* by Michael Pollan. Our brains are profoundly suffering in modern society right now, and I believe that anything that can safely increase neuroplasticity and ground us in more gratitude, awe, connection, and a sense of cosmic safety should be taken very seriously. Recently, *The Economist* ranked twenty drugs on their danger to individuals and society. At the top of the list were legal drugs: alcohol, opioids, amphetamines (Adderall), and tobacco. At the bottom of the list—the three safest drugs ranked—were MDMA, LSD, and magic mushrooms (psilocybin). Up to 25 percent of American adults are now on antidepressants, like SSRIs, or antianxiety meds, like benzodiazepines, that numb us and don't address the root-cause physiology (but produce recurring revenue for the medical system). Psilocybin and other psychedelics have been stigmatized. Today neuroscientists are almost universally calling research on psychedelics the most promising of their careers. Many of these natural compounds, like the psilocybin found in "magic mushrooms," come directly from the earth to induce profound, consciousness-expanding experiences.

A 2016 Johns Hopkins study showed that "67% of the volunteers rated the experience with psilocybin to be either the single most meaningful experience of his or her life or among the top five most meaningful experiences of his or her life . . . similar, for example, to the birth of a first child or death of a parent." I can't think of a more societally important research finding.

Recently, a UCSF study showed that a group with severe PTSD who "received MDMA during therapy experienced a significantly greater reduction in the severity of their symptoms compared with those who received therapy." Gül Dölen, a neuroscientist at Johns Hopkins, said, "There is nothing like this in clinical trial results for a neuropsychiatric disease." Scott Ostrom, a participant in the UCSF study who faced crippling PTSD from his time in Iraq, said the experience "stimulated my own consciousness's ability for self-healing . . . You understand why it's OK to experience unconditional love for yourself."

Just a week before I would learn of my mom's terminal diagnosis, I sat on the ground in the desert as the sun was going down. I had been inspired to try psilocybin mushrooms in what I can only describe as an internal voice that whispered: *it's time to prepare.* At the time, I didn't know consciously what I was preparing for, but as I basked in the moon's bright rays,

I experienced the embodiment of being one with the moon, every star, every atom in the grains of sand I was sitting on, and my mother in an inextricable and unbreakable chain of universal connectedness for which the human concept of "death" was no match. In that moment I was certain there was no separation between any of it. I felt myself as part of an infinite and unbroken series of cosmic nesting dolls of millions of mothers and babies before me from the beginning of life. I felt how I had been assembled out of the universe's building blocks through my mother as the creative portal who printed my ever-changing form from stardust deep inside her belly, and how that form became the lightning rod to channel my spirit or spark my consciousness, kicking off the duality of spirit/consciousness and body that defines our human experience and can cause psychological pain if unexamined.

In my experience, psilocybin can be a doorway to a different reality that is free from the limiting beliefs of my ego, feelings, and personal history. Because I was able to experience that limitlessness and peace—albeit transiently—I now know what is possible and can work to access that state through daily habits. I know that the mind is more powerful than we think and can conjure huge, positive, creative visions if we *simply allow* it to, and that this potential of thought shifts what's possible in our day-to-day lives.

TRUST THE PROCESS

Just after my mom died, I traveled to New York City. Late one night, I walked to the first-floor apartment on West Eleventh Street where she spent ten formative years of her young adult life. It's the apartment where I know she read Buddhist texts, built her business, played piano late into the night, and got ready to go out and dance at Studio 54. Sitting on the stoop, tears gently streaming down my cheeks, I visualized her walking through the door during her single years: six feet tall and fabulous—with me already living inside of her as an egg that had been present in her body since she was a fetus in my grandmother's body seventy-two years prior. I looked out on the street, the exact spot where she kissed my father on their first date in 1981, the man who would become the other part of the puzzle to unlock the life-giving potential within her and bring my form and consciousness to fruition.

From the corner of my eye, I noticed an old, tattered book lying on the ground. It was called *The Odd Woman* (a vintage term for an older single woman, like myself at the time), and it was written by Gail Godwin (my mother's name was also Gayle). I was compelled to walk over and pick it up. I opened the book. The page read,

> One day the whole universe will accept: that there isn't any struggle essentially, except what our self-created ego tells us is a struggle.
>
> All the disharmonies, conflicts, conversations, love affairs and failures and death are superficial events. None of them are significant, really.
>
> The only significant thing is how we enjoy the moment, our attitude toward the moment. One should simply give himself up to the moment, enjoy it, even if it is horrendous.
>
> Are you saying that if a person is getting murdered at a certain moment, he should enjoy that moment? Why not? Why not enjoy it? It's his last moment, the last personal, superficial event in his finite life. Sure, why not enjoy it? What else better is there to do?

Perhaps my mom was speaking to me. Even in the most extreme case—imminent death—we should have awe and appreciation for life and see the illusion of our ego and the reality of total connectedness. This is exactly what she did; as she faced her terminal cancer diagnosis—thirteen days of life, the final sands rapidly falling through the hourglass—she exuded joy, gratitude, and curiosity.

We have no control over so much. In the face of inevitable mortality, chronic stress triggers in our environment, and traumatic childhood experience with little cultural awareness of resilience or coping, an unshakable sense of safety can be elusive. Of course, we should take reasonable precautions for our own safety and our family's safety—but living in chronic stress or fear is neither optimal nor rational.

The road to maximal human well-being is not paved with more

pharmaceuticals and procedures for an increasing list of isolated conditions. Improving our health requires understanding that we are inextricably interconnected with everything else in the universe, including soil, plants, animals, people, air, water, and sunlight. To thrive, we must get back to having awe for our interdependent relationship with everything in the natural world. We also must recognize that every part of our own bodies is interconnected, not a fragmented set of isolated parts as the forty-two specialties of medicine might have us believe. The more advanced our understanding of life sciences gets, the more convinced I am that achieving our highest potential as humans involves recommitting to many natural basics that modern living has separated us from. This doesn't require us to reject modernity or re-create a bygone era; instead, we can use cutting-edge tools, technology, and diagnostics to empower us to understand more deeply our relationship to the world around us, and to help us align our daily choices and investments toward the metabolic needs coded deep within our cells. At this moment we have the understanding and the tools to live the longest, happiest, healthiest lives in human history. The foundation of this is helping our cells make Good Energy.

To view the scientific references cited in this chapter, please visit us online at caseymeans.com/goodenergy.

PART 3

THE GOOD ENERGY PLAN

Four Weeks to Good Energy

If simple habits (like eating whole foods, getting enough sleep, practicing regular movement, and managing stress) are so transformational, why do so few people consistently perform them? If these simple actions made people so happy and healthy, why aren't we all doing them?

I think this question hangs in our collective subconscious and fuels the insidious beliefs in the medical system that "patients are lazy," "lifestyle interventions fail," and "people want the easy way out." Or that more complex and "innovative" solutions must be the answer. These criticisms of patients conveniently ignore the fact that trillions of dollars of incentives are pushing us to eat ultra-processed food, be sedentary, sleep less, and live in chronic fear.

The truth: practicing *simple* Good Energy habits is an act of rebellion. This section outlines twenty-five of the most important ones, with a four-week plan to help integrate them into your life. By engaging with these simple habits, you can thrive and minimize your risk for so many of the conditions related to suboptimal cellular energy production spanning depression, obesity, high cholesterol, hypertension, infertility, and so many more.

The goal of this plan isn't to commit to all habits all at once; it is to instill a mindset shift and embark on a path of curiosity that is sustainable. In the pursuit of Good Energy, it can feel like you need to redesign your entire life around protecting yourself from all the toxic elements of modern culture while spending an inordinate amount of time engaged in healthy habits. Ultimately, we want to minimize the choices that overwhelm the body and bog down Good Energy processes (e.g., refined sugar, refined grains, seed oils, environmental toxins) and maximize the choices that build resilience and match the body's needs to support optimal function (e.g., quality sleep, omega-3s, regular movement).

When resilience and supportive choices consistently outweigh the stressors on the body, you're going to feel good and thrive. Each day I aim to cobble together as many Good Energy habits as I can to tune my engine, build biological capacity and resilience, and tip the scales toward cellular function and health. Simultaneously, I try to protect myself from excess *allostatic load*, a term that refers to the cumulative burden on the body of chronic stressors and life events. Each day, based on mood, circumstances, and motivation, the combination of Good Energy habits may look a little different, and that is OK—we are not robots, we are humans. The foundation for success is knowing which habits are going to be helpful to support metabolic health and trying to construct your days with as many as possible, as consistently as possible. Some habits will become second nature and feel effortless, while others may be a struggle every day to implement.

In week one of the four-week plan, we'll take a set of surveys to get a baseline assessment of where you are excelling with Good Energy habits and where you have the most room for improvement. We'll define your "why," start a food journal system, establish a measurement framework, and set up an accountability system. In week two, we'll focus on food, including adopting the first three Good Energy habits, which you will commit to for the following three weeks: clearing out the "Unholy Trinity" of Bad Energy foods (refined grains, refined sugars, and industrial seed oils). Additionally, you will be introduced to all the other food habits, so you can prepare for weeks three and four. In weeks three and four, you'll pick three Good Energy habits of your choosing, which you'll commit to in addition to the three baseline habits from week two.

Again, the goal of this month isn't to be perfect or to commit to every habit at once. It is to gain familiarity with the Good Energy habits and gain confidence in bringing more of them into your life. And ideally, during this month you'll move yourself up the "hierarchy of competence" curve when it comes to Good Energy actions (see the box below).

Hierarchy of Competence

The hierarchy of competence is a learning model popularized in the 1960s that describes the process of becoming effortlessly competent in a skill or habit. It is a helpful framework for understanding where you want to get to on your metabolic health journey. It is split into the following four levels:

1. Level One: Unconscious incompetence (the worst)
2. Level Two: Conscious incompetence
3. Level Three: Conscious competence
4. Level Four: Unconscious competence (the best)

Unconscious incompetence means that you are not living the behavior and don't even understand why it's important.

Conscious incompetence means you know what you need to do to be healthy but still are not regularly engaging in the behavior.

Conscious competence means that you are enacting the habit regularly and consistently but must make a conscious effort to make it happen and you still experience some friction and struggle.

Unconscious competence means that you are enacting the habit regularly and barely need to think about it. It's second nature and just part of your life!

We all want to eventually get to level four for every Good Energy habit, where doing each habit is just the way that we live, without it being a conscious effort. Unfortunately, most of us have been living at a level one or two for most habits because our culture (school, work, home life), food incentives, and health care incentives are designed to keep us incompetent at being healthy and to normalize destructive behaviors, environments, and habits. In level one, we're making consistent unhealthy habits but think they are fine and normal because we just don't know: we're *unconscious* of our incompetence. An example might be sleeping with a TV on in the background, not knowing that blue light may be severely impacting our melatonin secretion, or eating foods with artificial colorings because you aren't aware that many of these are likely neurotoxic and promote oxidative stress. As has been discussed throughout this book, several industries work hard to make you incompetent in your health behaviors, as well as unconscious about it, by normalizing unhealthy habits and choices, making them cheaper, and calling people elitist for attempting to be healthy, among many other tactics that keep us sick.

After reading this book, you will at least be at level two for all Good Energy habits: *consciously* incompetent. You know what you need to do to make Good Energy in your body and for radiant health, but you may not quite enact it every day for every habit. By the end of week four of Good Energy living, you want to start getting toward level three (conscious competence) for the three habits that you choose, as well as the three core Good Energy habits (eliminating refined grains, sugar, and seed oils). Over time and with consistent awareness and practice, you will move to level four, where healthy living is simply the way you live your life.

I recommend going through the full list of twenty-five Good Energy habits (see pages 283–301) and rating your competence level for each. Some of us might be level four for a few of them and level two for others. I am a level two for mindful eating and heat therapy. (I know it would be good for my cells if I did them, but I don't regularly.) I waver between level two and level three for sleep consistency and sleep quantity. (I am usually solid on these habits, but they are a big challenge and I must think about them and plan every day.) And I have just recently moved from level three to level four with 10,000 steps a day and resistance training. (I achieve them without much difficulty and have systems in my day to build them in, like walking meetings, a treadmill desk, and resistance training classes on the schedule that I've prepaid for). My strong level four habits are getting enough fiber; not eating refined grains, sugars, and seed oils; and getting into nature regularly. These things are now unconscious habits in my life; I would struggle to *not* do them. Try choosing your three Good Energy habits in weeks three and four from those habits for which you are currently level two (consciously incompetent) and see if you can work up to level three (consciously competent) during the two weeks.

WEEK ONE—ESTABLISH BASELINE METRICS AND CREATE ACCOUNTABILITY

The first step in the Good Energy journey is determining your *why*. If you cannot articulate specific aspirations for the person you aspire to be in your one precious life, you will find that making consistent healthful choices is much harder. But if you know you are building toward an identity that is very clear, motivation will come much easier.

Being thinner isn't an identity or a value, and I can guarantee you that this goal isn't enough to get you to a truly healthier place. Living longer isn't even an identity or a value. These principles motivated me in the past, and from my experience, they are not as sustainable as values that touch on deeper themes of purpose.

Values reflect your personal, unique judgment on what is important in life and why you want to be alive. Your choices and behaviors are how you show the world—and more importantly, yourself—what those values are. Behaviors and choices dictate whether your body will be functional and well powered. Misalignment between choices and values is the foundation of a more difficult life.

In my case, I choose to make Good Energy choices because I am building toward the identity of a person who:

- Values the precious gift of life, my body, and my consciousness
- Wants to have the energy and biologic capacity to be a positive force for my family, close friends, and the world
- Lives and thinks for myself and does not want my body to be controlled by industry forces that make money by keeping me and the global population sick and dependent

- Makes choices that respect the biodiversity and integrity of the soil, the earth, air, and animals

What are your reasons? What identity does having your cells make Good Energy bring to your life? What values do you want to live by?

Take fifteen minutes now to make a list of *why* you want your cells to function better and be powered well.

Next, take stock of what levers you need to pull to give your cells the best chance of making cellular energy properly. What are the factors in your life that are particularly hurting—or helping—your cells? For you versus for me, it may look very different. I might need to dial in sleep and more frequent movement throughout the day, while you may need to get rid of the environmental toxins in your house and move away from ultra-processed foods. The set of quizzes below will help you identify where you are on the Good Energy spectrum and zero in on which areas of your life may have the most room for optimization with Good Energy habits.

Metrics: Are You in the 6.8 Percent?

Note: These numbers should all be available for free at your annual physical:

1.___ Fasting glucose is less than 100 mg/dL
2.___ Triglycerides are less than 150 mg/dL
3.___ HDL is above 40 mg/dL (men) or 50 mg/dL (women)
4.___ Waist circumference is less than or equal to 102 cm (40 inches) for men and less than or equal to 88 cm (35 inches) for women
5.___ Blood pressure is less than 120/80 mmHg

Total: ___/5

If you do not score 100 percent on this section, you are part of the 93.2 percent of Americans who have work to do to optimize energy production in the cells.

OPTIONAL: I also recommend requesting the following tests be performed and comparing your results to the guidelines in Chapter 4:

- Fasting insulin and calculation of HOMA-IR
- High-sensitivity CRP (hsCRP)
- Hemoglobin A1c
- Uric acid
- Liver enzymes: aspartate transaminase (AST), alanine transaminase (ALT), and gamma-glutamyl transferase (GGT)
- Vitamin D

If your doctor won't order tests for you, or you'd prefer to pursue this testing in a simpler way, I recommend signing up for Function Health's comprehensive lab panel for approximately $500.

If your doctor says you don't need any of these tests, you can use the following note to request them:

> *I am requesting the following tests be ordered for me so I can better understand my overall metabolic health. I am committed to knowing where I stand with key metabolic biomarkers and tracking them over time so I can work to keep them in a healthy range. I know that many markers can indicate subtle dysfunction long before they reach the clinical diagnostic thresholds, and I want to know earlier rather than later if these changes are occurring. I appreciate your support in helping me understand my health better, and I welcome the opportunity to work with you to optimize my results. Thank you.*

The Good Energy Baseline Quiz

The following quiz can help you zero in on where you may benefit from focusing your energy to move toward Good Energy. The goal is to spark awareness about where there are opportunities to best support your mitochondrial and cellular health.

FOOD

1.___ I currently use a food journal or food tracker consistently to monitor what foods and beverages I'm consuming.

2.___ If given a list of foods, I can accurately identify the difference between an unprocessed/minimally processed food and an ultra-processed food.

3.___ I read the food label very carefully on every packaged product I purchase.

4.___ I am confident that I eat fewer than 10 grams of *added refined* sugar per day. (This does not include fruit sugars or other naturally occurring sugars in their whole food unprocessed form.)

5.___ I am certain that I have consumed no high-fructose corn syrup in the last month.

6.___ I eat at restaurants, eat fast food, or get takeout for fewer than three meals per week.

7.___ I am certain that I eat at least 30 grams of fiber per day.

8.___ I am certain that I eat at least thirty different plant foods per week (between fruits, vegetables, spices, herbs, nuts, seeds, and legumes).

9.___ I prepare the majority of my meals at home.

10.___ I eat at least one unsweetened probiotic food every day (such as unsweetened yogurt, kimchi, sauerkraut, natto, tempeh, or miso).

11.___ I eat at least one serving of cruciferous vegetables every day (such as broccoli, brussels sprouts, cauliflower, bok choy, kale, arugula, cabbage, radishes, rutabaga, or kohlrabi).

12.___ I eat at least 3 cups of dark leafy greens every day (like spinach, mixed greens, or kale).

13.___ If I eat outside of the house, I ask about what oils are used and avoid foods with refined seed oils.

14.___ I do not eat foods made with white flour (like flour tortillas, white bread, hamburger or hot dog buns, pastries, doughnuts, cookies, and most crackers).

15.___ I do not drink sodas of any kind (sweetened or diet).

16.___ I do not have a big "sweet tooth" and don't tend to crave sugar excessively.

17.___ When they're offered to me, it is easy for me to say no to foods with ultra-processed grains like bread, crackers, cookies, cakes, pastries, and doughnuts. I do not crave these foods.

18.___ When offered to me, it is easy for me to decline eating desserts with added sugars, like cakes, cookies, and ice cream.

19.___ It is easy for me to avoid and decline refined liquid sugars like soda, sweet tea, lemonade, fruit juices, Frappuccinos, sweetened coffee beverages, slushies, and chocolate milk. I rarely, if ever, drink these.

20.___ I drink coffee or tea without any natural or artificial sweeteners.

21.___ I do not eat artificial sweeteners like aspartame, Equal, or sucralose.

22.___ I can go more than four hours without eating during the day and feel fine, without excess hunger or cravings.

23.___ I avoid conventional/nonorganic foods and buy mostly organic food or food directly from farmers' markets.

FOR OMNIVORES:

24.___ I avoid farm-raised fish and eat mostly wild-caught fish.

25.___ I avoid conventional meats and mostly eat organic pasture-raised grass-fed meats.

26.___ I avoid conventional eggs and mostly eat organic pasture-raised eggs.

27.___ I buy organic milk and cheese originating from pasture-raised grass-fed cows.

Total: ___/23

or ___/27 for omnivores

If you scored less than 18/23 (or 21/27 for omnivores), you still have significant room for improvement in your diet to enable Good Energy. This is an area you should focus on as you choose which areas to prioritize.

CIRCADIAN RHYTHM

SLEEP

1.___ I consistently use a sleep-tracking device.

2.___ I sleep between seven and eight hours every night.

3.___ I have a consistent bedtime and usually am asleep within a one-hour window every night.

4.___ I have a consistent wake time and wake within a one-hour window every morning.

5.___ I can fall asleep easily nearly every night.

6.___ I can stay asleep throughout the night and fall back to sleep easily.

7.___ I do not have insomnia.

8.___ I feel rested and energetic during the day and rarely feel sluggish or like I need a nap midday.

9.___ I do not snore.

10.___ I have not been diagnosed with sleep apnea.

11.___ I have not taken any prescription sleep medication in the last year.

12.___ I have not taken antihistamine-based sleep medication in the last year (e.g., Unisom, Excedrin PM, Tylenol PM, Benadryl).

13.___ My phone and other devices never interrupt my sleep with sounds, lights, or vibration.

Total: ___/13

If you scored less than 10/13, you still have significant room for improvement in your sleep behaviors to enable Good Energy. This is an area you should focus on as you choose which areas to prioritize.

MEAL TIMING AND HABITS

1.___ I can fast for fourteen hours without difficulty.

2.___ I eat at consistent meal times each day (e.g., having dinner between 5:00 and 7:00 p.m. most days).

3.___ I am intentional about when I eat and do not tend to mindlessly snack and graze throughout the day.

4.___ I pause before eating to be mindful of my food.

5.___ I express gratitude for my food before I eat.

6.___ I eat slowly and methodically, trying to chew every bite fully before swallowing.

7.___ I make a point to sit down while I'm eating.

8.___ I do not use my phone while eating.

9.___ I do not watch TV or use my computer while eating.

10.___ I eat most of my meals with other people, like friends, family, or colleagues.

11.___ I am cognizant of not eating just before bedtime, and I try to stop eating three hours before I go to sleep.

Total: ___/11

If you scored less than 8/11, you may still have significant room for improvement in your meal-timing behaviors to enable Good Energy.

LIGHT

1.___ I spend at least fifteen minutes outside within one hour of waking every day.

2.___ I go outside during daylight hours at least three times for more than five minutes each.

3.___ I watch the sunset outdoors at least three days per week.

4.___ I spend at least three cumulative hours outside per day (add up walks, gardening, eating outdoors, playing outdoors with children, etc.).

5.___ I consistently use red lights in my home at night or blue-light-blocking glasses after the sun goes down.

6.___ I consistently use dimmers on my lights at home and turn them down in the evening.

7.___ I do not view any screens in the evening without using blue-light-blocking glasses.

8.___ My phone, tablet, and computer turn to "night mode" or "dark mode" after dark.

9.___ My bedroom is completely dark, and I use blackout shades.

10.___ My bedroom is absent of TVs, computers, LED clocks, or other lit screens.

Total: ___/10

If you scored less than 8/10, it means that you still have significant room for improvement in your light-related behaviors to enable Good Energy.

STRESSING THE BODY
MOVEMENT
1.___ I use a wearable step tracker every day.
2.___ I am certain I get at least 7,000 steps each day based on wearable data.
3.___ I consistently use a wearable tracker to track my resting heart rate.
4.___ Based on my wearable data, I know that my resting heart rate has been less than 60 bpm on average over the last month.
5.___ I know that I get 150 minutes of moderate aerobic activity per week (the equivalent of brisk or more strenuous walking).
6.___ I lift weights at least twice per week for at least thirty minutes.
7.___ I do not sit for more than one hour at a time without standing up and intentionally moving my body for at least two minutes.
8.___ I find ways to play sports or physical games at least once per week (e.g., pickleball, table tennis, volleyball, soccer, Spikeball, basketball, Frisbee, or dodgeball).

Total: ___/8

If you scored less than 6/8, it means that you still have significant room for improvement in your movement-related behaviors to enable Good Energy.

TEMPERATURE
1.___ I expose myself to hot temperatures intentionally at least once per week (e.g., sauna or hot yoga).
2.___ I expose myself to cold temperatures intentionally at least three times per week for more than one minute (e.g., cold plunge, cryotherapy, or cold shower).
3.___ I seek out ways to get very cold or very hot for its health benefits.

Total: ___/3

If you scored less than 2/3, it means that there is still room for improvement in your movement-related behaviors to enable Good Energy.

MIND-BODY
STRESS, RELATIONSHIPS, AND EMOTIONAL HEALTH

1.___ I use a wearable tracker that indicates my heart rate variability.

2.___ Based on my wearable data, I know some of the factors that negatively impact my HRV, like alcohol or work stress.

3.___ I practice mindfulness habits, like intentional deep breathing, journaling, meditation, or prayer, every day.

4.___ I have worked with a practitioner (like a therapist or coach) or program to address suboptimal behavioral and thought patterns and have successfully improved these.

5.___ I have worked with a practitioner (like a therapist or coach) or program to address past traumas in my life from childhood and adulthood that may be overtly or subtly impacting my life and have significantly improved my relationship to these experiences.

6.___ I feel confident in my ability to use my body to calm my mind (e.g., walking, breathwork, or tapping, a method of stimulating acupressure points with the fingertips to manage emotions).

7.___ I feel confident in my ability to use my mind to calm my body (e.g., mantras, body scans, or visualizations).

8.___ I have at least one trusted person in my life with whom I can talk openly and honestly about most topics.

9.___ I am comfortable honestly and openly expressing my feelings to the important people in my life.

10.___ I have a set of clear strategies I can use when I get stressed or activated to calm myself down.

11.___ I have a sense of purpose bigger than myself.

12.___ I "ground" regularly by sitting or standing barefoot directly on the ground.

13.___ I consistently feel awe for my life and the world around me.

14.___ I am aware of my self-talk and intentionally communicate lovingly to myself and catch myself when I am not.

15.___ I intentionally focus on gratitude each day.

16.___ I feel hopeful and excited about the future.

17.___ I feel that I am authentically expressing myself most of the time and do not need to suppress my personality or true self.

18.___ I have outlets that let me bring my creative visions to life (e.g., art, music, writing, crafts, cooking, decorating, or planning activities or trips) and engage with them regularly.

19.___ I feel that anything is possible and believe that I can cultivate the life that I want.

20.___ I feel limitless.

21.___ I feel a sense of connection to everything in the universe.

Total: ___/21

If you scored less than 16/21, it means that you still have room for improvement in your movement related to stress, relationships, and emotional health to enable Good Energy.

TOXINS

INGESTED TOXINS

1.___ I filter my tap water with a reverse osmosis filter or a high-efficacy charcoal filter (e.g., Berkey) and rarely ever drink unfiltered water.

2.___ I have checked my water quality against the Environmental Working Group (EWG) database and understand whether specific contaminants are above recommended levels.

3.___ I drink at least half an ounce of water per pound of body weight per day.

4.___ When I leave the house, I bring filtered water in a non-plastic (e.g., glass or metal) bottle.

5.___ I avoid drinking water out of single-use plastic bottles.

6.___ I avoid foods that have natural flavors or artificial flavors.

7.___ I do not eat foods with any artificial dyes in them.

8.___ I rarely store my food in plastic containers or buy food in plastic containers, and instead opt for metal or glass storage.

9.___ I do not drink more than one alcoholic beverage per day. (Note: A standard serving of alcohol in the United States is defined as 14 grams of alcohol, which is less than you might think. This is 5 ounces of wine, 12 ounces of beer, or a single 1.5-ounce shot of distilled spirits.)

10.___ I do not drink more than seven alcoholic beverages per week.

11.___ I do not smoke cigarettes or other tobacco products.

12.___ I do not use chewing tobacco or similar forms of chewable nicotine.

13.___ I do not smoke cigars.

14.___ I do not vape.

15.___ I avoid over-the-counter medications, like acetaminophen, ibuprofen, diphenhydramine, and/or acid-suppressing medications; I take them cumulatively fewer than five times per year.

16.___ I have not taken oral antibiotics in the past two years.

17.___ I do not take oral hormonal contraceptives.

18.___ I do not eat high-mercury fish (tuna, lobster, bass, swordfish, halibut, or marlin) more than once per week.

Total: ___/18

If you scored less than 14/18, you still have significant room for improvement related to limiting toxin exposure to enable Good Energy.

ENVIRONMENTAL TOXINS

1.___ I filter my shower water with a whole-house water filter or attached shower head filter.

2.___ I filter the air in my house with a HEPA filter.

3.___ I do not use scented candles in my home.

4.___ I do not use air fresheners, scent diffusers, plug-in scents, or scented room sprays in my car, bathrooms, or other parts of my home.

5.___ I read the labels of any home care or personal care products I buy to ensure clean, nontoxic, non–artificially scented ingredients.

6.___ My shampoo and conditioner are unscented (i.e., do not include ingredients "parfum," "natural fragrance," or "fragrance") or only scented with essential oils.

7.___ My laundry detergent is unscented and has no colorings or dyes.

8.___ My dish soap is unscented and has no colorings.

9.___ I do not use scented laundry sheets or fabric softener.

10.___ My cleaning supplies (like all-purpose cleaner sprays or concentrates) are unscented and have no colorings or dyes.

11.___ I do not use perfume or cologne.

12.___ My deodorant is unscented (or only scented with essential oils).

13.___ My deodorant is aluminum-free.

14.___ My lotion is unscented (or only scented with essential oils) and has no colorings or dyes.

15.___ My soap or body wash is unscented (or only scented with essential oils).

16.___ My toothpaste is fluoride-free and has no colorings or dyes.

17.___ I check the toxicity ratings of my home care and personal care products on websites like the EWG.

18.___ The majority of my clothing, underwear, sheets, and other linens are made from natural, organic materials like cotton or bamboo rather than polyester or fabrics treated with synthetic dyes and chemicals.

Total: ___/18

If you scored less than 15/18, you still have room for improvement related to reducing environmental toxin exposure to enable Good Energy.

———

Now that we've taken stock of the several categories in our lives that can help us achieve Good Energy, we are going to prepare to take action.

Create a Food Journal and Start Logging on Day One

As we learned in Chapter 4, food journaling has been shown to significantly enhance weight-loss efforts and adherence to healthy eating. Whether you choose to do this with a smartphone application, in a digital note or document, or in a paper journal, the key point is to have a record of what went into your body so that you are certain of what your body is made of and whether it has what it needs to make Good Energy.

You will want to write down every single bite you take, even if it's a nibble of bread, a single french fry, or a tiny square of chocolate. As you work toward your best health, you want to be clear about your relationship with food and where you have room for improvement.

Log the times of each intake, at least a rough estimate of the amount, and the brands of any packaged foods eaten.

I recommend using one of the three following methods:

- Use a dedicated paper journal to manually write your food logs and take it with you everywhere.
- Keep a running digital note on your smartphone or in a Google Doc.
- Use an app like MacroFactor, MyFitnessPal, or Levels.

Using food logging apps like MacroFactor is simple because they utilize a barcode scanner that will pull in ingredients, serving size, and nutritional information. Most products (even a lot of fresh produce) have barcodes, and you can simply scan and log. If you are cooking more complex meals from whole foods, you may find that keeping a digital note or Google Doc, and simply voice dictating what was in your meal, is easier.

ACTION:
- Create a food journal and start logging all food and beverage intake on day one and continue throughout the month.
- Each Saturday, review your food journal for thirty minutes and assess what's going into your body. Identify if you have areas where you are struggling with Good Energy eating, and assess what the barriers are to making it happen.

Order Wearable Devices

Activity, Heart Rate, and Sleep Tracking

I cannot recommend highly enough getting an inexpensive wearable activity tracker that measures sleep, steps, heart rate, and HRV. When you put on a wearable tracker, you will see how different your perception is of what you do each day and what actually happens. In Chapter 4, you read data about how people, on average, estimate they are doing six times more physical activity per week than they actually are. And recall from Chapter 8 that simply walking 10,000 steps per day is associated with 50 percent lower dementia risk, 44 percent lower risk of getting type 2 diabetes, and much lower risk of cancer and depression.

Wearables allow us to know *for certain* that we are hitting our marks on key pillars like sleep and activity. Without that certainty, you can *think* you're living a Good Energy lifestyle when you're not.

ACTION:

- Order a Fitbit Inspire 2 (available from Amazon, Fitbit, Best Buy, Target, and Walmart), Apple Watch, Oura Ring, or Garmin Tracker.

I have tried many wearable trackers, and the Fitbit Inspire 2 is my favorite because it is simple, affordable, holds a long charge (usually over a week), and has a screen that shows you in real time how many steps you've taken and what your heart rate is. It costs $55 to $60 at most retailers. The Fitbit app shows long-term and real-time trends for steps, heart rate, amount of moderate and vigorous physical activity, sleep data, active hours, and HRV, among many other metrics. Apple Watch has many similar features but is much more expensive and needs to be charged every day. I have not used a Garmin Tracker or Oura Ring, but they have similar features to the Fitbit. The Whoop strap is an incredible product for tracking workouts, recovery, sleep, and HRV but does not include step counting.

Optional: Glucose Monitoring

As discussed in previous chapters, tracking blood sugar can be extremely helpful as you work toward Good Energy. You have two options: a standard glucometer, for which you would prick your finger each morning as well as forty-five minutes and then two hours after eating, and manually log your findings in your food journal. A simpler method that is less painful and will give you much more data is to use a continuous glucose monitor (CGM). A CGM gives you much more granularity into the cause-and-effect relationship between your actions and your blood sugar response. While glucometers are available at any pharmacy, as well as at retailers like Amazon, CGMs require a prescription in the United States (but not in most other countries). Unless you have type 1 or type 2 diabetes, you will likely have to pay out of pocket for a CGM, and your doctor may push back about writing you a prescription. The cost will likely be between $75 to $150 per month for CGM sensors. A more streamlined approach is to get a CGM through Levels, which offers the physician consultation, CGM prescriptions sent to your home, and software that interprets glucose data.

ACTION:

- Purchase a glucometer (I recommend Keto-Mojo GK+, available on Amazon, which measures glucose and ketones) or obtain a prescription for a CGM (through your physician or Levels).

Set Up an Accountability System

Accountability and community support can significantly amplify health efforts—a fact that is supported by abundant scientific research. The effect is dramatic: a meta-analysis of all studies looking at adherence to weight-loss interventions showed that two of the three main factors associated with success were supervised attendance and social support. Simply having others involved means you're more likely to stick with habits.

One way to build accountability into your life is partnering with a friend or colleague who is also on a health journey or who is willing to be a witness and supporter of your journey and commit to checking in with you regularly about your progress.

In the one month after setting up a relationship with an accountability partner:

- I went from an average of 49,601 steps per week to 80,966.
- I went from an average of 6 hours 42 minutes of sleep per night to 7 hours 35 minutes.
- My resting heart rate went from 63 to 52 bpm.

A second helpful way to ensure accountability is to prepay for wellness experiences so that there is a real cost to not doing it. If I am traveling to a city for work, I'll often schedule several workout classes at local studios in that city. Since I must pay for these classes in advance, it almost guarantees that I am going to go. I also prepay for a package of therapy or coaching sessions every few months so that all I must do is schedule them. And when I travel, I like to stay in an Airbnb rather than a hotel, so I have a refrigerator. I always pick up groceries or have them delivered on day one (which is invariably cheaper than eating all of my meals at restaurants).

A third key to accountability is planning as many activities as possible around Good Energy habits, like social, work, and family events and meals. When I'm heading to a city where I know I'll be catching up with several people, I plan morning coffee walks with friends or organize a hike. During a family holiday, offer to cook a few of the meals and prepare a Good Energy–aligned feast for everyone. When staying with friends, have a box of healthy food (I like Daily Harvest) or groceries delivered as a generous contribution, but also to ensure that you have the food you need to be healthy. When I have visitors, I plan almost every event to check off "Good Energy" boxes, like taking a neighborhood walk or local hike, walking through a park or botanical garden, taking friends to try cold plunging in the ocean or a local body of water, doing breathwork together, going to a concert where we'll be standing, streaming an online workout class on the TV and doing it together, mountain biking, paddleboarding, snow-shoeing, or going to a meditative sound bath together. If you're invited to a party, commit to bringing a few healthy food and beverage items to ensure you'll have unprocessed, Good Energy food to eat.

ACTION:

- Choose an accountability partner whom you trust and who is willing to support you with daily text messages, emails, or check-ins. Ask them to commit to this role for at least four weeks.
- Schedule a thirty-minute accountability meeting once a week to go over food journals and habit tracking.
- Prepay for wellness activities.
- Organize social and work activities around Good Energy habits.

WEEK TWO—FOCUS ON FOOD

While all metabolic habits are important, getting food right is the base of the pyramid. In week two, you'll adopt the first three Good Energy habits and audit the labels of your food to remove the Unholy Trinity of ingredients: added sugar, refined grains, and seed oils. Everyone on the Good Energy four-week program should eliminate these three ingredients in weeks two, three, and four. Additionally, you'll learn about habits four through seven, which are all focused on what to bring *into* the diet, and which you can choose to implement in weeks three and four as part of your additional Good Energy habits.

Good Energy Habits

Nutrition

1	Eliminate refined added sugars	• Eliminate all foods, drinks, and condiments with refined or liquid sugars. • Added sugars may include the following names: white sugar, brown sugar, powdered sugar, cane sugar, evaporated cane juice, raw sugar, turbinado sugar, demerara sugar, coconut sugar, maple syrup, honey, molasses, agave nectar, corn syrup, high-fructose corn syrup, glucose, dextrose, fructose, maltose, sucrose, galactose, maltodextrin, lactose, caramel, barley malt, rice syrup, date sugar, beet sugar, invert sugar, and golden syrup. • Read all labels for any "added sugars," and do not buy any products with them. • Remove anything with added sugar from your home and throw them away. • Track this through your food journal.
2	Eliminate refined grains	• Eliminate all foods with ultra-processed refined flour or grain. • These include all standard breads (white, wheat, and whole wheat), rice (white and brown), pasta, bagels, tortillas, crackers, cereals, pretzels, doughnuts, cookies, cakes, pastries, pizza crusts, waffles, pancakes, croissants, English muffins, hamburger buns, hot dog buns, and muffins. • Ingredients on packaged food might include: wheat flour, all-purpose flour, self-rising flour, bread flour, cake flour, pastry flour, whole wheat flour, semolina flour, farina, durum wheat flour, spelt flour, barley flour, rye flour, rice flour, oat flour, or buckwheat flour. • Read all labels closely. • Track this through your food journal.
3	Eliminate industrial seed oils	• Eliminate all foods, drinks, and condiments with refined industrially manufactured seed oils. • These include: soybean oil, corn oil, cottonseed oil, sunflower oil, safflower oil, peanut oil, grapeseed oil, and any oil that says "hydrogenated."

- Refined seed oils are found in a wide variety of foods, including many store-bought salad dressings, mayonnaise, hummus, dips, potato chips, peanut butter, corn chips, crackers, granola bars, cookies, pastries, muffins, doughnuts, fried chicken, chicken nuggets, chicken tenders, fish sticks, frozen pizza, french fries, packaged popcorn, tortilla chips, cheese puffs, snack mixes, vegetable chips, canned soups, instant noodles, cakes, brownies, pancakes, waffles, butter alternatives, packaged muffins, cookies, croissants, biscuits, and roasted nuts.
- Track this through your food journal.

ACTION:

- Adopt the first three Good Energy habits by getting rid of *every single* food in your house that includes added sugar, refined grains, or industrial seed oils, and eliminate all these foods for the next three weeks.
- Start learning about the additional food habits four through seven and how to incorporate Good Energy eating into your life, below (however, you won't need to incorporate these habits until weeks three and four). Purchase any foods, cookbooks, or tools you need for weeks three and four.

| 4 | Eat over 50 grams of fiber per day | <ul><li>Track fiber intake daily and aim to get 50 grams per day or more from food sources. If getting 50 grams of fiber initially causes bloating or stomach upset, you may want to start slow, with 30 grams per day from foods like avocados, raspberries, and chia seeds, and work up to beans and legumes (which some people find "gassy") and higher quantities of fiber.</li><li>Using a barcode-scanning app like MacroFactor can make this extremely simple, as it will automatically pull in the fiber content.</li><li>Best sources to maximize fiber are beans, legumes, nuts and seeds, and certain fruits.</li><li>Specific foods with high fiber include:<ul><li>Navy beans (~10 grams per ½ cup)</li><li>Black beans (~7.5 grams per ½ cup)</li><li>Chia seeds (8 grams per 2 tablespoons)</li><li>Basil seeds (15 grams per 2 tablespoons; I use Zen Basil brand)</li><li>Flaxseeds (8 grams per 1 ounce)</li><li>Lentils (~15 grams per 1 cooked cup)</li><li>Raspberries and blackberries (~8 grams per 1 cup)</li><li>Brussels sprouts (6 grams per 1 cooked cup)</li></ul></li></ul> |

		• Broccoli (5 grams per 1 cooked cup) • Avocados (~13 grams per avocado) • Track fiber intake in your food journal.
5	Eat three or more servings of probiotic foods per day	• Ensure you are getting three or more servings of probiotic-rich foods that do not have added sugar every day. • Sources include yogurt, kefir, sauerkraut, kimchi, miso, tempeh, natto, kvass, and apple cider vinegar. • Make sure that any yogurt and kefir is unsweetened and says "live active cultures" on the label. • While kombucha is a probiotic-rich food, read the label very carefully. Most commercial kombucha brands are now using excessive amounts of sugar or fruit juice to sweeten, making conventional kombucha more like a soda than a health drink. The brand with the lowest sugar on the market I have found is Lion Heart, with just 2 grams of sugar per serving. Kvass (e.g., from Biotic Ferments), a fermented drink that uses vegetables (like carrots or beets) as the carbohydrate source for fermentation, is a fantastic alternative to kombucha. • Track this through your food journal.

6	Increase omega-3 intake to a minimum of 2 grams per day	• Ensure you are getting a minimum of 2 grams (2,000 mg) of omega-3 fats each day.
		• The best animal-based sources of omega-3s are:
		  • Wild-caught salmon (1.5–2.0 grams per 3-ounce serving)
		  • Sardines (1.3 grams per 2-ounce serving)
		  • Atlantic mackerel (1.1 grams per 3-ounce serving)
		  • Rainbow trout (0.8 gram per 3-ounce serving)
		  • Anchovies (1.1 grams per 2-ounce serving)
		  • Organic pasture-raised eggs (0.33 gram per 1 egg)
		• The best plant-based sources are:
		  • Chia seeds (5.9 grams per 2.5 tablespoons)
		  • Basil seeds (2.8 grams per 2 tablespoons)
		  • Flaxseeds (2.3 grams per tablespoon)
		  • Hemp seeds (1.2 grams per tablespoon)
		  • Walnuts (2.6 grams per 1-ounce serving)
		  • Algal oil (up to 1.3 grams per serving). Algal oil is generally taken in supplement form and is one of the only plant-based sources of DHA and EPA.
		• Tip: I always keep cans of wild-caught fish from Wild Planet in my pantry and add the fish on top of salads or on flaxseed crackers for a quick and nutritious snack.
		• I like to keep seeds and nuts handy and sprinkle them on top of all my meals for an easy and delicious way to boost my omega-3 intake.
		• If choosing to use omega-3 supplements, buy from a high-quality source like WeNatal, Nordic Naturals, Thorne, or Pure Encapsulations.
		• Keep track of this quantity in your food journal.

| 7 | Increase antioxidants, micronutrients, and polyphenols through plant diversity | • Incorporate thirty different types of organic plant foods into your diet each week, coming from organic or regenerative fruits, vegetables, nuts, seeds, beans, legumes, herbs, and spices.
• Of these thirty different types per week, eat at least two servings of cruciferous vegetables per day. These include broccoli, cauliflower, brussels sprouts, kale, bok choy, arugula, watercress, collard greens, mustard greens, turnip greens, radishes, horseradish, rutabaga, kohlrabi, and cabbage.
  • Chop cruciferous vegetables and let sit for thirty to forty-five minutes to activate a key Good Energy component, sulforaphane, and make it more heat stable.
• Keep track of this quantity in your food journal. |
| 8 | Eat at least 30 grams of protein per meal | • Aim to eat 30 grams of protein at each meal, for a total of at least 90 grams of protein per day.
• Good sources include:
  • Meats: beef, chicken, turkey, pork, and game meats like elk and bison
  • Fish and seafood
  • Dairy products: milk, cheese, and Greek yogurt
  • Eggs
  • Legumes: beans, lentils, and peas
  • Soy products: edamame, tofu, and tempeh
  • Nuts and seeds: hemp seeds, chia seeds, pumpkin seeds, almonds, sunflower seeds, flaxseeds, cashews, pistachios
  • If using protein powders, choose organic and/or grass-fed or regenerative (if animal-based) with minimal ingredients, no added sugars, no colorings, no "natural flavors" or artificial flavors, no gums, and no ingredient names you aren't familiar with. I like Truvani, Equip Prime Protein (Unflavored), Garden of Life Grass Fed Collagen, and Be Well.
• Keep track of this quantity in your food journal.
• Note: If you have kidney problems, talk to your physician before changing your protein quantity. |

How can you follow these dietary principles as simply, cheaply, and easily as possible, based on your current lifestyle, time constraints, and cooking abilities?

Below we'll explore a variety of packaged and grab-and-go food options that adhere to Good Energy principles, as well as strategies for preparing simple or more complex home-cooked meals.

Packaged Food

Cooking your meals at home from whole-food ingredients sets you up for the best success at Good Energy eating because you can control the quality of the raw ingredients, ensure that the food is organic, minimize additives and industrial seed oils, and maximize health-supporting additions (like a dollop of fermented foods or chia seeds atop your meals!). Since it is nearly impossible to cook every meal from scratch, I've included a list of ideas for packaged or grab-and-go snacks for busy days.

Some of my favorite packaged or grab-and-go foods that meet Good Energy standards and can be found at many major grocery stores or online:

- Daily Harvest frozen soups, Harvest Bakes, and Harvest Bowls (I top these with a few chia seeds, a tin of sardines, black beans, and sauerkraut for a perfect Good Energy lunch!)
- Organic whole fruits that are easy to transport, like apples, oranges, and pears
- Organic precut vegetables, like carrot sticks
- Natierra Organic Freeze-Dried fruit packs
- Unroasted organic nuts (make sure to check the label to ensure they do not have any added oils)
- Organic coconut flakes, like Let's Do Organic brand
- HOPE hummus (this is the only hummus brand I have found that is organic and does not contain refined seed oils)
- Wholly Guacamole organic classic minis
- Gaea Organic Olive snack pack
- Brami Italian Snacking Lupini Beans (lupini beans are special because they are extremely high in fiber and have zero net carbohydrates, while having lots of protein)
- Flackers Flaxseed crackers
- Ella's Flats seed crackers
- Brad's Veggie Chips and Kale Chips
- gimMe Organic Roasted Seaweed Snacks with sea salt and avocado oil
- Artisana Organics Raw Almond Butter snack packs

- Stonyfield Organic 100% Grassfed Organic Yogurt Cups
- Cocojune unsweetened coconut milk yogurt cups
- Straus Organic Whole Milk Plain Greek Yogurt
- Epic bars (choose the versions that have no added sugar, like Chicken Sriracha and Salt and Pepper Venison)
- Paleovalley or Chomps 100% Grass Fed Beef Sticks
- Hard Boiled Eggs from Vital Farms
- Organic Valley string cheese
- Wild Planet Wild Sardines in Extra Virgin Olive Oil
- Wild Planet packets: Wild Pink Salmon, Albacore Tuna, Skipjack Tuna
- Kettle & Fire Bone Broth
- Organic nuPasta Konjac Root noodles
- Malk Almond Milk
- Three Trees Organic Almond Milk
- Alexandre Family Farms A2 100% Grass-Fed Organic Milk
- Choi's Organic Nori, 50 sheets (great as a tortilla alternative)
- NuttZo Organic nut butter
- Sweet Nothings Organic Spoonable Smoothie Cups
- Arizona Pepper's Hot Sauce
- Yellowbird Hot Sauce
- Muir Glen Organic Salsa
- Wildbrine Raw Organic Sauerkraut
- Serenity Kids pouches

Preparing Simple Good Energy Meals at Home

Cooking healthy meals needn't be complicated. A Good Energy kitchen has an abundance of fresh produce, a variety of proteins, and several different probiotic, omega-3, and fiber sources always handy. Preparing a meal then simply becomes mixing and matching these *components* into an infinite variety of options. Learning a few simple techniques, like roasting vegetables and a protein source at 425°F on a baking sheet, or sautéing protein and vegetables in a stovetop pan, and learning a few spice combinations and toppings that you like means that you can go forward with a huge variety of recipe-free easy meals.

Here are some of the main foods that check off the various Good Energy components while also being low glycemic. (Many of these fit into multiple categories and can be counted toward different Good Energy habits. For example, ground venison has a huge amount of micronutrients, but I categorize it as a healthy protein for the purposes of designing my meals. Similarly, sauerkraut is filled with phytonutrients, but I categorize it below as a fermented food.)

Building Good Energy Meals: Components

MICRONUTRIENTS/ ANTIOXIDANTS	FIBER	PROTEIN	OMEGA-3 FATS	FERMENTED FOODS
Roasting or sautéing vegetables (all can be cooked at 425°F till browned): • Asparagus, bottom 2 inches of stems removed, remaining chopped into 1-inch pieces • Bell peppers, cut into 1-inch squares or slices • Broccoli florets • Brussels sprouts, quartered with rough ends cut off • Cabbage (red, green, or napa), thinly sliced • Carrots, whole or chopped into ½- to 1-inch cubes • Cauliflower florets • Celery root, chopped into ½- to 1-inch cubes • Cherry tomatoes, whole • Eggplant, chopped into 1-inch cubes • Fennel, thinly sliced • Green beans, whole • Kohlrabi, chopped into 1-inch cubes • Leeks, sliced into ¼-inch rings • Mushrooms, sliced	• Chia seeds • Basil seeds • Flaxseeds • Lentils • Split peas • Beans • Konjac root products • Raspberries • Blackberries • Tahini • Brazil nuts • Almonds • Walnuts • Pecans • Hazelnuts • Pistachios • Avocados	• Chicken breasts • Turkey cutlets • Pork (loin, tenderloin, etc.) • Beef (flank steak, sirloin, etc.) • Tofu • Tempeh • Ground pork • Ground lamb • Ground turkey • Ground beef • Ground venison • Ground bison • Shrimp • Scallops • Salmon • Sardines • Mackerel • Unsweetened Greek yogurt • Pastured eggs • Beans • Lentils	• Salmon • Anchovies • Sardines • Mackerel • Chia seeds • Basil seeds • Flaxseeds • Hemp seeds • Pasture-raised eggs	• Sauerkraut • Kimchi • Unsweetened yogurt • Kefir • Tempeh • Miso • Natto • Apple cider vinegar

MICRONUTRIENTS/ ANTIOXIDANTS	FIBER	PROTEIN	OMEGA-3 FATS	FERMENTED FOODS
• Okra, whole or sliced into ½-inch rounds				
• Onions, quartered or sliced into ¼-inch half-moon slices				
• Parsnips, chopped into ½- to 1-inch cubes				
• Radishes, quartered				
• Romanesco, cut coarsely into 1-inch cubes/florets				
• Shallots, quartered or sliced into ¼-inch half-moon slices				
• Zucchini, cut into quartered spears or ½-inch cubes				
Salad vegetables:				
• Canned artichoke hearts, chopped				
• Avocados, cubed				
• Bean sprouts				
• Bell peppers (red, green, yellow, or orange), chopped into ½-inch slices or small ¼-inch squares				
• Broccoli florets				
• Cabbage (red, green, or napa), sliced very thinly				
• Carrots, chopped				
• Cauliflower florets				
• Celery, chopped				
• Cucumbers, chopped				
• Fennel, thinly sliced				
• Green beans, whole or cut into 1-inch pieces				
• Jicama, cut into ½-inch cubes or spears				
• Mushrooms, chopped into small squares				
• Onions (red, yellow, or white), thinly sliced or chopped into ¼-inch squares				

MICRONUTRIENTS/ ANTIOXIDANTS	FIBER	PROTEIN	OMEGA-3 FATS	FERMENTED FOODS
• Radishes, quartered • Snap peas, whole or cut into 1-inch pieces • Tomatoes, chopped into small cubes or halved if cherry				
Greens: • Arugula • Collard greens • Kale • Lettuce (romaine, butter, iceberg, etc.) • Mixed greens • Spinach • Swiss chard				
Fruits: • Apples • Berries (blueberries, raspberries, strawberries, blackberries) • Cherries • Kiwis • Lemons • Limes • Oranges • Papaya • Peaches • Pears • Pomegranate seeds				
Nuts and seeds: • Almonds • Basil seeds • Brazil nuts • Chia seeds • Hazelnuts • Hemp seeds • Pecans • Pistachios • Pumpkin seeds • Walnuts				
All spices and herbs				

Looking at these lists, you can see how many easy meals you can throw together with foods from all five elements.

1. **Breakfast Yogurt Parfait:** Unsweetened whole milk Greek yogurt with chia seeds, raspberries, and blackberries
   Micronutrients/Phytonutrients: Raspberries and blackberries
   Fiber: Chia seeds
   Protein: Greek yogurt; can also add 1 scoop of grass-fed collagen
   Omega-3 Fats: Chia seeds
   Fermented Food: Greek yogurt

2. **Egg Scramble:** Three pasture-raised eggs, 3 ounces ground grass-fed beef, sauerkraut, sautéed spinach, avocado, and hot sauce
   Micronutrients/Phytonutrients: Spinach, hot sauce
   Fiber: Avocado
   Protein: Eggs and beef
   Omega-3 Fats: Eggs
   Fermented Food: Sauerkraut

3. **Baked Salmon and Vegetables:** Baked salmon with a side of baked brussels sprouts seasoned with paprika, salt, pepper, and garlic powder, and beet sauerkraut
   Micronutrients/Phytonutrients: Brussels sprouts, garlic powder
   Fiber: Brussels sprouts
   Protein: Salmon
   Omega-3 Fats: Salmon
   Fermented Food: Sauerkraut

4. **Southwestern Tofu Scramble:** Tofu with black beans, red bell peppers, onions, cumin, and garlic powder, topped with sauerkraut, avocado, hot sauce, and hemp seeds
   Micronutrients/Phytonutrients: Red bell peppers, onions, garlic powder
   Fiber: Black beans, avocado
   Protein: Tofu, black beans
   Omega-3 Fats: Hemp seeds
   Fermented Food: Sauerkraut

5. **Chicken Stir-Fry:** Chicken breast, broccoli, carrots, and red bell peppers, sautéed on the stove top with miso and tamari, topped with beet sauerkraut and drizzled with tahini and ground flaxseeds
    Micronutrients/Phytonutrients: Red bell peppers
    Fiber: Tahini, flaxseeds
    Protein: Chicken breast
    Omega-3 Fats: Flaxseeds
    Fermented Food: Miso, sauerkraut

Cooking More Complex Good Energy Meals

Prepare any meals from the recipes at the back of this book, or from the following cookbooks (most recipes are Good Energy–friendly, but make sure to double-check the absence of refined grains):

*   *Food Food Food* by The Ranch Malibu
*   *Whole30 Cookbook* by Melissa Hartwig Urban
*   *Whole Food Cooking Every Day* by Amy Chaplin
*   *It's All Good* by Gwyneth Paltrow
*   *I Am Grateful* by Terces Engelhart
*   *Inspiralize Everything* by Ali Mafucci

WEEKS THREE AND FOUR—ENACT THREE PERSONALIZED GOOD ENERGY HABITS

While maintaining the elimination of refined grains, refined added sugars, and industrial seed oils (Good Energy Habits one through three), it's time to add in three additional habits in weeks three and four.

Pick three habits (from habits four through twenty-five) that you don't already perform regularly that you will make a commitment to perform over these next two weeks. As you go into weeks three and four, the following habit formation best practices from authors James Clear and BJ Fogg can be helpful.

Habit Tips from the Experts

Tiny Habits

Tiny Habits is a behavior change method and book developed by Stanford University professor BJ Fogg. The key concept of *Tiny Habits* is to make small, incremental changes to your daily routine that are easy to do and require minimal effort. The idea is that by starting with tiny habits, you can create lasting change in your life without feeling overwhelmed or discouraged.

To apply the *Tiny Habits* method, you start by identifying a behavior that you want to change or develop. Then, you break that behavior down into tiny, specific actions that can be completed in just a few seconds. For example, if you want to start flossing your teeth regularly, your tiny habit might be to floss just one tooth after brushing your teeth in the morning. After successfully completing your *tiny* habit, you celebrate your achievement with a positive emotion, like saying "I'm awesome!" or doing a small fist pump. Over time, these tiny habits build momentum and can lead to bigger changes in your behavior and your life.

As you think about developing big positive habits in your life, like improving sleep consistency, reflect on how to break them down into tiny pieces that you can achieve consistently and build confidence and momentum. For instance, you might currently go to bed at vastly different times each night, so it would seem too hard to immediately try to set a bedtime and stick to it. Instead, think about small ways to break this up to develop confidence and competence. You might:

- Start by creating a very lenient cutoff for bedtime that you think you can achieve most nights. Once you hit this goal every day for a week or two, move it up by thirty minutes for another two weeks.
- Start wearing a sleep tracker every night to objectively understand your sleep baseline.
- Have your phone send you a reminder to get ready for bed at a certain time each night.
- Get a sleep accountability coach through an online service like Crescent Health.

- Start wearing blue-light-blocking glasses after dark each night and view sunlight first thing in the morning so that you're more likely to be tired at night, and have functional circadian rhythms.
- Stop drinking caffeine after noon.

Habit Stacking

James Clear's bestselling book *Atomic Habits* provides practical strategies for building good habits and breaking bad ones. One of the key practical takeaways from *Atomic Habits* is the concept of habit stacking, which involves linking a new habit to an existing habit. For example, if you want to start doing push-ups every day, you might link this habit to your existing habit of brushing your teeth in the morning. After brushing your teeth, you do three push-ups. Another example of habit stacking is that every time you open the front door, you think of one thing you're grateful for. This makes it easier to remember to do the new habit and makes it more likely that you will follow through consistently.

The Habit Loop Requires Reward!

According to James Clear, triggers are important because they provide a cue for your brain to start the habit loop. The habit loop consists of three parts: the trigger, the behavior (the habit itself), and the reward. When you consistently follow this loop, your brain learns to associate the trigger with the behavior and the reward, making the habit easier to maintain over time.

One key to building new habits is to create clear and consistent triggers. For example, the sound of your alarm clock in the morning might trigger you to get out of bed and start your morning routine.

It's also important to note that triggers can be both internal (such as a feeling of hunger) and external (such as a notification on your phone), and they can be positive (such as a reminder to drink water) or negative (such as a stressful situation that triggers an unhealthy coping mechanism). By understanding and controlling your triggers, you can take control of your habits and create positive changes in your life.

Don't underestimate the power of small rewards. When I text my sleep data to my accountability buddy each week, and she responds with enthusiasm when I've adhered to the sleep habits that matter to me, I feel really, really good. This reinforces the behavior immensely!

Additional Good Energy Habits (Commit to at Least Three)
Movement

9	Engage in moderate-intensity movement for at least 150 minutes per week	• Calculate your maximum heart rate by subtracting your age from 220, and then determine what 64 percent of that number is, which is the floor for moderate-intensity movement. For me, that would be $220 - 35 = 185 \times 0.64 = 118$ bpm. For me, this means I need to get my heart rate above 118 bpm for 150 minutes a week at a minimum. • Trying out different activities with your wearable tracker can help you learn what "moderate" activity feels like. For me, a brisk flat walk does not get me to 118 bpm, but a brisk walk up a hill or a flat jog does. • Verify your time at a specific heart rate range with your wearable, and log your time each day in your Good Energy tracker.
10	Resistance train three times per week	• Commit to resistance training twice per week or more for at least thirty minutes each session. • Incorporate exercises that fatigue the arms, legs, *and* core every week. This can be done with body-weight exercises or with weights. There are numerous options for starting a resistance training program with online classes, in-person classes, personal training, and resistance-focused gyms. I've recommended several in the supplementary materials at caseymeans.com/goodenergy. • Make sure that the sessions are planned and scheduled before week three begins. This may mean signing up for classes at a local gym, finding a free YouTube series you like that uses just body-weight training, signing up for an online resistance training program, or other avenues. • Log your resistance training in your Good Energy tracker.
11	Take 10,000 steps per day	• For the month, commit to getting 10,000 steps a day, verified by a wearable tracker. • Tip: Splitting walks up into short spurts throughout the day makes this very simple. If you walk around the block twice in the morning while drinking your coffee, you'll likely accrue around 1,000 steps. Walking the perimeter of your house or apartment while brushing your teeth for two or three minutes can get you 300 to 500 steps. Walking while taking a thirty-minute phone call will accrue anywhere from 2,000 to 4,000 steps. Taking a thirty-minute light jog can get you 4,000 or more steps. Walking around the grocery store can get you 1,000 steps. • Log your total steps per day in the Good Energy tracker.

12	Move regularly throughout the day	• Commit to getting up and moving around for at least ninety seconds every hour for eight waking hours per day. This is surprisingly hard if you have a desk job, where it's easy to let hours go by without standing up. One of the best parts of wearables like the Apple Watch and Fitbit is that they specifically tell you how many hours you got up and moved. Based on this information, you can see if any parts of your day are particularly sedentary. For me, my wearables have shown me that my most sedentary hours are from 2:00 to 5:00 p.m., so now I can troubleshoot those hours.
		• You can set a timer on your phone to remind you to get up every hour, or set your wearable to alert you that you need to stand up.
		• Log active hours per day in the Good Energy tracker.

Sleep

13	Get seven to eight hours of sleep per night, confirmed by a sleep tracker	• You will aim to get between seven and eight hours of total sleep every single night, as tracked by a wearable tracker. Wearables will show you how much of the night you were awake, tossing and turning, which is subtracted from total sleep time and is important to account for. Going to bed at 11:00 p.m and getting up at 7:00 a.m. does not translate to eight hours of sleep.
		• This is a habit that may take extreme levels of boundary setting, like going to bed earlier than other people in your household or sleeping in longer. It may require you to keep pets out of your bedroom or sleep in a different bedroom from your partner if they tend to wake you up.
		• Track your sleep amount based on wearable data and log it in the Good Energy tracker.
14	Get consistent sleep, with regular bedtimes and wake times	• Adhere to a set one-hour bedtime and wake time window to minimize social jet lag. This could be a bedtime between 10:00 and 11:00 p.m. and a wake time between 7:30 and 8:30 a.m., verified by your sleep tracker.
		• Track this amount from your wearable data and log it in the Good Energy tracker.

Stress, Relationships, and Emotional Health

15	Meditate daily	• For the month, practice meditation with a guided app or meditation group every day, for a minimum of ten minutes per day.
		• In doing this practice, you build the powerful capacity to understand that you are an observer of your thoughts, and that they are not your identity. This awareness is a liberating first step in getting out of the "autopilot" of thought patterns that many of us are in and suffer from. Additionally, meditations focused on the breath can be extremely relaxing.
		• Suggestions for apps and meditation opportunities are in the supplementary materials at caseymeans.com/goodenergy.
		• Log the daily practice in your Good Energy tracker.

| 16 | Examine reactivity and maladaptive patterns (self-exploration and therapy) | • For the month, read at least two books from our suggested reading list and also form a relationship with a licensed mental health provider and have at least one session. Suggestions are in the supplementary materials.
• Log the progress in your Good Energy tracker. |

Meal Timing and Habits

| 17 | Adhere to a defined eating window | • Aim to eat within a ten-hour window each day and fast for at least fourteen hours. Choose what window you want to adhere to, like 10:00 a.m. to 8:00 p.m. or 8:00 a.m. to 6:00 p.m.
• Tip: If it is a struggle for you to *not* eat late at night, try to have a sizable snack right before the end of your eating window, even if it's soon after dinner. (For instance, if you had dinner at 6:00 p.m. and the end of your eating window is 8:00 p.m., have a few flaxseed crackers, bites of cheese, or almond butter on celery sticks at 7:50 p.m.)
• Log whether you were able to adhere to this window in your Good Energy tracker. |
| 18 | Practice mindful eating | • Eat all main meals (breakfast, lunch, and dinner) sitting down, without engaging with any screens (phone, computer, TV, tablet, etc.).
• Once your food is in front of you, take ten deep breaths before eating while reflecting on gratitude for the meal.
• While chewing each bite, put your silverware down and chew the bite at least fifteen times.
• Log whether you were able to adhere to mindful eating habits in your Good Energy tracker. |

Light

| 19 | Maximize sunlight exposure in the daytime | • Spend at least fifteen minutes outdoors without sunglasses on during the first hour after waking every day.
• If the sun is not up when you wake, then you should aim to be outside for fifteen minutes during or just after sunrise, and/or turn on bright lights or a light box upon waking.
• Get outside in the daylight for at least fifteen minutes four additional times per day, for a total of at least one cumulative hour outside per day. This could look like working out outside, eating breakfast and/or lunch outdoors, taking a walk, gardening, or taking phone calls outside. It is so easy to let a day go by without spending a full hour outside in at least four fifteen-minute chunks.
• Find ways to move your indoor activities to the outdoors, or front-load your outdoor activities to the first hour of the day.
• Log whether you were able to adhere to morning sunlight in your Good Energy tracker. |

| 20 | Minimize nighttime blue light | • Wear blue-light-blocking glasses between sundown and bedtime. (See recommendations for glasses at caseymeans.com/goodenergy)
• After the sun goes down, turn off any unnecessary lights and dim necessary lights to a low level. Add dimmers to your home lights if you can.
• Turn all screens (computer, phone, tablet) to "dark mode" or "night shift" after the sun goes down.
• Log whether you were able to adhere to minimizing nighttime blue light in your Good Energy tracker. |

Temperature

| 21 | Get heat exposure for at least one cumulative hour per week | • Aim to get one cumulative hour of very hot heat exposure per week.
• This can be through a dry sauna, infrared sauna, or a heated exercise class like hot yoga.
• In weeks one and two, find a facility or gym that has access to a sauna or heat therapy and arrange for your sessions for weeks three and four.
• The heat should be hot enough that you feel uncomfortable and are sweating significantly.
• Log hot minutes per day in the Good Energy tracker. |
| 22 | Get cold exposure for at least twelve cumulative minutes per week | • Aim to get twelve cumulative minutes of very cold exposure per week.
• This can be through cryotherapy, cold showers, or cold immersion in a cold plunge tub or cold body of water (like a lake, river, or pool in winter).
• If you choose to do cryotherapy or cold immersion, you'll want to find a facility to do so and arrange this before weeks three and four. If you go into a body of water for a cold plunge, don't go alone. Make sure you are safe! When I moved to Oregon, I found a group on Meetup that cold plunged together several days per week, and I joined in.
• How cold should it be? It should feel like an extreme challenge that you want to escape. Aim for an eventual goal temperature of 35°F to 45°F for three minutes per session.
• Log cold minutes per day in the Good Energy tracker. |

Ingested Toxins

23	Get sufficient clean water per day	• Purchase a reverse osmosis water filter (for either countertop or under the sink) or a high-grade carbon filter, like Berkey, and drink at least ½ ounce of clean water per pound of body weight per day. • Do not drink tap water or water from a plastic bottle. • Tip: I recommend purchasing a glass or metal water bottle that you love and know how many ounces of water it holds. I like to fill three 32-ounce glass mason jars for 96 ounces total, which is what I need to drink each day at a minimum for my weight. I fill them each night with reverse osmosis water and have them out on my counter when I wake up, so that I know the exact minimum I need to drink that day. • Log the clean water intake (in ounces) in your Good Energy tracker.

If you smoke (cigarettes, cigars, marijuana, etc.) or vape any products, stop these completely. They will hurt your mitochondria and vastly diminish your ability to make Good Energy.

Environmental Toxins

24	Clean personal care and home care products	• Overhaul the products used in your home and on your body to greatly minimize your daily toxic exposures.
		• The following products should be swapped out for unscented,* nontoxic versions that have no colorings or dyes:
		  • Personal care products: shampoo, conditioner, body wash, body soap, shaving cream, deodorant, body lotion, hand lotion, makeup, lip balm, nail polish, hand soap, hand sanitizers, perfume, and cologne.
		  • Home products: laundry detergent, fabric softener, laundry sheets, stain-remover sprays, counter spray, disinfectants, floor cleaners, bleach, scented candles, plug-in air fresheners, car air fresheners, and room sprays.
		• Products can be very sneaky with fragrance. Even products labeled "nontoxic," "green," or "natural" may still include fragrance, which should be avoided.
		• Verify your products on the EWG website, looking for "EWG verified" products or products scoring a 1 or a 2.
		
		*Products that are scented exclusively with essential oils are OK. These are extremely rare and need to be sought out from specialty retailers and have the specific essential oils listed in the ingredients. Remove anything with the words "fragrance," "natural fragrance," or "parfum" in the ingredient list.

		• Tip: This does not need to be expensive!
		  • For home care, a simple and cheap way to adhere to this rule is to make a multipurpose cleaning spray from one part white vinegar to five parts filtered water, plus any essential oils you like, all mixed in a glass spray bottle. This solution can clean counters, showers, toilets, and many types of durable floors, and baking soda can be sprinkled on surfaces for extra cleaning capability.
		  • For multipurpose soap (hand soap, dish soap, body soap, and general cleaning soap), I recommend diluting Dr. Bronner's Baby Unscented Pure-Castile Liquid Soap into glass pump bottles and putting them in the kitchen and all bathrooms.
		  • For face and body lotion and makeup remover, you can use organic jojoba oil or organic coconut oil.
		• See full product recommendations in the supplementary materials online at caseymeans.com/goodenergy. Prepare your home and products before week three begins so that weeks three and four involve as many clean and nontoxic products as possible.
		• Log your swaps in your Good Energy tracker.

25	Get nature exposure for four hours per week	• Spend four cumulative hours per week in a natural or green space. In a city, this could be a park, botanical garden, or riverfront trail. Outside of cities, this could be a local trail, or a full excursion into the mountains or wilderness. Ideally, you should get as deep into nature as possible, away from cars and roads, where you are immersed in natural plant life. • In weeks one and two, make sure to schedule your four hours of time in nature on your calendar (and in your tracker) in preparation for weeks three and four. Determine which locations you are going to go to for your nature time, and make it specific. • Log your minutes in nature per day in your Good Energy tracker.

Before starting your two weeks of living out additional Good Energy habits, reflect on how you're going to make the habits fit into your life and how you might move from level two to level three or from level three to level four on the hierarchy of competence. What must be true in your life to go from conscious incompetence to conscious competence, or from conscious competence to unconscious competence? I urge you to reflect on creative ways to make them happen and the realities that would prevent them. Don't limit yourself with reasons why it *won't* work for you or your life; think big and let yourself imagine how that habit could be possible. For instance, if your goal is to minimize refined grains in your diet, you might need to do the following to get to level three, conscious competence:

- Start following grain-free food blogs and social media accounts to learn new recipes and keep them front of mind.
- Get a grain-free cookbook with recipes that look yummy to you.
- Sign up for a grain-free meal kit delivery service or a grain-free frozen food delivery service like Daily Harvest.
- Throw away all refined grains in your house.
- Sign up for grocery delivery so you aren't tempted to buy grains at the grocery store.
- Look at menus before you go to a restaurant to figure out a meal that doesn't have refined grains.
- Ask waiters not to bring bread before the meal.
- Learn how to bake with grain-free flours.
- Read all labels on products from the grocery store.
- Learn grain-free, minimally processed swaps for your favorite grain-based products and purchase them, like lentil pasta and cauliflower pizza crust.
- Figure out a few bread and dessert alternatives that you like a lot that don't have refined grains.
- When making plans with friends, family, or coworkers to share a meal, have a list of healthy restaurants and cafés handy that you can suggest.
- Bring a grain-free healthy dessert or side dish to a dinner party or family holiday.

REFLECTIONS

After each week of the four-week plan, set aside a half hour to look at your Good Energy tracker and food journal and take stock of how you did. If you didn't meet your goals, write a few sentences about what barriers might have gotten in the way. Try to connect with your accountability partner to talk these through and troubleshoot to improve your success in the next week. What *would* you need to change for you to be more successful?

At the end of week four, reflect on whether you improved your level of competence across the food habits and the additional three habits you chose. Were you able to move from conscious incompetence to conscious competence? What were the strategies you used to make the habits happen? Do you need to try to break the habit into even smaller habits to build confidence and make progress? Doing this cycle of action, tracking, reflection, and recommitment is a powerful exercise that you will do throughout your life until every habit becomes second nature: unconscious competence.

Most important, check in on how it felt to create some of these habits. Do you notice anything different in the way you feel? Do you feel proud of yourself for starting this journey? Was it helpful to have accountability?

ACTION:

- Choose three additional Good Energy habits from habits four through twenty-five to fully commit to for weeks three and four.
- Reflect and journal on the ways that you are going to build those habits into your life for weeks three and four.
- Fill these out in your Good Energy tracker in preparation for weeks three and four, scheduling every activity into the tracker.
- At the end of each week, reflect on the Good Energy tracker and food journal to take stock of how things went.

GET OUT OF THE MATRIX

During this month, I am hoping you proved that you can add new habits to your life and that they make you feel better. I also hope you improved your mindset, realizing there is meaning in consciously giving your cells the biological needs that modern industrial life has stolen.

As the months go on, work to stack additional habits in this plan. There is no destination—but I am convinced the commitment to daily actions that respect our cells is the secret to a happy life.

The Good Energy tracker and other resources can be found online in the supplementary materials at caseymeans.com/goodenergy.

GOOD ENERGY RECIPES

Breakfast

Summer Bounty Frittata with Simple Mixed Greens
Nut-Free, Gluten-Free

Time: 40 minutes

SERVINGS: 4

This frittata is an easy make-ahead meal for breakfasts throughout the week. Blending spinach with the eggs adds a bright green color to the frittata and also sneaks in a great source of Good Energy micronutrients like magnesium and vitamins A, E, C, K, folate, B_1, B_6, and B_{12}. Each egg provides 6 grams of whole food protein as well as about 330 milligrams of omega-3 fatty acids. A pasture-raised egg has about double the omega-3s that a conventionally raised egg has. Serve the frittata alongside my simple mixed green salad for an extra dose of thylakoids (which help with feeling full!) and micronutrients.

While many recipes work well with frozen cauliflower rice, this frittata is best with fresh. I make fresh cauliflower rice by putting cauliflower florets in a large food processor with an "S" blade and pulsing a few times until the cauliflower becomes a coarse rice-like consistency. Don't overpulse or the cauliflower will get grainy and watery when cooked.

6 large eggs

2 cups baby spinach, tightly packed

¼ teaspoon sea salt, plus more as needed

1 tablespoon extra-virgin olive oil

1 medium leek, white and light green parts, thinly sliced and thoroughly rinsed

1 small zucchini, halved lengthwise and cut into ½-inch cubes (about 1½ cups)

1 cup fresh cauliflower rice (see headnote)

Freshly ground black pepper

2 tablespoons chopped fresh dill, plus more for garnish

1 cup grape tomatoes

2 ounces feta cheese, crumbled (optional)

Simple Mixed Greens

4 to 6 handfuls of greens, like arugula, spinach, or mesclun

Juice of ½ lemon, or more to taste

3 tablespoons high-quality extra-virgin olive oil

Flaky salt and freshly ground black pepper

1. Preheat the oven to 350°F. Place the eggs, spinach, and salt in a blender. Cover and blend for 30 seconds, or until the mixture is thoroughly incorporated and bright green.

2. In a 10-inch cast-iron skillet, heat the olive oil over medium heat. Add the leeks and cook for 3 to 4 minutes, or until just beginning to soften. Add the zucchini and cauliflower rice and season with salt and pepper to taste. Cook for 4 to 5 minutes, or until the zucchini is tender-crisp and golden brown. Sprinkle with the chopped dill.

3. Pour the eggs into the skillet with the vegetables. Tilt the skillet to evenly distribute the eggs around the zucchini mixture. Top with the tomatoes and feta crumbles, if using, and place the skillet in the oven. Bake for 13 to 15 minutes, or until the eggs are set and solid to the touch in the center.

4. While the frittata cools, prepare the salad: In a large mixing bowl, toss the salad greens with the lemon juice and olive oil. Season with salt and pepper to taste.

5. Serve a slice of warm frittata with the salad. Garnish with additional dill.

STORAGE: Store in an airtight container in the refrigerator for 3 to 4 days.

Strawberry Chia Smoothie

Gluten-Free, Dairy-Free, Soy-Free

Time: 5 minutes

SERVINGS: 1

This smoothie is a nutrient powerhouse thanks partly to Brazil nuts, which add around 270 micrograms of selenium, a hefty dose of this essential trace mineral. Selenium acts as an antioxidant and assists in healthy glucose metabolism. And the best part? You don't need any milk to achieve that creamy texture; the water and nuts will emulsify in a high-speed blender to make nut milk and save time and cost!

½ cup frozen strawberries

¼ cup frozen raspberries

½ cup frozen cauliflower florets

4 Brazil nuts

1 tablespoon chia seeds

1 tablespoon maca powder

2 teaspoons beet powder

¼ teaspoon vanilla extract

¼ teaspoon ground cardamom

Juice of ½ lemon

Place all of the ingredients in a blender with 1 cup water and blend on high speed for 30 seconds, or until smooth. Serve immediately.

Maca Smoothie, 2 Ways
Gluten-Free, Soy-Free, Nut-Free, Dairy-Free
Time: 5 minutes

SERVINGS: 1

The blood sugar–spiking potential of frozen banana in this smoothie is balanced with fat and fiber. Ingredients like avocado and hemp seeds bring the fiber total up to 11 grams. Maca is a cruciferous root vegetable with potent antioxidant properties, helping mitigate oxidative stress in the body. I've included two of my favorite variations for this powerhouse smoothie.

TROPICAL

½ frozen banana

¼ cup frozen avocado (about ¼ fresh avocado)

¼ cup frozen pineapple chunks

½ cup baby kale, lightly packed

1 tablespoon hemp seeds

1 tablespoon tahini

1 tablespoon maca powder

¼ teaspoon vanilla extract

BERRY

½ frozen banana

½ cup frozen blueberries

¼ cup frozen avocado (about ¼ fresh avocado)

½ cup baby kale, lightly packed

1 tablespoon hemp seeds

1 tablespoon tahini

1 tablespoon maca powder

Juice of ½ lime

Place all of the ingredients (for either the Tropical or Berry variation) in a blender with 1 cup water. Blend on high speed for 30 seconds, or until smooth. Serve immediately.

Good Energy Milk

Gluten-Free, Dairy-Free, Soy-Free

Time: 5 minutes, plus 8 to 10 hours for soaking

SERVINGS: 4 (8-OUNCE) CUPS

Walnuts and hemp seeds are rich in omega-3 fatty acids, which are connected to reduced levels of pro-inflammatory biomarkers, plaque buildup in arteries, and blood pressure. Each glass of this nut and seed milk provides 3.5 grams of omega-3s. Making your own nut milk at home is also a great way to avoid hidden sugars and other additives that are often found in store-bought options. Plus, it's a fun and simple project that can save you money in the long run.

½ cup walnuts

1 teaspoon sea salt

½ cup hemp seeds

1 teaspoon vanilla extract

1. Place the walnuts in a medium bowl. Cover the nuts with a few inches of water and add the salt. Cover and set aside to soak for 8 to 10 hours.
2. Drain the nuts and rinse thoroughly.
3. In a blender, place the walnuts, hemp seeds, and vanilla with 4 cups filtered water. Use a little less water for a creamier consistency or a little more for a thinner milk. Blend on high speed for 2 to 3 minutes, or until thoroughly combined, white, and frothy.
4. Line a pitcher with a nut milk bag or place a colander lined with cheesecloth over a bowl. Pour the milk into the nut milk bag or colander to strain the nut and seed pulp. Squeeze or press with clean hands to extract as much milk as possible.
5. Shake before using, as the milk will naturally separate.

STORAGE: Store in a clean container in the refrigerator for 3 to 4 days.

Spinach-Chickpea Wraps with Creamy Scrambled Eggs and Spicy Mushrooms

Gluten-Free, Soy-Free, Nut-Free

Time: 45 minutes

SERVINGS: 3 (2 WRAPS PER SERVING)

The sautéed mushrooms in this recipe are a fantastic source of beta-glucans, a compound that acts as a prebiotic fiber. Beneficial bacteria in the gut break down the beta-glucans to produce short-chain fatty acids, which can reduce insulin resistance. Pro tip: You can make the wraps in bulk and freeze them for a more leisurely morning.

Spinach-Chickpea Wraps

½ cup chickpea flour

¼ cup cassava flour

1 cup baby spinach, tightly packed

3 or 4 fresh basil leaves

¼ teaspoon sea salt

Extra-virgin olive oil, as needed

Spicy Mushrooms

1 tablespoon extra-virgin olive oil

3 cups cremini mushrooms, sliced

Sea salt and freshly ground black pepper

Pinch of crushed red pepper flakes

Creamy Scrambled Eggs

1 tablespoon grass-fed butter

6 large eggs, beaten

Sea salt and freshly ground black pepper

6 basil leaves, for garnish

Hot sauce (optional)

1. **Make the wraps:** In a blender, place the chickpea flour, cassava flour, spinach, basil, salt, and 1 cup water. Blend on high speed for 30 seconds, or until smooth and vibrant green.

2. Heat a medium cast-iron skillet over medium heat. Pour ¼ cup of the batter into the heated skillet. Rotate the skillet in a circular motion to spread the batter, as if making a crepe. Cook for 1 to 2 minutes on each side, or until the wrap is pliable. If the batter sticks, use a few drops of olive oil to grease the pan. Repeat until 6 wraps are complete. Set aside.

3. **Sauté the mushrooms:** Heat the olive oil in the same skillet over medium heat. Add the mushrooms and season with salt, black pepper, and red pepper flakes to taste. Cook for 5 to 6 minutes, or until the mushrooms are tender and golden brown. Set aside.

4. **Make the creamy scrambled eggs:** Add the butter to the same skillet over medium-low heat. Once melted, add the beaten eggs and season with salt and pepper. Gently scramble the eggs for 2 to 3 minutes, or until just set.

5. To assemble, place two wraps on a plate, line each with two basil leaves, and add some scrambled eggs and spicy mushrooms. If desired, top with hot sauce.

STORAGE: The wraps can be prepared in bulk and stored in the freezer for up to 3 months. To reheat, simply warm the wraps in a dry pan over medium heat for 30 seconds on each side, or until warm and pliable.

Chia or Basil Seed Pudding 3 Ways
Gluten-Free, Dairy-Free, Soy-Free
Time: 10 minutes, plus soaking overnight

SERVINGS: 1

Chia and basil seeds are potent sources of metabolic-friendly fiber. When soaked in liquid, basil and chia seeds swell and gelatinize, creating a pudding texture. This is due to mucilage, a soluble fiber that allows the seeds to absorb ten to twenty times their weight in water. Here are three delicious pudding base and topping flavor combinations.

TROPICAL COCONUT
Base
3 tablespoons chia or basil seeds, or a combination

⅔ cup Good Energy Milk (page 311) or preferred milk

½ teaspoon blue spirulina

¼ teaspoon lime zest

¼ cup fresh pineapple, finely diced

1 tablespoon shredded coconut

Pinch of sea salt

Toppers
¼ cup chopped fresh pineapple

1 teaspoon hemp seeds

Freshly squeezed lime juice

RASPBERRY AND ALMOND
Base
3 tablespoons chia or basil seeds, or a combination

⅔ cup Good Energy Milk (page 311) or preferred milk

¼ cup raspberries, finely diced

⅛ teaspoon vanilla extract

¼ teaspoon beet powder

Pinch of sea salt

Toppers

¼ cup blackberries

1 tablespoon chopped almonds

Squeeze of fresh lemon juice

DARK CHOCOLATE AND ORANGE

Base

3 tablespoons chia or basil seeds, or a combination

⅔ cup Good Energy Milk (page 311) or preferred milk

¼ cup orange segments, finely chopped

1½ teaspoons cocoa powder

⅛ teaspoon vanilla extract

¼ teaspoon ground cinnamon

½ teaspoon maca

Pinch of sea salt

Toppers

¼ cup orange segments

1 tablespoon chopped hazelnuts, lightly toasted

1 teaspoon pumpkin seeds

In a medium bowl, mix the base ingredients with a whisk until well incorporated, then cover. (Alternatively, add the ingredients to a large mason jar and shake until combined, then leave on the lid.) After 2 to 3 minutes, rewhisk (or reshake). Refrigerate overnight to soak. Garnish with the toppers just before serving.

Spiced Almond Flour Pancakes with Stewed Apples

Gluten-Free, Dairy-Free, Soy-Free

Time: 30 minutes

SERVINGS: 2

Cinnamon, an essential ingredient in this recipe, may regulate blood glucose levels and exhibit antioxidant and anti-inflammatory properties. The stewed apples are a great substitute for sugary syrup—they provide a little sweetness along with vitamin C, potassium, and vitamin K.

Stewed Apples

1 apple, peeled and diced

1 teaspoon unrefined coconut oil

¼ teaspoon ground cinnamon

⅛ teaspoon sea salt

1 teaspoon freshly squeezed lemon juice

Pancakes

1 cup blanched fine-ground almond flour

1 teaspoon baking powder

⅛ teaspoon sea salt

½ teaspoon ground cinnamon

⅛ teaspoon ground nutmeg

⅛ teaspoon ground ginger

⅛ teaspoon ground allspice

½ cup canned full-fat coconut milk

2 large eggs

½ teaspoon vanilla extract

Unrefined coconut oil, for the pan, to prevent the pancakes from sticking

1. **Make the stewed apples:** In a small saucepan, add the diced apple, coconut oil, cinnamon, salt, lemon juice, and ½ cup water and bring to a simmer over medium heat. Cook for 10 minutes, or until

the apples become tender and fragrant and the water reduces to a syrupy consistency.

2. **Meanwhile, make the pancakes:** In a medium bowl, combine the almond flour, baking powder, salt, cinnamon, nutmeg, ginger, and allspice. In a separate bowl, whisk together the coconut milk, eggs, vanilla, and ¼ cup water. Stir the coconut milk mixture into the dry ingredients.

3. Heat a cast-iron skillet or griddle over medium-low heat. Reduce the heat to low and add a little coconut oil to prevent the batter from sticking. Pour ¼ cup of the batter into the skillet and cook for about 2 minutes on each side, or until golden brown and fluffy. Adjust the heat as necessary while the pancakes cook.

4. Serve the pancakes warm with the stewed apples.

Sardine-Scallion Fritters with Tzatziki
Gluten-Free, Soy-Free
Time: 25 minutes

SERVINGS: 3 (6 MEDIUM FRITTERS)

Sardines, a great source of omega-3 fatty acids, are also a low-mercury fish, making them a safe seafood choice. Scallions are a member of the allium family, which contains compounds that may have cancer-preventive properties.

5 ounces frozen spinach, thawed (about 1 cup)

1 (4-ounce) tin sardines, drained and mashed

4 scallions, green and white portions thinly sliced

4 large eggs, beaten

2 tablespoons coconut flour

½ teaspoon sea salt

Freshly ground black pepper

Extra-virgin olive oil, for frying

1 tablespoon chopped fresh dill, plus more for
   garnish

Tzatziki
1 cup plain whole-milk yogurt

2 tablespoons chopped fresh dill

1 tablespoon freshly squeezed lemon juice

1 garlic clove, minced

Sea salt and freshly ground black pepper

1. Squeeze the excess water out of the spinach. In a medium mixing bowl, combine the spinach, sardines, scallions, and eggs. Add the coconut flour, salt, and pepper to taste and stir until well combined.

2. Heat a skillet over medium heat and add a small swirl of olive oil. Working in batches, scoop the batter into the skillet, forming medium

fritters. Cook the fritters for 3 to 4 minutes per side, or until golden brown and cooked through.

3. **Make the tzatziki:** In a small bowl, whisk together the yogurt, dill, lemon juice, and garlic. Season generously with salt and pepper.

4. Garnish the fritters with additional dill and serve with the tzatziki.

Lunch

Fennel and Apple Salad with Lemon-Dijon Dressing and Smoked Salmon
Gluten-Free, Dairy-Free
Time: 20 minutes

SERVINGS: 4

Salmon supplies our bodies with omega-3s, vitamin D, vitamin B_{12}, potassium, and selenium while being relatively low in mercury. It's also worth noting that choosing unsweetened smoked salmon is important to avoid added sugars.

1 small red onion, thinly sliced

2 medium bulbs fennel, quartered, cored, and thinly sliced

1 Granny Smith apple, thinly sliced

4 ribs celery, thinly sliced

½ cup green olives, pitted and sliced

¼ cup chopped fresh dill

½ cup Lemon-Dijon Dressing (page 353) or to taste

½ cup fennel fronds, if available

6 ounces smoked salmon, sliced

2 tablespoons finely chopped toasted pecans

1. In a large mixing bowl, toss the onion, fennel, apple, celery, olives, and dill with the Lemon-Dijon Dressing. Allow to sit for 5 to 10 minutes to marinate.

2. To serve, divide the salad equally among four plates. Garnish with fennel fronds, smoked salmon, and toasted pecans.

Rainbow Salad with Lemon-Dijon Dressing and Soft-Boiled Eggs

Gluten-Free, Soy-Free, Nut-Free

Time: 15 minutes, plus 1 hour for marinating

SERVINGS: 4

Cruciferous vegetables like kale, red cabbage, and sauerkraut are rich in isothiocyanates—molecules that fight oxidative stress by increasing the gene expression of the antioxidant-promoting gene, Nrf2. The marinated chickpeas are a great source of whole food protein and can be made ahead of time, making meal prep a breeze. Soft-boiled eggs, pumpkin seeds, and optional crumbled feta cheese bring the protein total of this salad up to 24 grams.

Za'atar-Marinated Chickpeas

1 (15-ounce) can chickpeas, drained, rinsed, and patted dry

2 teaspoons extra-virgin olive oil

1 shallot, thinly sliced

1 garlic clove, finely minced

2 tablespoons red wine vinegar

1 teaspoon za'atar spice blend

¼ teaspoon sea salt

Soft-Boiled Eggs

4 large eggs

Salad

4 cups arugula, tightly packed

1 orange bell pepper, ribs and seeds removed and sliced

1 medium yellow squash, diced

4 cups sliced red cabbage

½ cup beet sauerkraut

Lemon-Dijon Dressing (page 353)

Sea salt and freshly ground black pepper

¼ cup pumpkin seeds

¼ cup crumbled feta cheese (optional)

1. **Make the marinated chickpeas:** In a medium mixing bowl, add the chickpeas, olive oil, shallot, garlic, vinegar, za'atar, and salt and stir until combined. Cover and marinate for at least 1 hour. The chickpeas may be made up to 5 days in advance.

2. **Make the soft-boiled eggs:** Bring a medium saucepan of water to a gentle boil over medium-high heat. Carefully lower the eggs into the water and cook for 7 minutes. Once done, place the eggs in a bowl of ice water until they are cool enough to handle. Peel the eggs and set aside.

3. **Make the salad:** In a large mixing bowl, toss the arugula, bell pepper, yellow squash, red cabbage, and sauerkraut with a desired amount of Lemon-Dijon Dressing. Season the salad components with salt and black pepper to taste.

4. To serve, divide the salad evenly among four bowls. Sprinkle with the pumpkin seeds, marinated chickpeas, and feta, if using. Top with halved soft-boiled eggs.

STORAGE: Store the undressed salad and its components in the refrigerator for up to 5 days.

Curried Roasted Vegetables with Coconut Flour Flatbread
Gluten-Free, Soy-Free
Time: 35 minutes

SERVINGS: 2 TO 3

The spices in curry powder have some of the highest antioxidant levels of any food, including turmeric, a potent anti-inflammatory spice. Turmeric acts as both an antioxidant and an anti-inflammatory substance, directly inhibiting the expression of inflammatory gene NF-κB. Coconut flour and psyllium husks in the flatbread add 17 grams of fiber per serving and can be found at most health food stores, although psyllium is sometimes in the supplements area. Cassava flour is a grain-free gluten-free alternative flour made from the cassava plant root, sometimes called yuca.

Coconut Flour Flatbread

½ cup coconut flour

¼ cup cassava flour

2 tablespoons whole psyllium husks

½ teaspoon baking powder

¼ teaspoon sea salt

¼ cup canned full-fat coconut milk

Curried Roasted Vegetables

1 medium head cauliflower, cut into small florets

1 large tomato, cut into wedges

1 small yellow onion, sliced

3 medium carrots, coarsely chopped

1 tablespoon curry powder

2 tablespoons extra-virgin olive oil, plus more for frying

Sea salt and freshly ground black pepper

½ cup frozen peas

Cilantro

Plain whole-milk yogurt

1 lime, cut into wedges

1. **Make the flatbread dough:** Preheat the oven to 400°F. In a medium bowl, whisk together the coconut flour, cassava flour, psyllium husks, baking powder, and salt. Add the coconut milk and 1½ cups warm water and mix until well combined. Set aside for at least 10 minutes.

2. **Make the curried roasted vegetables:** On a large rimmed baking sheet, toss the cauliflower, tomatoes, onion, and carrots with the curry powder, olive oil, salt, and pepper until well coated. Roast for 20 to 25 minutes, tossing occasionally, until the vegetables are golden brown and tender. During the last 5 minutes of roasting, add the frozen peas and toss with the vegetable mixture. Roast until the peas are bright green.

3. Divide the flatbread dough into 6 equal pieces. Roll each piece into a ball. Place a ball between two sheets of parchment paper. Using a rolling pin, roll out the dough to about ½ inch thickness. Repeat for the remaining dough balls.

4. Heat a cast-iron skillet over medium heat. Add a little olive oil and place one rolled-out flatbread in the heated skillet. Cook for 3 to 4 minutes on each side, or until golden and starting to puff. Transfer to a plate, and repeat with the remaining flatbread.

5. Serve the curried roasted vegetables with the warm flatbread, cilantro, yogurt, and lime wedges.

Cauliflower Rice Hand Rolls
Gluten-Free, Dairy-Free, Soy-Free, Nut-Free
Time: 30 minutes

SERVINGS: 2

The cauliflower sushi rice, made with omega-3-rich flaxseeds and tangy rice wine vinegar, adds a nutritious and blood sugar–balancing twist to typical white sushi rice. Roasted nori sheets are rich in iodine, an essential trace mineral that supports thyroid and metabolic health.

Spicy Salmon

1 (6-ounce) can wild salmon, drained and flaked with a fork

1 tablespoon Herbed Aioli (see page 361) or avocado oil mayonnaise

1 pinch crushed red pepper flakes (optional)

Sea salt and freshly ground black pepper

Cauliflower Sushi Rice

½ recipe Simple Cauliflower Rice (page 354), warm

1 teaspoon rice wine vinegar

1 tablespoon sesame seeds

2 teaspoons ground flaxseeds

Miso-Tahini Sauce

1 date, pitted

3 tablespoons tahini

1 teaspoon tamari

1 teaspoon red miso

2 teaspoons rice wine vinegar

1 garlic clove, minced

1 teaspoon freshly grated ginger

3 to 4 roasted nori sheets, cut into quarters

1 ripe but firm Hass avocado, halved, pitted, peeled, and sliced

1 small cucumber, diced

1. **Make the spicy salmon:** In a medium bowl, mix the salmon, aioli, and red pepper flakes, if using, until well combined. Season with salt and black pepper to taste. Set aside.

2. **Make the cauliflower sushi rice:** In a separate bowl, mix together the warm cauliflower rice, vinegar, sesame seeds, and flaxseeds. Set aside.

3. **Make the miso-tahini sauce:** Soak the date in hot water for 10 to 15 minutes to soften, and then drain. In a miniature food processor, blend together the tahini, tamari, miso, date, vinegar, garlic, and ginger. Thin with 1 to 2 tablespoons of water, or until the dip is thick but pourable.

4. To assemble the hand rolls, top a sheet of nori with some cauliflower rice, spicy salmon, sliced avocado, and cucumber. Wrap and serve with miso-tahini sauce.

Classic Chicken and Celery Salad Wraps
Gluten-Free, Dairy-Free, Soy-Free, Nut-Free
Time: 50 minutes

SERVINGS: 2 TO 4

Homemade Herbed Aioli (see page 361) or avocado oil mayonnaise
(Primal Kitchen brand is available at most major grocers) provides
richness without the use of inflammatory seed oil–based mayonnaise.
Using collard leaves instead of traditional wheat wraps or bread is
a Good Energy swap. With components that can be prepared ahead
of time and stored in the refrigerator, these wraps are great for a quick
lunch.

1½ pounds skinless, boneless chicken breasts

Sea salt

4 to 8 large collard leaves

¼ cup Herbed Aioli (see page 361) or avocado oil mayonnaise

Juice of ½ lemon

¼ cup finely diced red onion

2 ribs celery, diced

2 tablespoons dried sour cherries (optional)

1 cup thinly sliced red cabbage

1 cucumber, cut into spears

1. In a medium bowl, season the chicken breasts with salt and refrigerate
for 20 to 30 minutes.
2. Meanwhile, bring a wide pot of water to a boil over high heat. Using a
sharp knife, trim the thickest part of each collard leaf stem to create an
even thickness. Season the water generously with salt. Add the collard to
the water to blanch the leaves for about 1 minute, or until pliable and
bright green. Submerge the cooked leaves in ice water to halt the cooking
process. Place on a clean towel to dry.
3. Remove the chicken from the refrigerator. Add 3 cups water to a
medium saucepan with a lid and bring to a simmer over medium-high

heat. Add the chicken and cover. Reduce the heat to low and simmer until the chicken is cooked through, 15 to 20 minutes, depending on the thickness.

4. In a large bowl, whisk together the aioli, lemon juice, onion, celery, and sour cherries, if using.

5. Remove the chicken breasts from the water and pat dry. Finely dice the chicken and add to the mayonnaise mixture. Stir until well combined.

6. To assemble the wraps, top a blanched collard leaf with some chicken salad, sliced red cabbage, and cucumber spears. Wrap and enjoy.

Dinner

———

Pork and Cauliflower Fried Rice
Nut-Free, Gluten-Free, Dairy-Free

Time: 30 minutes

SERVINGS: 2

Swapping cauliflower rice for white rice taps into the beneficial compounds in cruciferous vegetables, including a range of micronutrients like vitamin C, vitamin K, folate, vitamin B_6, and potassium.

1 tablespoon plus 1 teaspoon tamari

1 tablespoon rice wine vinegar, plus more for serving

1 tablespoon almond butter

3 garlic cloves, minced

½ pound ground pork

Sea salt and freshly ground black pepper

2 cups diced cremini mushrooms

3 cups fresh cauliflower rice (about 10 ounces)

1 carrot, diced

½ medium red onion, diced

2 cup chopped kale

2 large eggs, beaten and lightly seasoned with salt and pepper

2 scallions, green and white portions thinly sliced

1. In a small bowl, whisk together the tamari, vinegar, almond butter, and garlic. Set aside.

2. Heat a large skillet over medium-high heat. Add the ground pork and cook, breaking up large lumps with a wooden spoon, for 5 to 7 minutes, or until golden brown. Season with salt and pepper to taste.

3. Add the mushrooms and cook for 4 to 5 minutes, or until tender and golden brown. Add the cauliflower rice, carrot, onion, kale, and the tamari-vinegar mixture. Cook for 2 to 3 minutes, or until tender-crisp.

4. Make a small well in the center of the skillet ingredients and add the beaten eggs. Gently scramble the eggs for 2 to 3 minutes, or until just set, and then combine with the cauliflower rice mixture. Remove from the heat.

5. Garnish with sliced scallions and a few shakes of vinegar to taste.

Seared Wild Salmon with Chive Salsa and Creamy Cauliflower and Celery Root Puree
Gluten-Free, Dairy-Free, Soy-Free, Nut-Free

Time: 20 minutes

SERVINGS: 2

Wild salmon is a great source of powerful long-chain omega-3 fatty acids eicosapentaenoic acid (EPA) and docosahexaenoic acid (DHA). If you choose wild salmon over farmed, you will take advantage of the diverse diet and nutrition benefits that wild salmon delivers.

2 (6- to 8-ounce) wild salmon fillets, skin on

Sea salt and freshly ground black pepper

1 tablespoon avocado oil

Chive Salsa

3 tablespoons sliced fresh chives

¼ cup finely diced tomatoes

1 tablespoon freshly squeezed lime juice

½ teaspoon extra-virgin olive oil

Sea salt and freshly ground black pepper

⅓ recipe Creamy Cauliflower and Celery Root Puree (page 347)

1. Pat the salmon fillets dry and season with salt and pepper. In a 10-inch cast-iron or medium oven-proof skillet, heat the avocado oil over medium-high heat, until just shimmering but not smoking. Add the fillets skin-side down and sear for 3 to 4 minutes undisturbed, or until the skin is well browned. Flip the salmon and cook for 2 to 3 minutes more, or until just cooked through. Remove from the heat.

2. Meanwhile, prepare the salsa. In a small mixing bowl, add the chives, tomatoes, lime juice, olive oil, and salt and pepper to taste.

3. To serve, spoon equal amounts of the cauliflower puree on the center of each plate. Place salmon on top, skin-side up. Divide equal amounts of the salsa between the plates.

Mushroom and Creamy Cauliflower Bake
Gluten-Free, Dairy-Free
Time: 1 hour 30 minutes

SERVINGS: 4 TO 6

Instead of using mashed potatoes as a topping in this ode to shepherd's pie, I use my Creamy Cauliflower and Celery Root Puree (page 347), just as enjoyable but with more fiber and micronutrient density. Making low-carb swaps like this is an easy way to minimize glycemic variability.

2 tablespoons extra-virgin olive oil

8 ounces mixed wild mushrooms, sliced

1 large onion, sliced

1 black garlic clove, mashed

1 tablespoon red miso

Freshly ground black pepper

3 cups chicken bone broth or stock, or vegetable stock

1 cup brown lentils

¼ teaspoon dried thyme

Sea salt

½ cup chopped walnuts

2 cups baby spinach

Creamy Cauliflower and Celery Root Puree (page 347)

1. Preheat the oven to 400°F. In a wide, oven-safe sauté pan with a lid, heat the olive oil over medium-high heat. Add the mushrooms and cook for 4 to 5 minutes, or until tender and browned. Reduce the heat to medium. Add the onion and cook, stirring frequently, for 8 to 10 minutes, or until golden brown and fragrant.

2. Add the black garlic, miso, pepper to taste, and ½ cup broth. Using a wooden spoon, release any browned bits from the bottom of the pan and mix well. Bring the mushroom mixture to a simmer and continue to cook for 3 to 4 minutes, or until half of the liquid has evaporated and the mushrooms are covered in a glossy, brown glaze.

3. Add the lentils, thyme, and remaining 2½ cups broth. Season the broth with salt and more pepper if needed. Bring the lentils to a simmer and cover. Cook for 25 to 30 minutes, or until the lentils are tender and most of the liquid is absorbed. Remove from the heat, add the walnuts, and mix in the baby spinach until just wilted.

4. Smooth the Creamy Cauliflower and Celery Root Puree over the top of the lentil filling. Place the uncovered pan in the oven and bake for 25 to 30 minutes, or until golden brown. Serve hot.

Spiced Turkey and Mushroom Lettuce Wraps
Gluten-Free, Soy-Free, Nut-Free
Time: 30 minutes

SERVINGS: 3

Typical wheat flour wraps are made with ultra-refined white flour, which can contribute to big swings in glucose levels. Using lettuce leaves in place of wheat wraps is an easy Good Energy swap to reduce processed food intake. The ground turkey in this recipe provides about 40 grams of protein per serving, making this a satiating dinner.

1 tablespoon extra-virgin olive oil

¼ teaspoon ground cumin

¼ teaspoon ground cinnamon

¼ teaspoon ground allspice

¼ teaspoon crushed red pepper flakes

1 medium red onion, diced

3 garlic cloves, minced

1 teaspoon freshly grated ginger

3 cups cremini mushrooms, coarsely chopped into ¼-inch pieces

¾ teaspoon sea salt, plus more to taste

Freshly ground black pepper

1 medium tomato, finely chopped

1 pound ground turkey

1 tablespoon plain whole-milk yogurt

½ cup chopped fresh cilantro, plus more for garnish

¼ cup chopped fresh mint

1 tablespoon red wine vinegar

1 head butter lettuce (about 5 ounces)

¼ cup crumbled feta cheese, for garnish

1. In a 10-inch cast-iron skillet, heat the olive oil over medium heat. Add the cumin, cinnamon, allspice, and red pepper flakes and cook for about 15 seconds, or until fragrant but not burnt. Add ¾ cup of the onion (reserve

the rest for garnish), garlic, and ginger to the skillet. Cook, stirring occasionally, for 2 to 3 minutes, or until the onion begins to pick up color and soften.

2. Add the mushrooms and season with ¼ teaspoon salt and black pepper to taste. Cook for 5 to 6 minutes, or until the mushrooms begin to brown and become tender. Add the diced tomato and mix well.

3. Raise the heat to medium-high and add the turkey. Season with the remaining ½ teaspoon salt or to taste. Cook for 6 to 8 minutes, or until fully cooked, breaking up large lumps with a wooden spoon. Remove from the heat.

4. Add the yogurt, cilantro, mint, and vinegar and mix until the yogurt has fully dissolved into the pan juices. Serve with the butter lettuce leaves for wrapping and the cilantro, reserved red onion, and feta for garnish.

Tofu Masala with Toasted Cashews and Cucumber-Mint Raita

Gluten-Free, Soy-Free

Time: 1 hour

SERVINGS: 2 TO 3

Reducing oxidative stress is a key factor for Good Energy, and including spices like cumin and turmeric provides significant antioxidant power to this recipe.

Cucumber-Mint Raita

½ cup plain whole-milk yogurt

½ cup grated cucumber and juices

¼ teaspoon sea salt

⅛ teaspoon ground cumin

2 tablespoons chopped fresh mint

2 teaspoons freshly squeezed lemon juice

Turmeric Tofu

1 tablespoon unrefined coconut oil

1 (14-ounce) package extra-firm tofu, drained, cubed, and patted dry

Freshly ground black pepper, to taste

¼ teaspoon ground turmeric

¼ teaspoon salt, or to taste

Masala Sauce

1 tablespoon grass-fed butter

½ teaspoon ground cumin

½ teaspoon ground coriander

1 teaspoon sea salt

Freshly ground black pepper

1 large yellow onion, sliced

1 teaspoon freshly grated ginger

3 garlic cloves, minced

1 serrano chili, sliced

1 (14.5-ounce) can diced tomatoes

½ cup canned full-fat coconut milk

½ teaspoon garam masala

¼ cup raw cashews

Simple Cauliflower Rice (page 354)

Cilantro, for garnish

1. **Make the cucumber-mint raita:** In a small mixing bowl, whisk together the yogurt, grated cucumber, salt, cumin, mint, and lemon juice. Taste and adjust the seasoning if necessary. Cover and refrigerate until ready to serve.

2. **Prepare the turmeric tofu:** In a wide sauté pan over medium-high heat, heat the coconut oil. Add the tofu and lightly fry for 4 to 5 minutes, or until golden on all sides. Season with pepper, turmeric, and salt. Remove the tofu to a plate and set aside.

3. **Make the sauce:** In the same wide sauté pan, melt the butter over medium heat. Add the cumin, coriander, salt, and pepper to taste and cook for 15 to 30 seconds, or until fragrant but not burnt. Add the onion, ginger, garlic, and serrano chili and cook for 8 to 10 minutes, or until the onion mixture is tender and golden brown. Remove from the heat and allow to cool.

4. Add the onion mixture to a high-speed blender with the diced tomatoes, coconut milk, and garam masala. Blend until smooth.

5. Return the sauce to the sauté pan. Cook the sauce for 4 to 5 minutes over medium heat, or until bubbling and fragrant. Taste and adjust the seasonings if necessary. Add the tofu and simmer for 3 to 4 minutes, or until the tofu is coated and flavorful and the sauce is slightly thickened.

6. In a small skillet over medium-low heat, toast the cashews, tossing frequently for even color, for 3 to 4 minutes, or until golden.

7. Serve with Simple Cauliflower Rice, raita, toasted cashews, and cilantro for garnish.

Hearts of Palm "Crab Cakes" with Rainbow Slaw
Gluten-Free, Soy-Free
Time: 1 hour

SERVINGS: 4 (2 CAKES PER SERVING)

These "crab cakes" made with hearts of palm are an affordable alternative to traditional crab cakes. The combination of hearts of palm, chickpea flour, and aromatics provides 15 grams of protein and 10 grams of fiber per serving, with no refined carbohydrates.

Rainbow Slaw

1 large carrot

1 medium beet

1 Granny Smith apple

½ medium red onion, thinly sliced

Juice of ½ lemon

Sea salt

Yogurt-Caper Dipping Sauce

1 cup plain whole-milk Greek yogurt

2 tablespoons sauerkraut

1 tablespoon capers, coarsely chopped

1 tablespoon Dijon mustard

Juice of ½ lemon

Sea salt, as needed

Hearts of Palm "Crab Cakes"

2 (14-ounce) cans hearts of palm, drained, rinsed, and finely chopped

1 cup chickpea flour

2 large eggs, beaten

1 rib celery, finely diced

½ red bell pepper, ribs and seeds removed and diced

½ medium red onion, finely diced

¼ cup fresh flat-leaf parsley, finely chopped

2 tablespoons ground flaxseeds

1 teaspoon Old Bay Seasoning

½ teaspoon garlic powder

¼ teaspoon coarse sea salt

Unrefined coconut oil, for frying

1. **Make the slaw:** Cut the carrot, beet, and apple into matchsticks with a spiralizer, by grating on the large holes of a box grater, or with a sharp knife. In a medium bowl, mix the shredded vegetables and onion with the lemon juice and season with salt to taste. Refrigerate until ready to use.

2. **Make the dipping sauce:** In a medium bowl, mix the yogurt, sauerkraut, capers, mustard, and lemon juice. If needed, season with salt. Refrigerate until ready to use.

3. **Make the "crab cakes":** In a large bowl, combine the hearts of palm, chickpea flour, eggs, celery, bell pepper, onion, parsley, flaxseeds, Old Bay Seasoning, garlic powder, and salt.

4. In a large skillet, heat a small amount of coconut oil over medium heat. Working in batches, drop the batter into the skillet forming medium patties (8 total), and cook for 3 to 4 minutes on each side, or until golden brown and crispy.

5. Serve hot with the rainbow slaw and dipping sauce.

Cheesy Cauliflower Rice Bowl

Gluten-Free, Dairy-Free

Time: 40 minutes

SERVINGS: 4

The "cheesy" sauce gets its flavor from gut-friendly fermented miso and nutritional yeast. Nutritional yeast is a yeast fungus (similar to what you would use for bread or beer making) that has been "deactivated" by heat. It is often used to add depth of flavor and umami to plant-based dishes, and it is a good source of several B vitamins and protein. Use the sauce in this recipe, mixed with your favorite hot sauce as a spicy dip, or as a cheese sauce for a lentil or vegetable pasta.

1 (15-ounce) can black beans, drained and rinsed

2 medium tomatoes, diced

½ cup diced red onion

½ cup chopped fresh cilantro, plus more for garnish

Juice of 1 lime

Sea salt and freshly ground black pepper

"Cheesy" Sauce

2 cups chopped cauliflower, florets and stems, fresh or frozen

1 medium carrot, chopped

½ small yellow onion, chopped

½ cup canned full-fat coconut milk

¼ cup nutritional yeast

1 teaspoon Dijon mustard

1 teaspoon apple cider vinegar

¾ teaspoon sea salt

½ teaspoon red miso

Simple Cauliflower Rice (page 354)

1 ripe but firm Hass avocado, halved, pitted, peeled, and sliced

¼ cup chopped or sliced almonds

1. In a large bowl, mix the black beans, tomatoes, red onion, cilantro, and lime juice. Generously season with salt and pepper. Set aside.

2. **Make the "cheesy" sauce:** Fill a wide pot with 2 inches of water. Set a steamer basket in the pot, then bring the water to a simmer over medium-high heat. Add the cauliflower, carrot, and onion to the basket and cover. Steam for 10 to 12 minutes, or until very tender when pierced with a fork.

3. Drain the vegetables and add to the bowl of a food processor or a blender. Add the coconut milk, nutritional yeast, mustard, vinegar, salt, and miso and blend until smooth.

4. To serve, toss the cauliflower rice with the black bean mixture and divide equally among four bowls. Top with sliced avocado, almonds, and a drizzle of "cheesy" sauce.

Pesto Zucchini Noodles with Walnut Gremolata
Gluten-Free, Soy-Free
Time: 35 minutes

SERVINGS: 4

Zucchini noodles stand in for traditional semolina-based pasta in this recipe, increasing the nutrient and fiber content of the dish while eliminating the processed carbohydrates.

Zucchini Noodles

6 medium zucchini (about 3 pounds)

Sea salt

Walnut Gremolata

¼ cup finely chopped walnuts

¼ cup finely chopped sun-dried tomatoes

1 tablespoon chopped fresh basil

Zest of 1 lemon

Sea salt and freshly ground black pepper

Basil-Arugula Pesto

½ cup fresh basil, tightly packed

½ cup arugula

¼ cup chopped walnuts

¼ cup grated Parmesan cheese or nutritional yeast, plus more for serving

1 garlic clove

¼ cup extra-virgin olive oil

Juice of 1 lemon

½ teaspoon sea salt

¼ teaspoon freshly ground black pepper

1 tablespoon extra-virgin olive oil

1½ cups grape tomatoes, halved

2 cups arugula

1. **Make the zucchini noodles:** Using a spiralizer, cut the zucchini into noodles. If you don't have a spiralizer, you can use a vegetable peeler to make thin ribbons instead. Place the zucchini noodles in a large colander and season with salt. Set the zucchini aside for at least 10 minutes to release excess moisture.

2. **Make the gremolata:** In a small bowl, combine the walnuts, sun-dried tomatoes, basil, and lemon zest. Season lightly with salt and pepper. Set aside.

3. **Make the pesto:** In the bowl of a food processor, combine the basil, arugula, walnuts, Parmesan, garlic, olive oil, lemon juice, salt, and pepper. Pulse until the mixture is smooth. Set aside.

4. In a large skillet, heat the olive oil over medium-high heat. Add the tomatoes and cook for 4 to 5 minutes, or until just blistering. Add the zucchini noodles and arugula and cook, stirring occasionally, for 2 to 3 minutes, or until tender-crisp. Season with salt and pepper to taste. Remove from the heat and toss the zucchini mixture with the pesto until evenly coated.

5. To serve, divide the zucchini noodles among four plates. Top each plate with a sprinkle of the gremolata and grated Parmesan.

Snacks/Sauces/Sides/Desserts

Creamy Cauliflower and Celery Root Puree
Gluten-Free, Dairy-Free, Soy-Free, Nut-Free

Time: 30 minutes

SERVINGS: 4 TO 6

This puree is an easy swap for mashed potatoes, while packing many Good Energy benefits. Sulforaphane compounds in cauliflower have been shown to upregulate the Nrf2 pathway, a cellular defense system that helps protect against oxidative stress and inflammation, making it a Good Energy powerhouse recipe.

6 cups chopped cauliflower, florets and stems

2 cups chopped celery root

2 medium carrots, chopped

2 garlic cloves

¼ cup nutritional yeast

1 tablespoon extra-virgin olive oil

2 tablespoons hemp seeds

2 teaspoons freshly squeezed lemon juice

½ teaspoon sea salt

Freshly ground black pepper

1. Fill a wide pot with 2 inches of water. Set a steamer basket in the pot, then bring the water to a simmer over medium-high heat. Add the cauliflower, celery root, carrots, and garlic to the basket and cover. Steam for 10 to 12 minutes, or until very tender.

2. Once cooled, drain the vegetables and add them to the bowl of a food processor or a high-speed blender. Add the nutritional yeast, olive oil, hemp seeds, lemon juice, salt, and pepper to taste. Blend until smooth and creamy.

STORAGE: Creamy Cauliflower and Celery Root Puree can be prepared in advance and stored in an airtight container in the refrigerator for up to 3 days.

Smoky Carrot-Harissa Dip
Gluten-Free, Dairy-Free, Soy-Free
Time: 20 minutes

MAKES: 4 CUPS DIP

This dip uses toasted caraway and cumin seeds, which are among the foods with the highest antioxidant levels. Pair this dip with protein- and omega-3-rich Herbed Flax Crackers (page 358) for a well-balanced snack plate.

2 pounds carrots, chopped

½ teaspoon caraway seeds

1 teaspoon cumin seeds

¼ cup harissa paste

1 teaspoon smoked paprika

2 garlic cloves

½ cup cashews

2 tablespoons extra-virgin olive oil, plus more for drizzling

2 teaspoons red wine vinegar

Sea salt and freshly ground black pepper

1. Fill a wide pot with 2 inches of water. Set a steamer basket in the pot, then bring the water to a simmer over medium-high heat. Add the carrots to the basket and cover. Steam for about 10 minutes, or until tender.
2. While the carrots steam, add the caraway and cumin seeds to a small dry pan over medium heat. Toast, moving the spices frequently, for 2 to 3 minutes, or until fragrant. Using a mortar and pestle, a spice grinder, or a clean coffee grinder, coarsely grind the caraway and cumin seeds.
3. In the bowl of a food processor or a high-speed blender, add the carrots, cumin and caraway seeds, harissa paste, paprika, garlic, cashews, olive oil, vinegar, salt, and pepper and blend until thoroughly combined. Drizzle with olive oil and serve with Herbed Flax Crackers (page 358) and seasonal crudités.

Beet-Lupini Dip

Gluten-Free, Dairy-Free, Soy-Free, Nut-Free

Time: 25 minutes, plus up to 90 minutes for roasting

MAKES: 4 CUPS DIP

Lupini beans are typically available pickled and are linked to improved blood sugar control because they have significant fiber and protein and zero net carbohydrates (calculated by subtracting fiber from total carbohydrates). Fermented sauerkraut supports a healthy gut microbiome and pairs well with the prebiotic fiber found in lupini beans.
Beets are a Good Energy powerhouse, containing high levels of nitrate that can be converted to blood vessel–dilating nitric oxide. Enjoy them in this dip with Herbed Flax Crackers (page 358) and seasonal vegetables.

2 large beets (about 1¼ pounds) or 16 ounces cooked

1 (15-ounce) can chickpeas, drained and rinsed

1 cup cooked lupini beans (like Brami brand), or additional chickpeas if lupini
    beans are unavailable

½ cup tahini

4 garlic cloves

2 tablespoons extra-virgin olive oil, plus more for drizzling

½ cup beet sauerkraut, plus juices, or traditional sauerkraut

½ teaspoon ground cumin

Sea salt and freshly ground black pepper

1. If using cooked beets, skip to step 2. Preheat the oven to 400°F. Cover the beets in foil and place on a small rimmed baking sheet. Roast for 60 to 90 minutes, or until the beets are tender and give little resistance when pierced with a knife. Remove from the oven and allow to cool.
2. Once cooled, peel and coarsely chop the beets and add to the bowl of a food processor. Add the chickpeas, lupini beans, tahini, garlic, olive oil, sauerkraut, and cumin and blend until smooth. Season with salt and

pepper to taste. To serve, drizzle with olive oil and sprinkle with additional ground pepper. Serve the dip with Herbed Flax Crackers (page 358) and seasonal crudités.

STORAGE: Store in an airtight container in the refrigerator for up to 7 days.

Cheesy Broccoli-Chive Biscuits
Gluten-Free, Soy-Free
Time: 45 minutes

MAKES: 8 BISCUITS

A Good Energy biscuit with no refined carbohydrates! Similar to cauliflower, broccoli is a potent source of isothiocyanates, powerful compounds that activate key genes involved in Good Energy and combat oxidative stress.

2½ cups broccoli rice, fresh or frozen*

3 tablespoons sliced chives

3 large eggs

⅔ cup shredded cheddar cheese or nutritional yeast

1½ cups almond flour

1 teaspoon baking powder

¼ teaspoon garlic powder

½ teaspoon sea salt

Freshly ground black pepper

1. Preheat the oven to 350°F. Line a rimmed baking sheet with parchment paper.
2. In a large bowl, combine the broccoli rice, chives, eggs, and cheese.
3. In a separate bowl, mix the almond flour, baking powder, garlic powder, salt, and pepper. Fold the dry ingredients into the wet ingredients until thoroughly combined.
4. Using an ice cream scoop or large spoon, drop the biscuits in 8 even portions. Bake for 30 to 35 minutes, or until the biscuit tops are golden.

*NOTE: If using frozen broccoli rice, bake for an additional 5 to 10 minutes.

STORAGE: Store in an airtight container in the refrigerator for up to 5 days.

Lemon-Dijon Dressing
Gluten-Free, Dairy-Free, Nut-Free

Time: 5 minutes

MAKES: I CUP (EIGHT 2-TABLESPOON SERVINGS)

I like to shake up a jar of this dressing and use it throughout the week on my Fennel and Apple Salad (page 321), Rainbow Salad (page 323), and others. Making your own salad dressing is a great way to avoid hidden sugars and other additives in store-bought versions.

2 tablespoons freshly squeezed lemon juice

2 tablespoons apple cider vinegar

2 tablespoons freshly squeezed orange juice

1 tablespoon Dijon mustard

1 tablespoon tamari

Sea salt and freshly ground black pepper

½ cup extra-virgin olive oil

1. In a medium bowl, add the lemon juice, vinegar, orange juice, mustard, tamari, and salt and pepper to taste.
2. While continuously whisking, drizzle in the olive oil and mix until the dressing is emulsified. Alternatively, add all of the ingredients to a jar with a tight-fitting lid and shake for 30 seconds, or until well combined.

STORAGE: Store in an airtight container in the refrigerator for up to 7 days.

Simple Cauliflower Rice
Gluten-Free, Dairy-Free, Soy-Free, Nut-Free

Time: 15 minutes

SERVINGS: 2 TO 4

Cauliflower rice is a fantastic low-carb, high-fiber base for a meal and has over triple the fiber of white rice.

1 large head cauliflower, leaves removed

2 teaspoons extra-virgin olive oil

Sea salt

1. Coarsely chop the cauliflower florets and stems and place in the bowl of a food processor. Pulse until the cauliflower pieces are approximately the size of grains of rice.

2. In a medium saucepan with a lid, heat the olive oil over medium heat. Add the cauliflower rice and salt to taste and mix well.

3. Cover, reduce the heat to low, and steam for 4 to 6 minutes, or until tender-crisp. Serve immediately.

Black Bean Brownies
Gluten-Free, Dairy-Free, Soy-Free
Time: 45 minutes, plus chilling overnight

SERVINGS: 12

Beneficial polyphenols in cocoa powder may support healthy insulin levels, and fiber-rich black beans help to balance the sugar in the dates.

Sugar-free chocolate chips sweetened with monk fruit are an optional addition that makes these brownies extra indulgent.

8 dates, pitted and coarsely chopped

¾ cup cocoa powder

1 (15-ounce) can black beans, drained and rinsed

½ cup canned full-fat coconut milk

2 tablespoons ground flaxseeds

1 teaspoon vanilla extract

1 teaspoon baking powder

1 tablespoon beet powder

¼ teaspoon sea salt

Unrefined coconut oil

½ cup sugar-free chocolate chips sweetened with monk fruit (optional)

Flaky Maldon salt

1. Preheat the oven to 350°F. If the dates are dry, soak them in hot water for 10 to 15 minutes to soften.
2. In the bowl of a large food processor, add the dates and cocoa powder and pulse until the dates are broken down. Add the black beans, coconut milk, flaxseeds, vanilla, baking powder, beet powder, and salt. Pulse the ingredients until a batter forms, taking time to scrape down the sides of the bowl with a spatula.
3. Grease an 8 × 8-inch baking dish with coconut oil. If using the chocolate chips, combine the batter and chips in a large mixing bowl. Spread the batter evenly in the baking dish using a spatula.

4. Bake for 35 minutes. The brownies will be quite soft and spongy when they first come out of the oven, but their consistency will transform to dense and fudgy overnight. Sprinkle with the flaky salt. Chill overnight in the refrigerator and serve the next day.

STORAGE: Store in an airtight container in the refrigerator for up to 5 days.

Mixed Berry Crumble with Toasted Pecans
Gluten-Free, Soy-Free
Time: 55 minutes

SERVINGS: 8

This crumble topping is a combination of tiger nut flour, a high-fiber flour, and high-antioxidant pecans, making it a great alternative to a traditional crumble made with white flour.

6 cups frozen mixed berries, such as raspberries, blueberries, and strawberries

¾ cup tiger nut flour

½ cup chopped pecans

4 tablespoons (½ stick) cold grass-fed unsalted butter, cubed, or coconut oil

3 tablespoons maple syrup

1 teaspoon vanilla extract

¼ teaspoon sea salt

¼ teaspoon ground cinnamon

1. Preheat the oven to 350°F. Add the frozen berries to a 10-inch cast-iron skillet or baking dish.
2. In a large mixing bowl, combine the tiger nut flour, pecans, butter, syrup, vanilla, salt, and cinnamon. Using a fork, break up the pieces of butter or oil until the consistency is sandy.
3. Spoon the topping mixture evenly over the berries and bake for 40 to 45 minutes, or until the top is golden brown and the berries are bubbling.
4. Allow the crumble to cool slightly before serving.

Herbed Flax Crackers
Dairy-Free, Gluten-Free, Soy-Free, Nut-Free
Time: 1 hour 30 minutes

MAKES: ABOUT 80 CRACKERS

Unlike traditional crackers, these Herbed Flax Crackers will leave you
feeling energized by stabilizing your blood sugar and giving you Good
Energy benefits of fiber, omega-3s, protein, and micronutrients! Flaxseeds
are packed with omega-3 fatty acids, which are anti-inflammatory and
promote cell membrane elasticity. I use oregano in this recipe, but feel free
to swap in your favorite dried herbs, such as rosemary, thyme, or sage.

2 cups whole flaxseeds, finely ground in a spice grinder or food processor

½ cup sesame seeds

¼ cup nutritional yeast

¼ cup whole psyllium husks

½ teaspoon garlic powder

1 teaspoon sea salt

1 teaspoon dried oregano

1. Preheat the oven to 325°F. In a large bowl, combine the ground
flaxseeds, sesame seeds, nutritional yeast, psyllium husks, garlic powder,
salt, and oregano. Add 1 cup water and stir until the mixture is fully
combined.
2. Prepare two sheets of parchment paper to fit either one large baking
sheet or two medium baking sheets. Place half of the dough on one of the
sheets of parchment and cover with an additional sheet. Using a rolling
pin, roll the batter to an even thickness, about ⅛ inch thick. Repeat with
the remaining half of the dough. Cut the crackers with a knife to your
desired size. If a more organic shape is preferred, the crackers can be
broken apart after cooking.
3. Bake for 1 hour 15 minutes, or until crisp and slightly darkened. The
crackers will continue to firm as they cool.

Lemon-Almond Cake with Jammy Strawberries

Gluten-Free, Soy-Free

Time: 45 minutes

SERVINGS: 12

Almond flour, a nutritious alternative to ultra-refined white flour found in most cakes, is high in protein, healthy fats, and vital nutrients like vitamin E and magnesium. The high-antioxidant strawberry topping leans on strawberries' natural sweetness instead of sugar.

4 tablespoons (½ stick) grass-fed unsalted butter, melted, plus more for
   preparing the cake pan

2 cups blanched superfine almond flour

½ cup monk fruit sweetener, like Lakanto

1 teaspoon baking powder

½ teaspoon baking soda

¼ teaspoon salt

4 large eggs

1 teaspoon vanilla extract

Zest and juice of 2 lemons

Jammy Strawberries

3 cups strawberries, stemmed and quartered

Pinch of salt

½ teaspoon vanilla extract

½ teaspoon rose powder (optional)

1. Preheat the oven to 350°F. Line the bottom of a 9-inch springform pan or cake pan with parchment paper. Grease the sides of the pan with butter.

2. In a large bowl, whisk the almond flour, sweetener, baking powder, baking soda, and salt. In a medium bowl, whisk the eggs, then add the melted butter, vanilla, lemon zest, and lemon juice. Add the wet

mixture to the dry mixture and whisk until the cake batter is well combined.

3. Pour the cake batter into the prepared pan. Bake on the center rack for 25 to 30 minutes, or until a toothpick or knife inserted in the center comes out clean.

4. **Meanwhile, make the jammy strawberries:** In a medium saucepan, add the strawberries, salt, vanilla, and ¼ cup water, and bring to a simmer over medium-high heat. Cook for 15 to 18 minutes, or until the strawberries are soft and the liquid has reduced to a syrupy consistency. Remove from the heat and add the rose powder, if using.

5. Allow the cake to cool for about 25 minutes. Remove the cake from the springform pan or flip it onto a serving plate. Serve slices with a spoonful or two of jammy strawberries.

TIP: Use the cake batter for muffins! Simply bake in a lined muffin tin for 18 to 22 minutes, or until a toothpick inserted into the center of each muffin comes out clean.

Baked Jicama Fries with Homemade Ketchup and Herbed Aioli

Gluten-Free, Dairy-Free, Soy-Free, Nut-Free

Time: 45 minutes

SERVINGS: 2 TO 4

Jicama is a root vegetable that's high in inulin fiber, which is beneficial for the gut microbiome diversity. With my homemade ketchup and herbed aioli, you can enjoy all the flavor of your favorite condiments without any of the hidden processed sugars or unhealthy seed oils found in store-bought versions.

1 medium jicama (about 1½ pounds), peeled and cut into ¼-inch-thick

    fries

1 tablespoon extra-virgin olive oil

½ teaspoon sea salt

¼ teaspoon freshly ground black pepper

Herbed Aioli

1 large egg yolk

1 garlic clove, minced and mashed into a paste

1 teaspoon freshly squeezed lemon juice

1 teaspoon Dijon mustard

1 tablespoon finely chopped fresh flat-leaf parsley

¼ teaspoon sea salt

⅓ cup unrefined avocado oil

Ketchup

1 date, pitted

¼ cup tomato paste

1 tablespoon red wine vinegar

¼ teaspoon garlic powder

¼ teaspoon sea salt

1. Preheat the oven to 425°F. Fill a wide pot with 2 inches of water. Set a steamer basket in the pot, then bring the water to a simmer over medium-high heat. Add the jicama and steam for 8 to 10 minutes, or until tender-crisp. Drain.

2. On a large rimmed baking sheet, toss the jicama with the olive oil, salt, and pepper. Spread the jicama into a single layer. Bake for about 30 minutes, flipping halfway through, until the fries are golden brown and crisp around the edges.

3. **Make the herbed aioli:** In a medium bowl, whisk together the egg yolk, garlic paste, lemon juice, mustard, parsley, and salt. Whisking continuously, slowly drizzle in the avocado oil until the mayonnaise thickens and the oil is well incorporated.

4. **Make the ketchup:** Soak the date in hot water for 10 to 15 minutes to soften, and then drain. In a small food processor, blend together the tomato paste, ¼ cup water, vinegar, date, garlic powder, and salt.

5. Serve the fries hot out of the oven with the herbed aioli and ketchup.

Salt and Vinegar Golden Beet Chips
Gluten-Free, Dairy-Free, Soy-Free, Nut-Free
Time: 1 hour

SERVINGS: 6

These chips are a perfect substitute for potato chips. Beets are loaded with folate, manganese, potassium, and fiber. Plus, baking them in extra-virgin olive oil instead of frying them in vegetable oil reduces the chance of inflammation and oxidative stress in the body.

3 or 4 medium-sized golden beets (about 1½ pounds), scrubbed or peeled

Extra-virgin olive oil

1 teaspoon apple cider vinegar

¼ teaspoon garlic powder

¼ teaspoon onion powder

Sea salt and freshly ground black pepper

1. Preheat the oven to 300°F. Slice the beets as thinly as possible, about ¹⁄₁₆ inch thick, using a mandoline or a sharp knife.

2. Lightly grease two rimmed baking sheets with olive oil, just enough to prevent the beets from sticking while they bake. In a large bowl, toss the beet slices with the vinegar, garlic powder, onion powder, and salt and pepper to taste. Arrange the beet slices in a single layer on the baking sheets.

3. Bake for 40 to 55 minutes, or until the beet chips are crispy and golden brown. Remove from the oven and cool completely before serving.

Acknowledgments

We first want to thank Gayle Means, our beloved mother. We decided to write this book in the days after she died, full of passion to carry forward her example of Good Energy and emboldened to help others become empowered to understand their health and how to avoid premature, preventable deaths.

Thank you to our dad, Grady Means, for being our inspiration of how to live the principles outlined in this book: exercising, writing, sailing, bodysurfing, hiking, laughing, growing, gardening, learning, and practicing gratitude at seventy-seven. You are our hero—thank you. This book would not exist without Leslie, Calley's wife and Casey's best friend. Thank you for being our tireless supporter, counselor, and therapist throughout this process—and for being our model of Good Energy with the love and constant growth trajectory you exhibit every day. Leslie also gave birth during the writing process to Roark, who inspires us with his joy and awe for the world that we should all aspire to. Thank you to Casey's incredible partner, Brian, who has been her rock over the past year and brings nonstop Good Energy into her life.

Thank you to our agent, Richard Pine, for believing in us and for foundational advice in molding this book, and to Eliza Rothstein for support. Thank you to Lucia Watson for being a model for us of what a talented and collaborative editor is.

We wrote this book while launching startups tied to the mission of metabolic health—and couldn't have done this without the support of our cofounders and teams. For Casey at Levels: Sam Corcos, Josh Clemente, and the tireless team who amplify the message of metabolic health daily (Mike H., Jackie,

Tony, Tom, Mike D., Support, Growth, Product, Engineering, R&D, Athena, and everyone else who has been part of the journey—the world is metabolically healthier because of you). For Calley at TrueMed: Justin Mares and team.

Thank you to our friends who read the book and provided invaluable feedback and support, including Carrie Denning, Fiona O'Donnell McCarthy, Steph Bell, Emily Azer, Ann Voorhees, and Nick Alexander. Thank you to Sonja Manning for your friendship and support on so many aspects of the book. Thank you to Kimber Crowe and Sally Nicholson for giving early book feedback and a lifetime of love and support. Thank you to Dhru Purohit for your continual support and inspiration to us in navigating business, health, writing, and life.

This book would not have been possible without forward-thinking medical leaders who inspired us to devote our lives to this cause—particularly Drs. Mark Hyman, Robert Lustig, David Perlmutter, Sara Gottfried, Dom D'Agostino, Terry Wahls, Ben Bikman, Molly Maloof, and David Sinclair.

We so admire the work of the countless health, nutrition, biohacking, and regenerative farming pioneers who have forged their own path, deeply inspired us, and created meaningful content with us, including Drs. Rick Johnson, Will Cole, Tyna Moore, Austin Perlmutter, Gabrielle Lyon, Steve Gundry, Chris Palmer, Howard Luks, Kevin Jubbal, Philip Ovadia, Ken Berry, David Cistola, and Bret Scher, as well as Jeff Krasno, Shawn Stevenson, Kayla Barnes, Chase Chewning, Louisa Nicola, Kelly LeVeque, Mona Sharma, Jason and Colleen Wachob, Jillian Michaels, Dave Asprey, Carrie Jones, Kara Fitzgerald, Kimberly Snyder (and Jon Bier), Ben Greenfield, Ronit Menashe, Vida Delrahim, Kristen Holmes, Nora LaTorre, Courtney Swan, Sarah Villafranco, Michael Brandt, Mariza Snyder, Molly Chester, Will Harris, Lewis Howes, Max Lugavere, Tom Bilyeu, Liz Moody, and so many other heroes in the media, podcasting, food, wellness, health, and entrepreneurial spaces working to create a better world. You've all helped us spread the message of foundational health over the last several years and we are inordinately grateful to you.

Thank you to Amely Greeven for early help on the book, Ashley Lonsdale for collaborating with us on delicious recipes, Jen Chesak for copyediting, and Monica Nelson, Nina Bautista, Vika Miller, Sabrina Horn, Robbie Crabtree, and Ezzie Spencer for various forms of life-changing personal coaching and support during the writing and publishing process.

And most importantly, thank you to the readers who are on a mission (like we are) to be empowered in their health. We can't think of a more important journey than to reach our limitless potential and maximal Good Energy in life.

Index